# Quantum Computing for the Brain

## Between Science and Economics

**ISSN: 2051-6304**

**Series Editor:** Frank Witte *(University College London, UK)*

---

The series *Between Science and Economics* aims at providing a mix of undergraduate and graduate textbooks, research monographs and essay and paper collections to serve as a library and resource for teachers, students, graduate students and experts studying fields in which economic and science issues and problems come together. The thrust of the series is to demonstrate that the contributing disciplines can benefit from learning from one another as well as contributing to the resolution of multi- and interdisciplinary questions. This involves the economic principles at work in science and technology as well as the roots of economic processes in biological, chemical and physical fundamentals in nature. It also encompasses the problems associated with complexity, order-to-disorder transitions, uncertainty, deterministic chaos and geometric principles faced by economics as well as many of the natural sciences.

*Published*

Vol. 3 *Quantum Computing for the Brain*
by Melanie Swan, Renato P. dos Santos, Mikhail Lebedev and Frank Witte

Vol. 2 *Quantum Computing: Physics, Blockchains, and Deep Learning Smart Networks*
by Melanie Swan, Renato P. dos Santos and Frank Witte

Vol. 1 *Blockchain Economics: Implications of Distributed Ledgers: Markets, Communications Networks, and Algorithmic Reality*
edited by Melanie Swan, Jason Potts, Soichiro Takagi, Frank Witte and Paolo Tasca

Between **Science** and **Economics** – Vol. 3

# Quantum Computing for the Brain


Melanie Swan
University College London, UK

Renato P. dos Santos
Lutheran University of Brazil, Brazil

Mikhail Lebedev
National Research University Higher School of Economics, Russia

Frank Witte
University College London, UK



**World Scientific**

NEW JERSEY • LONDON • SINGAPORE • BEIJING • SHANGHAI • HONG KONG • TAIPEI • CHENNAI • TOKYO

*Published by*

World Scientific Publishing Europe Ltd.

57 Shelton Street, Covent Garden, London WC2H 9HE

*Head office:* 5 Toh Tuck Link, Singapore 596224

*USA office:* 27 Warren Street, Suite 401-402, Hackensack, NJ 07601

**Library of Congress Cataloging-in-Publication Data**
Names: Swan, Melanie, author. | Dos Santos, Renato P., author. |
Lebedev, Mikhail, author. | Witte, Frank, author.
Title: Quantum computing for the brain / Melanie Swan, University College London, UK,
Renato P. dos Santos, Lutheran University of Brazil, Brazil,
Mikhail Lebedev, National Research University Higher School of Economics,
Russia, Frank Witte, University College London, UK.
Description: New Jersey : World Scientific, [2022] | Series: Between science and economics,
2051-6304 ; 3 | Includes bibliographical references and index.
Identifiers: LCCN 2021035837 | ISBN 9781800610613 (hardcover) |
ISBN 9781800610620 (ebook) | ISBN 9781800610637 (ebook other)
Subjects: LCSH: Quantum computing. | Neurosciences.
Classification: LCC QA76.889 .S92 2022 | DDC 006.3/843--dc23
LC record available at https://lccn.loc.gov/2021035837

**British Library Cataloguing-in-Publication Data**
A catalogue record for this book is available from the British Library.



For any available supplementary material, please visit
https://www.worldscientific.com/worldscibooks/10.1142/Q0313#t=suppl

Desk Editors: Jayanthi Muthuswamy/Michael Beale/Shi Ying Koe

Typeset by Stallion Press
Email: enquiries@stallionpress.com

# Preface

*Quantum Computing for the Brain* is intended as a comprehensive resource with practically usable high-level descriptions of quantum information methods, as directed towards the specific yet portable context of computational neuroscience (specifically, neural signaling). The book arose from the need for a guide to the entirety of the emerging quantum information science field, in plain language, for all levels of participants. A concise toolkit is provided for quantum engineers, researchers, executives, business strategists, product managers, policy-makers, investors, and students to become immediately effective in applying quantum strategies to solving real-life problems.

The book can be treated as two separate lines of material, either as quantum information science or quantum neuroscience on its own, or as the integration of the two as quantum information science applied to computational neuroscience. As standalone components, Chapter 3 serves as a comprehensive guide to AdS/Studies, Chapters 16–18 can be employed as a quantum machine learning module, and Chapters 10–11 as a quantum optical networks module. Computational neuroscience is a representative problem area as one of science's most complex undertakings, with extensibility in approach and methods to many other fields with similar problem structures such as quantum finance, quantum cryptography, and quantum machine learning. The book is appropriate for all levels of interest without any background in the underlying areas.

As with other fields, computational neuroscience may migrate to the more capacious platforms of quantum computing. Such platforms offer scalable energy-efficient computation that surpasses supercomputing and more naturally corresponds to the three-dimensional structure of atomic reality. New classes of complex problems can be addressed more fully such as the modeling of neural signaling in which two central challenges are synaptic integration (aggregating thousands of incoming spikes from dendrites and other neurons) and electrical-chemical signaling (incorporating neuron–glia interactions at the molecular scale).

Many technical requirements of neural signaling cannot be fully accommodated classically, including spatial interactions and partial differential equations (PDEs). Neurons are typically modeled only in their electrical activity with ordinary differential equations (ODEs) instead of via diffusion-based electrical-to-chemical neurotransmitter conversions across the synaptic cleft that are received as molecular ions at dendritic arbors, with flexible geometries and ongoing dendritic spikes. The AdS/Brain theory is proposed as a composite model of neural signaling based on recent advances in quantum information science related to many-body dynamics, information scrambling (spread), entropy-based short-and-long-range (UV–IR) correlations between subsystems, renormalization, continuous-time quantum walks, entanglement generation, and quantum teleportation. Linking quantum methods to computational neuroscience, a list of Millennium Prize-type quantum neural circuits is elaborated in the final chapter. The overall focus of the book is to operationalize quantum concepts into a standardized toolkit to apply to quantum neuroscience and beyond. Towards this goal, the AdS/Brain platform aims to serve as a generic quantum neural field theory model in which to easily incorporate ongoing foundational physics findings in neuroscience interpretations.

Quantum computing is an emerging physics-driven research frontier whose complexity is rooted in quantum mechanics. The exciting news is that the mysteries of the counterintuitive behavior of the quantum mechanical world (namely, superposition and entanglement) can be harnessed in quantum machines for computation, communication, and sensing, and directed towards the goals of improving human quality of life through the continued understanding and treatment of neuropathologies.

# About the Authors

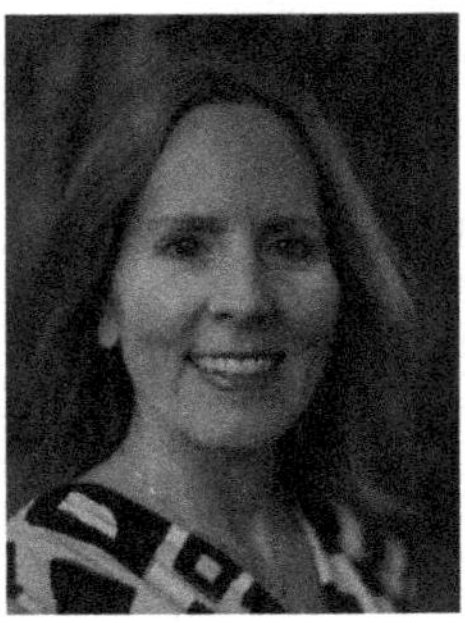

**Melanie Swan** is a Research Associate at the Centre for Blockchain Technologies at University College London. She has a PhD from Purdue University, an MBA from the Wharton School of the University of Pennsylvania, and a BA from Georgetown University. Her previous academic affiliations include Kingston University London and Université Paris 8. With research interests in emerging science and technology as related to biology, she pioneered the crowdsourced health research study in genomics, participated in brain–cloud interface research, and led the Telecom Economics Program at the optical networking boutique Ovum-RHK. She is an Affiliate Scholar with the Institute for Ethics and Emerging Technologies and a participant in FQXi's foundational physics Essay Contest. She is the author of the best-selling book *Blockchain: Blueprint for a New Economy*, and coauthor of two other books, *Blockchain Economics* and *Quantum Computing: Physics, Blockchains, and Deep Learning Smart Networks*.

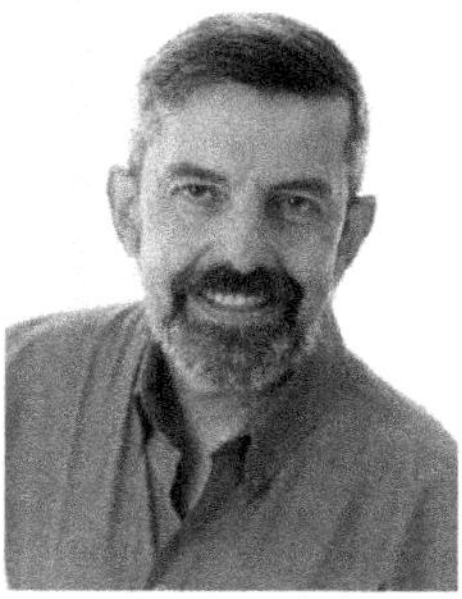

**Renato P. dos Santos** is a researcher on blockchain technologies and Graduate Professor at the Lutheran University of Brazil. He is a member of the British Blockchain Association, holds a DSc (Physics) degree, and did postdoc work in artificial intelligence and specializations in data science and blockchain technologies. He is also the author of more than 100 scientific papers on philosophy of cryptocurrencies, data science in STEM education, second life in STEM education, Web 2.0 technologies, ethnoscience, physics teaching, artificial intelligence and computer algebra in physics, and quantum field theory. He is a reviewer and editor of prestigious scientific periodicals and conferences around the world and has developed systems for second life, forex market, qualitative physics, and computer algebra.

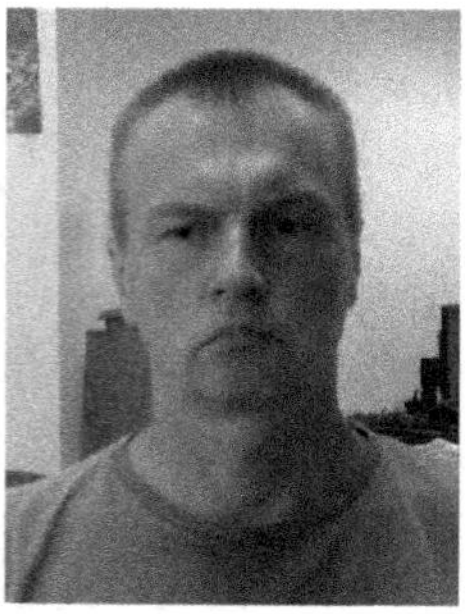

**Mikhail Lebedev** is a Full Professor at the National Research University Higher School of Economics (HSE University) in Moscow, Russia. Other affiliations include Full Professor at Skolkovo Institute of Science and Technology, Moscow, Russia, a Professor and Scientific Head at the Center for Bioelectric Interfaces, HSE University, Moscow, Russia, and a Professor at I.M. Sechenov First Moscow State Medical University, Moscow, Russia. Lebedev is a neurophysiologist, developer of brain–machine interfaces, author of more than 100 papers, and editor of journals and books. He has an MSc in biophysics from Moscow Institute of Physics and Technology (MIPT), a PhD in Neurobiology from University of Tennessee, Memphis, and postdocs from the International School for Advanced Studies, Trieste (SISSA), and National Institute of Mental Health, Bethesda (NIMH); he is Senior Research Scientist at the Duke University Center for Neuroengineering. His research interests include motor control, electrocorticography, neurophysiology of the cortex and basal ganglia, and neural prostheses. Lebedev won the Spotlight Award, a Megagrant from the government of Russia, the Russian Science Foundation grant to support a world-class laboratory, and the Visiting Professor Award at the Technical University of Munich.

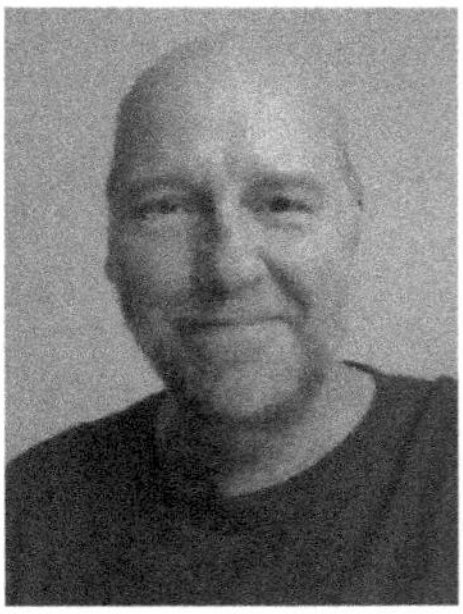

**Frank Witte** received his PhD in Theoretical Physics (1995) from the University of Heidelberg, Germany. He worked as an Assistant and Associate Professor in Physics & Astronomy at Utrecht University and University College Utrecht, in the Netherlands, from 1996 to 2010, publishing on problems in elementary particle theory, (quantum) gravitational theory, and quantum game theory. In 2010, he accepted a position in the Department of Economics of University College London. He is currently an Associate Professor in Economics there and teaches Economics of Science, Environmental Economics, and Computational Methods in Economics. Frank has been a visiting fellow at St. John's College, Cambridge (UK, 2002), academic visitor at the Quantum Optics & Laser Science group of Imperial College London (UK, 2009), and International Visiting Fellow at Grinnell College (US, 2012). His current research focuses on the applications of physics-inspired methods to problems in environmental economics, economics of science, and the economics of networks.

# Contents

# List of Figures

# List of Tables

# Chapter 1

# Introduction to Quantum Neuroscience

*In the contemporary study of the brain, nearly all of the domains of physics are not only relevant but truly essential*

— Lynn and Bassett (2019, p. 3)

**Abstract**

Quantum Neuroscience has the possibility of bringing the modeling of the human brain's 86 billion neurons and 242 trillion synapses within reach, even with existing quantum systems (for example, a 53-qubit system has nine quadrillion states ($2^{53}$)). Available cloud-based quantum computing services could extend their offerings to tools for the study of the brain such as quantum machine learning, high-dimensional photonic entanglement, and spiking neural networks. Contemporary advances in foundational physics and information theory are informing the development of standardized neural circuits and quantum neuroscience applications in wavefunction modeling, quantum biology, and neuroscience physics.

## 1.1 The Brain Is the "Killer Application" of Quantum Computing

The thesis of this book is that the brain is the "killer application" of quantum computing. The many earlier applications are impressive but are not the main attraction. The "killer application" for quantum computing is not the rapidly emerging field of quantum finance, or quantum cryptography based on Shor's factoring algorithm, Grover's search algorithm, variational quantum eigensolvers (VQE), quantum approximate optimization algorithms (QAOA), quantum machine learning, continuous-time quantum walks, quantum chemistry models of atomically-precise protein docking, Majorana fermion braiding, the discovery of new superconducting materials to produce quantum processing units (QPUs), boson sampling, demonstrations of quantum advantage over classical systems, global quantum clocks, end-to-end qubit delivery with quantum teleportation, qudit-based high-dimensional entanglement heralding and distillation in photonic quantum networks, or even the study of superconducting black holes with scalar hair, thermofield double states, information scrambling, black hole interiors, spacetime superfluid crystals, and the complexity equals volume or action conjecture. No, the "killer application" of quantum computing is the brain.

The brain is tailor-made to exploit the possibilities of quantum computing. No other system is as complex, as multidimensional in time and space, as dynamical, as less well understood, as of peak interest, and as in need of three-dimensional modeling as it appears and functions in real-life as is the human brain. The high level of foundational physics progress, together with real-life data accruing in connectomics and high-volume brain scanning, suggests that now is precisely the moment of opportunity to define the emerging field of quantum neuroscience. Brain modeling is the limits-case application that defines the requirements for the quantum computing platform.

The five themes of this book are as follows:

1. The brain inexorably coming under greater scientific scrutiny.
2. Entropy and information-theoretic formulations (including short-range (UV) and long-range (IR) correlations in multiscalar domains).
3. Machine learning (classical and quantum) as a core infrastructural technology.
4. Global photonic networks for computation, communication, and sensing.
5. Energy-efficient computation and superconducting materials.

These themes come together to hint at universal problem-solving methods that extend across disciplines. The biggest overall trend of the information-theoretic formulation of problems for digitized and quantized computation is likely to persist. Entropy and short-long range correlations (UV-IR) are powerful conceptual tools that can help to address long-standing problems in neuroscience such as fluctuations. The challenge is to produce neural dynamics models in which each network node incorporates activity from both the local neural population, and influences from farther regions in the form of stochastic fluctuations (correlations). Physics-based models of entropy and short-long range correlations within a multi-tier system accommodate this requirement.

Another persistency across disciplines is the structural model of alternating linear-nonlinear activation. Whole-brain neural field theories exhibit an alternating linear (input function) and nonlinear (output function) activation structure (Amari, 1977), attempting to explain how stable periodic network states give way to discontinuous firing behavior (Coombes *et al.*, 2018). This structural pattern is seen in other advanced analytical methods such as the alternating linear-nonlinear structures of machine learning (max pooling, and convolutions-activations (LeCun *et al.*, 2015)), tensor networks (disentanglers and isometries (Vidal, 2008)), quantum optical networking with high-dimensional entanglement (path-encoded qudits (Wang *et al.*, 2018)), and matrix quantum mechanics (Han & Hartnoll, 2020).

### 1.1.1 *The complexity of the brain*

The brain is recognized as a complex system (Bassett & Gazzaniga, 2011). The central components, neurons, are themselves complex dynamical systems with a wide range of internal time scales (Sejnowski, 2020, p. 30036). The brain exhibits complexity via nonlocal interactions in which dynamic activity at one location influences distant locations without affecting intermediate regions (Nunez *et al.*, 2015, p. 7). Each scale tier of the brain has its own spatial and temporal processes and dynamics (Breakspear, 2017, p. 340). The brain operates by way of dynamical coordination and on-the-fly synaptic rewiring across twelve orders of magnitude at nine levels of organization ranging from the

Table 1.1. Levels of organization in the brain.

| No. | Level | Size (Decimal) | Size | Size (m) |
|---|---|---|---|---|
| 1 | Nervous system | 1 | >1 m | $10^{0}$ |
| 2 | Subsystem | 0.1 | 10 cm | $10^{-1}$ |
| 3 | Neural network | 0.01 | 1 cm | $10^{-2}$ |
| 4 | Microcircuit | 0.001 | 1 mm | $10^{-3}$ |
| 5 | Neuron | 0.000 1 | 100 $\mu$m | $10^{-4}$ |
| 6 | Dendritic arbor | 0.000 01 | 10 $\mu$m | $10^{-5}$ |
| 7 | Synapse | 0.000 001 | 1 $\mu$m | $10^{-6}$ |
| 8 | Signaling pathway | 0.000 000 001 | 1 nm | $10^{-9}$ |
| 9 | Ion channel | 0.000 000 000 001 | 1 pm | $10^{-12}$ |

central nervous system ($10^{0}$ m) to minute ion channels ($10^{-12}$ m) (Sterratt *et al.* (2011) and similarly indicated by Sejnowski (2020, p. 30037)) (Table 1.1).

The brain is complex but not intractable. The problem is a lack of data. Mathematical physics can likely explain phenomena once uncovered. The main issue is obtaining a fuller dataset of the brain's live activity at different scales and interactions. Advanced data collection efforts suggest that basic wiring diagrams of the human brain are no longer the gating factor as much as three-dimensional whole-brain models.

## 1.2 The Brain and Quantum Computing

There are 86 billion neurons in the human brain and 242 trillion synapses, meaning roughly 2,800 synapses per neuron (Martins *et al.*, 2019, p. 4). The population of glial cells in the human brain is slightly lower than neurons, about 85 billion (von Bartheld *et al.*, 2016). Avogadro's number typically refers to the number of particles (molecules, atoms, or ions) in a sample. Once unthinkably large (0.6 of a trillion × one trillion), Avogadro's number is now coming into computational reach. A simple heuristic is that $n$-qubits can store $2^n$ bits of information, which means that 79 qubits can store on the order of $2^{79}$ or

$6.04 \times 10^{23}$ bits of information, which is in the range of Avogadro's number. From the standpoint of modern computing, 86 billion and 242 trillion are not big numbers, but what is not yet fully understood is how neurons and synapses operate on an interlinked basis in the brain.

In quantum computing, one of the first standard gate-model systems released was the 19-qubit chip from Rigetti (Otterbach *et al.*, 2017). Available to customers as of August 2020 was the 27-qubit IBM Quantum Falcon processor (Jurcevic *et al.*, 2020). Research scientists not affiliated with vendors have been using state-of-the-art quantum computers for various tasks including IBM's Q 20 Tokyo processor with 20 superconducting qubits (Hamilton *et al.*, 2019), the Rigetti 16Q Aspen-1 processor with 16 qubits (Leyton-Ortega *et al.*, 2019), and the 7-qubit fully programmable trapped ion quantum computer (Zhu *et al.*, 2019). Google produced a research demonstration with a 53-qubit chip (Sycamore) in 2019 (Arute *et al.*, 2019), later confirming the chip's performance by simulating it on a supercomputer (Villalonga *et al.*, 2020). CERN indicates that a 79-qubit level (an Avogadro's number) of computation is needed for the LHC's upgrade to the High-Luminosity Large Hadron Collider (HL-LHC) expected to begin operation in 2026 with 50–100 times more computing needed than available before (Carminati, 2018) (Table 1.2).

Some of the first quantum neuroscience applications use quantum machine learning to study EEG data with quantum neural networks (CNNs, Aishwarya *et al.*, 2020) and quantum wavelet neural networks

Table 1.2. Neural entities and quantum computation.

| Level | Estimated Size | |
|---|---|---|
| Neurons | $86 \times 10^9$ | 86,000,000,000 |
| Glia | $85 \times 10^9$ | 85,000,000,000 |
| Synapses | $2 \times 10^{14}$ | 242,000,000,000,000 |
| Avogadro's number | $6 \times 10^{23}$ | 602,214,076,000,000,000,000,000 |
| 19 Qubits (Rigetti-available) | $2^{19}$ | 524,288 |
| 27 Qubits (IBM-available) | $2^{27}$ | 134,217,728 |
| 53 Qubits (Google-research) | $2^{53}$ | 9,007,199,254,740,990 |
| 79 Qubits (needed at LHC) | $2^{79}$ | 604,462,909,807,315,000,000,000 |

(RNNs, Taha & Taha, 2018). Such an approach is conducive as EEG data are brain waves (Nunez, 1974) that are in the form of wavefunctions that can be readily analyzed with quantum methods. Kiani *et al.* (2020) have developed quantum algorithms to reconstruct medical images captured in MRI, CT, and PET scans.

## 1.3 Status of Neuroscience

The brain is a "big data" domain and, with quantum computing, might become a "really big data" science. Imaging is a central focus in neuroscience research, particularly whole-brain imaging. Connectome projects have led to new methods in high-throughput imaging and recording techniques such that neuroscience data acquisition outpaces that of most other biomedical fields (Motta *et al.*, 2019). In high-throughput connectomics, ongoing work from the Allen Institute for Brain Science demonstrates terabyte-scale processing for contemporary neuron reconstruction (Wang *et al.*, 2019a) and petabyte-scale next-generation dataset acquisition methods (Yin *et al.*, 2019). In many substantial microscopy advances, single-molecule-scale resolution has been obtained to capture synaptic proteins at dendritic spines, myelination along axons, and presynaptic densities at dopaminergic neurons with expansion light-sheet microscopy (Gao *et al.*, 2019). The general research aim of whole-brain neuroscience is full-volume, three-dimensional, whole-brain analysis at multiple spatial and temporal scales. One task is integrating real-life data obtained simultaneously from EEG, MEG, fMRI, and tractography techniques. The challenge is interpreting brain potentials and other data to articulate the simple bulk properties of the brain and develop a nonlinear dynamical systems theory of the brain.

As in other fields, computational power is a key contributor to the kinds of techniques and resulting knowledge that are possible. Graphics Processing Units (GPUs) have made a difference in neuroscience data acquisition processing times and analysis capabilities (Vescovi *et al.*, 2017). Neuroscience might continue to benefit from the computational chip progression suggested as CPU-GPU-TPU-QPU (Central, Graphics, Tensor, Quantum Processing Units). In quantum computing more generally, an industry tipping point may be reached if universal quantum computing chips become feasible. In machine learning, the advent of fast GPUs enabled researchers to train networks 10–20 times faster (LeCun *et al.*, 2015, p. 439). Tensor Processing Units (TPUs) provided a similar advance, allowing matrix multiplications to flow through without having to store interim values in memory. An independent benchmarking analysis of chips at peak FLOPs recorded state-of-the-art CPU-GPU-TPUs at 2, 125, and 420 teraFLOPs, respectively (Wang *et al.*, 2019b, p. 4). QPUs are implicated in being able to solve problems faster than existing chips by exploiting the quantum properties of superposition and entanglement.

To complete the human connectome (and even the mouse connectome (Abbott *et al.*, 2020)), a qualitatively different mode of computing is likely necessary, similar to the technology-driven inflection point in the sequencing of the human genome that allowed its completion in 2001 (Pennisi, 2001). Human connectomes are not an immediate prospect since the whole-brain fruit fly connectome was only completed in 2018 (Zheng *et al.*, 2018). The imaging, data processing, and storage requirements may be 1 zettabyte per human connectome (Lichtman *et al.*, 2014, p. 8), which compares to 59 zettabytes of data generated worldwide in 2020 (Reinsel, 2020). Quantum computing may be precisely the computational platform that is adequate to the study of the brain and might eventually lead to personalized connectome analysis and neuropathology prevention.

### 1.3.1 *Whole-brain simulation*

The need for quantum neuroscience can be seen in the status of whole-brain simulation projects. Although progress has been made with existing technology, human whole-brain simulation remains a distant target with nonquantum platforms, namely, neuromorphic hardware systems and supercomputers. The largest model using the SpiNNaker neuromorphic platform is a partial brain simulation of 80,000 neurons and 0.3 billion synapses (van Albada *et al.*, 2018). The simulation compares favorably with brain network simulations using the computational neuroscience platform NEST, but comprises only a small portion of the brain's estimated 86 billion neurons and 242 trillion synapses. A supercomputing project fares better, realizing the simulation of one-third of the human brain (Igarashi *et al.*, 2019). A spiking neuron structure uses

76% of the total capacity of the Japanese K supercomputer (63,504 of 82,944 computational nodes) to simulate one-third of the human brain.

The Blue Brain project continues towards its goal of simulating the entire mammalian brain, starting with the mouse and progressing to the human. A supercomputing platform upgrade, to Blue Brain 5, was completed in 2018. However, the biggest factor in brain simulation is not floating-point operations (the specialty of supercomputers), but rather memory, bandwidth, and input–output performance. Project leader Henry Markram notes that "Simulating the human brain is a big data challenge" (Feldman, 2018). Even modeling a single neuron in the Blue Brain architecture requires about 20,000 ordinary differential equations. The initial project was simulating a rat neocortical column as a basic functional unit of the cortex (Markram, 2006). In humans, neocortical columns are about 2 mm in length and 0.5 mm wide and contain about 60,000 neurons. In comparison, rat neocortical columns are similar in structure but only contain 10,000 neurons. Quantum computing might facilitate neocortical column modeling and human whole-brain simulation more generally.

## 1.4 Status of Quantum Computing

> *Living things are made of atoms according to the laws of physics, and the laws of physics present no barrier to reducing the size of computers until bits are the size of atoms and quantum behavior holds sway*
>
> — Feynman *et al.* (2005) and Feynman (1985)

Quantum systems, unlike having classical bits that exist in distinct values of zero or one (Figure 1.1), have qubits (quantum information bits (Schumacher, 1995)) that exist in a state of superposition of all possible values in the space until collapsed into a measurement. In general, the term "quantum" refers to atoms, which are on the scale of nanometers ($10^{-9}$), and subatomic ions, electrons, and photons, which are on the scale of picometers ($10^{-12}$). Feynman (1985) was the first to propose the idea for a universal quantum computer. Such a computer would model nature exactly as it is, in three-dimensional atomically accurate representations, which would be a more scalable and natural computational method.

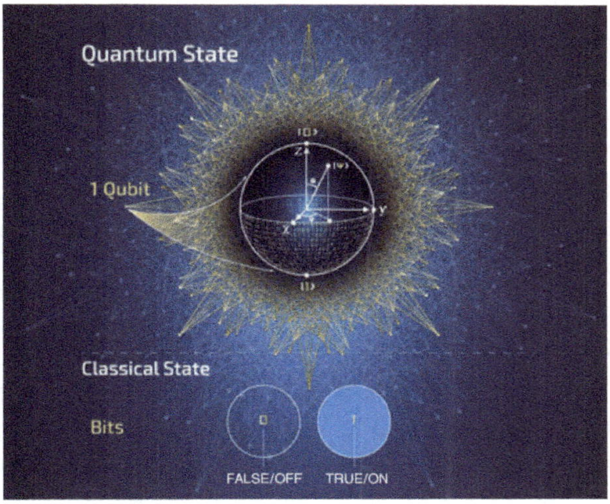


Figure 1.1. Quantum versus classical computing.
*Source*: Sandia National Laboratories.

Quantum computing is therefore defined as the use of engineered quantum systems to perform computation, typically the precise manipulation of quantum objects (atoms, ions, and photons) by means of external electromagnetic fields (Acin *et al.*, 2018). Quantum computing incorporates the principles of quantum physics as the approach to understanding quantum mechanical phenomena. Quantum mechanics describes the behavior of quantum objects that is stridently different from the macroscale classical domain through the properties of superposition, entanglement, and interference. Quantum communication involves the transmission of quantum state information between locations, and quantum information science is the field that provides an information-theoretic interpretation of quantum physics in the implementation of quantum computing and quantum communication networks. Each area has constituent domains of theoretical and experimental focus (Table 1.3).

The "big data" era is a substantial motivation towards the development of quantum computing. Data science applications are constrained by classical computing limitations. Quantum computers, however, have the potential to perform complex calculations and cycle through a series of

Table 1.3. Quantum terminology.

| Term | Description |
|---|---|
| Quantum computing | Computation with engineered quantum systems |
| Quantum communication | Transmission of quantum state information |
| Quantum physics | Foundational physics, quantum mechanics |
| Quantum information | Information-theoretic interpretation of physics |

permutations in ways that classical systems cannot. Modeling classical data as quantum wavefunctions allows more information to be incorporated in a complex format that is more scalable and (through entanglement) reveals otherwise unseen correlations in the classical data.

### 1.4.1 $2^n$ *scalability*

The biggest arguments in favor of quantum computing are its scalability as a next-generation computing platform, and its natural three-dimensional representational capability. Regarding scalability, a central feature of quantum mechanics is the $2^n$ problem. This is the issue that the number of possible particle states (the state space) grows exponentially as the size of the system grows. For example, a system consisting of $n$ 2-state quantum particles has $2^n$ possible states, and in general, might be in a superposition of all of them. The classical simulation of such a system requires one complex number per state, which means that simulating more than about 40 qubits in a general superposition state is beyond most classical capabilities (Kendon *et al.*, 2010, p. 3611).

With quantum computing's $2^n$ format, though, an exponentially large number of values can be encoded in a set of qubits for expedient information processing. Mathematically, the quantum state of $n$ qubits is a vector in a $2^n$-dimensional complex vector space. This means that performing a quantum logic operation or a qubit measurement multiplies the corresponding state vector by $2^n \times 2^n$ matrices (Biamonte *et al.*, 2017, p. 196). By building up these kinds of matrix transformations, quantum computers can execute common linear algebraic operations such as computing Fourier transforms (Shor, 1997), finding eigenvectors and eigenvalues

(Nielsen & Chuang, 2000), and solving linear sets of equations (Harrow *et al.*, 2009) exponentially faster than their best known classical counterparts.

In general, quantum computers have been shown to provide an exponential advantage over classical computers in solving both linear and nonlinear differential equations (Biamonte *et al.*, 2017; Lloyd *et al.*, 2020). The implication is that because quantum algorithms are better at performing algebra-related tasks, there could be many areas of quantum advantage over classical computing. The number of qubits required to implement various computational tasks suggests which kinds of problems may be tractable with currently available NISQ devices (noisy intermediate-scale quantum devices) with 50–100 qubits. The million-qubit quantum hardware needed for full-scale quantum neuroscience and other advanced applications is not immediately immanent. Technical breakthroughs are needed to deliver quantum error correction to progress from (non-error corrected) NISQ devices to FTQC (fault-tolerant quantum computing) (Preskill, 2021, p. 10). However, it is not too early to reformulate classical problems for the quantum domain and test them on simulation platforms.

### 1.4.2 *Three-dimensional format*

Aside from scalability, the other key benefit of quantum computing for modeling the brain is the ability to have three-dimensional representations of real-life systems. The organic molecules of life are three-dimensional, and also their representation in quantum computing. Feynman's vision to model nature as it actually is, with a universal quantum computer, becomes more prominent in quantum neuroscience applications. Brain entities and the chemical conversion processes that orchestrate their behavior are quantum mechanical in nature and an analogous computing environment for representing these processes is needed. The benefit of quantum computers is that they can store and process information about a simulated quantum system natively (NSF, 2016, p. 1). To perform such a quantum simulation, the Hilbert space of the underlying system is mapped directly onto the Hilbert space of the qubits in the quantum computer (Kendon *et al.*, 2010, p. 3609).

### 1.4.3 *Quantum advantage over classical computing*

An industry objective is demonstrating quantum advantage, applications in which quantum computers perform tasks that classical computers cannot. Quantum advantage is indicated differently based on the underlying platform. It could be demonstrated, for example, by sampling the output of random quantum circuits on gate-model platforms (Aaronson & Chen, 2016) or by conducting boson sampling on photonic platforms (Aaronson & Arkhipov, 2013). Google deployed the first method, sampling the output of random quantum circuits, to declare having achieved quantum advantage in October 2019 with a 53-qubit chip (Sycamore) (Arute *et al.*, 2019). IBM rebutted the claim (Pednault *et al.*, 2019). Google confirmed the computational result by simulating the random circuit sampling operation on the world's largest supercomputer at the time, Summit, in a 281-Pflop/s demonstration (Villalonga *et al.*, 2020). Notably, the quantum method was many orders of magnitude more energy-efficient than classical supercomputers.

A greater claim of quantum advantage, with no question of being unassailable with classical methods, occurred in December 2020 (Ball, 2020). The result in *Science* announced using a photon-based quantum computer to perform boson sampling (Zhong *et al.*, 2020). The work highlights the benefit of photonic platforms that operate at room temperature as opposed to the ultracold temperatures required by superconducting circuits. Debate continues as to which platform has more feasible near-term applications, the 53-qubit superconducting chip which is programmable but not commercially released, or the boson sampling method, which has already been applied in quantum chemistry (Sparrow *et al.*, 2018) and graph theory applications (Bromley *et al.*, 2020).

Indeed, perhaps the more important aim is not research demonstrations of quantum advantage, but progressing more quickly to scalable quantum computers for tackling real-life problems (Cirac, 2021). The status of end-user quantum computing is NISQ devices, used directly or via cloud-based services. NISQ devices can perform useful tasks and do not require error correction (Preskill, 2018). Such NISQ devices continue to be available from IBM and Rigetti (gate-model systems) and D-Wave Systems (quantum annealing machines with 5,000 qubits as of 2019). Researchers building their own boson sampling setups is another flavor of the NISQ device, and there are other platforms (Swan *et al.*, 2020, pp. 50–62).

The biggest threat of quantum computing is possibly being able to break existing cryptography. Shor's (1997) algorithm can factor large numbers expediently and is implicated in eventually forcing an evolution in cryptography standards (a sort of "Y2K for Crypto"). A 2019 U.S. National Academies of Sciences report estimates that this is unlikely within 10 years (Grumbling and Horowitz, 2019); however, methods are constantly improving. The U.S. NIST (National Institute of Standards and Technology) has a competition-based method to develop next-generation standards based on lattice cryptography (complex three-dimensional arrangements of atoms), as opposed to the difficulty of factoring large numbers, in a mathematical shift to group theory (lattices) from number theory (factoring) (Alagic *et al.*, 2019).

The vision is not that end users would have quantum desktop computers on which to open up an $N = 4$ Yang–Mills ground state, but rather would access it via cloud-based services as any other internet application. Gartner notes that the COVID-19 pandemic strengthened the demand for cloud services with worldwide public cloud end-user spending estimated to grow 18% in 2021 (Costello & Rimol, 2020). Cloud services are forecast to comprise 14.2% of the total global enterprise Information Technology (IT) spending market in 2024, up from 9.1% in 2020. The fastest-growing cloud service is application infrastructure services (PaaS) (more intelligent applications) as opposed to software as a service (SaaS) which has a larger share but a slower growth rate.

In 2019, Gartner estimated that by 2023, 20% of organizations will be budgeting for quantum computing and that 95% of organizations researching quantum computing strategies will use quantum computing as a service (QCaaS) (Panetta, 2019). To aid in this endeavor, 90% of enterprise quantum computing investments may turn to quantum consulting organizations, and employ an increasing number of degreed quantum physicists in product management roles. In an April 2021 survey, IDC similarly found that the number of organizations allocating about a fifth of their annual IT budgets to quantum computing is expected to rise from 7% in 2021 to an estimated 19% in 2023 (West, 2021). P&S Intelligence (2020) estimates the global market for quantum computing to grow from $507.1 million in 2019 to $64,988.3 million by 2030.

### 1.4.4 *Supercomputing versus quantum computing*

The question arises as to the relationship between supercomputing and quantum computing. On the one hand, the platforms can be complementary as they have different architectures and target different tasks. On the other hand, the bigger news is that quantum computing is likely to substantially leapfrog the capabilities of supercomputing. For example, state-of-the-art supercomputers (in 2018) were noted as already being limited in not being able to simulate universal random circuits of sufficient depth in a two-dimensional lattice of approximately $7 \times 7$ qubits (Boixo *et al.*, 2018, p. 595). Quantum computing is already demonstrating greater capability than 49-qubit systems ($7 \times 7$).

For understanding the complexity of the brain, a vastly more scalable platform beyond supercomputing such as quantum computing is necessary (Harris & Kendon, 2010, p. 3581). Supercomputers have only managed to simulate one-third of the human brain so far (Igarashi *et al.*, 2019). Quantum computing easily surmounts supercomputing with its scalability and three-dimensional problem instantiation as supercomputing remains constrained to massively parallelizable tasks. Further, a potential quantum revolution is indicated as a next-generation platform for computation in general, with cost-effective accessibility through cloud-based quantum computing applications, and as QPUs might be made in existing microprocessor fabrication facilities. Further, just as quantum computer simulations are run on supercomputers to the extent possible (Villalonga *et al.*, 2020), in the future, supercomputers might be simulated on quantum computers.

### 1.4.5 *Quantum finance and AdS/Finance*

One of the first applications of quantum computing that could enter the mainstream is quantum finance. Standardized quantum approaches and circuits could quickly extend to other fields such as neuroscience. Financial market participants are often early adopters of new technology, and individuals involved with J.P. Morgan, Goldman Sachs, Banco Santander, and other global financial institutions are publishing research discussing these efforts. Quantum finance is the branch of econophysics that applies theories and methods from quantum mechanics and economics to problems in finance, namely, option pricing, trading strategies, risk management, and portfolio optimization. Markets are complex nonlinear dynamical systems that do not have formal solutions, and hence quantum mechanical methods such as wavefunction modeling have been a mainstay in computational finance (Haven, 2002). What is new is the ability to more effectively model market behavior with quantum platforms that include wavefunctions and path integrals (Baaquie, 2004; Orus *et al.*, 2019).

A concrete application is implementing the traditional classical framework of the Black Scholes option pricing model with the Schrödinger wavefunction equation (option price is modeled as a state function). Such quantum finance methods may have been applied through topological quantum field theories such as the Chern-Simons 3-form as a form of quantum field theory on a three-dimensional manifold expressed with Lie algebra (Chern & Simons, 1974). These techniques may be responsible for the success of hedge funds such as Renaissance Technologies (founded by Simons) and its Medallion Fund, an effort which has resulted in the Simons Institute for the Theory of Computing.

Unlike disease, which ideally, is formally solvable and demonstrates ongoing progress towards this objective, markets have social feedback

Table 1.4. Quantum finance ecosystem.

| No. | *Analysis*<br>Quantum Finance | *Execution*<br>Quantum Blockchains | *Delivery*<br>Quantum Networks |
|---|---|---|---|
| 1 | Quantum amplitude estimation | Quantum key distribution | Heralded entanglement |
| 2 | Quantum Monte Carlo methods | Continuous-time quantum walks | End-to-end qubits |
| 3 | Anharmonic oscillators | Computational verification (zero-knowledge proofs) | Smart routing SLAs |
| 4 | Quantum kernel learning | GHZ-state optical blockchain | Benchmarking |

loops and are resistant to traditional formal solutions. Reflexivity is the term for participants modeling the potential behavior of other participants as hypothesized by George Soros (Davis & Hands, 2016). Reflexivity is an inherently quantum mechanical concept in that the role of the observer influences outcomes, but is difficult to model.

#### 1.4.5.1 *Classical-digital-quantum finance progression*

Conceptually, there is a progression from classical to digital (blockchains) to quantum finance. The potential future ecosystem for quantum finance can be seen in the structure of the deployment of quantum financial methods for analysis, quantum blockchains for execution, and quantum networks for delivery (Table 1.4).

Quantum blockchain applications focus on two areas, post-quantum cryptography and the instantiation of the underlying blockchain logic and protocol with quantum platforms (Li *et al.*, 2019). Post-quantum cryptography methods include quantum key distribution and lattice-based quantum cryptography, and are being extended to consider continuous-time quantum walks with Hadamard coins (Montero, 2017) and blind quantum computing (Flamini *et al.*, 2018). Continuous-time quantum walks with Hadamard coins (zero-one flips) enhance security as walks proceed on the basis of ballistic propagation through a lattice graph as opposed to classical algorithms which are constrained to diffusive spread. The faster the cryptographic algorithm, the safer it is, and in quantum finance, the faster a trading opportunity can be identified. In the application of instantiating blockchain logic in quantum networks, computational verification (zero-knowledge proof technology) (Swan, 2020) and optical networks are likely crucial to deployment. One project outlines a blockchain formulation with optical networks relying on entangled GHZ states (Rajan & Visser, 2019), similar to the use of GHZ states in a global quantum clock network proposal (Komar *et al.*, 2014). The execution of quantum financial analysis methods could be via quantum blockchains deployed on quantum networks and instantiating (anti-de Sitter) AdS/Finance as holographic option pricing (Treiblmaier *et al.*, 2021).

Quantum finance applications treat the analysis of financial markets. One of the main research activities in quantum finance is establishing standard quantum algorithms for deployment in financial analysis. So far, quantum finance methods demonstrate what is becoming the usual expected quadratic speedup of using quantum systems when benchmarked against classical methods (mainly classical Monte Carlo). The main applications of quantum finance target either individual instruments (with option pricing, trading, and risk management) or overall portfolio management.

Considering individual instruments, quantum amplitude estimation is a technique used to estimate the properties of random distributions such as risk measures (Woerner & Egger, 2019). In a quantum computing setup, the method is operationalized to estimate the probability of measuring a value of "1" in the last qubit. There are four steps in the quantum circuit execution. First, the system is defined to consist of a unitary operator acting on a register of qubits. Second, an estimation operator is created to operate on the system based on the unitary operator and quantum phase estimation (Kitaev, 1995) to approximate certain eigenvalues of the estimation operator. This requires additional qubits and additional applications of the estimation operator. Third, the additional qubits are put into equal superposition by applying Hadamard gates and used to control different powers of the estimation operator. Fourth, the system is evolved, an inverse quantum Fourier transform is applied, and the qubit state is measured. The result is an integer which is mapped to a classical estimation function. The quantum amplitude estimation method indicates a quadratic speedup compared to the convergence rate of classical Monte Carlo methods.

Research continues to improve the quantum amplitude estimation algorithm, for example, in the proposal of a version of amplitude estimation without phase estimation that requires fewer gates (Suzuki *et al.*, 2020). This method also results in a quadratic speedup compared to classical Monte Carlo methods and is tested by deploying option pricing circuits on an IBM Q Tokyo quantum device (Stamatopoulos *et al.*, 2020).

Another project also uses quantum amplitude estimation algorithms, and models the time evolution of interest rates with the Heath-Jarrow-Morton framework for stochastic dynamics (volatility-based) (Martin *et al.*, 2019). The successful deployment of the quantum finance circuit on a 5-qubit IBMQX2 quantum computer foresees the near-term practical applications of quantum computing in finance.

In portfolio optimization, a team simulated a quantum circuit Born machine for an ion-trap quantum computer (Alcazar *et al.*, 2020). A well-known portfolio management problem in finance was implemented using time-series pricing data from asset subsets of the S&P500 stock market index. The quantum model had superior performance as compared to classical machine learning methods (restricted Boltzmann machines). Other work also considers portfolio optimization with quantum Monte Carlo methods, quantum machine learning, and quantum annealing heuristics (Bouland *et al.*, 2020). In another project, a complete quantum finance field theory is proposed based on anharmonic (not simple harmonic) oscillators and energy, deployed through a Quantum Finance Forecast Center website (qffc.uic.edu.hk) (Lee, 2020). Finally, other work proposes quantum kernel learning based on reproducing kernel Hilbert spaces (Chatterjee & Yu, 2017).

The first step is that quantum finance enables better analysis of existing markets, and the second step could be that the quantum domain enables new financial instruments specific to its structure and parameters. Just as blockchain digital finance offers arbitrage possibilities between classical and digital instruments, for example, between a physical-world loan and a smart contract loan due in block time (the digital time regime of the blockchain) (Swan, 2016), the quantum domain likewise offers novel possibilities. Instead of Euclidean space and lockstep time, there could be a superpositioning of time and space. As in multiplexing in communications networks, time and space can be treated as different modes of "photonic finance". Instruments can measure in one space and many times (measure the same system at different times), or measure the system in different spaces at one time, with spacetime states created based on these measurement statistics (Zhang *et al.*, 2020). Thus, a loan on a Bloch sphere would not be a traditional 30-year mortgage and might have geodesic rather than linear pricing (an AdS/Finance application). Quantum methods access correlations not present in classical systems, and quantum finance might engage a new geometry of economic space with entropic connections (Potts, 2000, p. 47).

## 1.5 What This Book Does Not Cover

This book investigates the study of the brain using quantum computing. First, this means that the primary interest is in the most basic measurable physical-level behavior in the brain regarding neuronal and synaptic signaling. Higher-order behavior such as learning, attention, memory, and cognition are not examined in any specificity (these are addressed in other quantum neuroscience applications research such as using the quantum machine learning of EEG data to model decision-making (Aishwarya *et al.*, 2020)). Other such higher-level behaviors are assumed to exist, but the focus here is on the basic tiers of neural behavior as they may be modeled computationally most readily from available data and how these physical aspects may be addressable indicators of disease.

Second, this book does not discuss the hypothesis called quantum consciousness (that consciousness is caused by quantum effects). Koch and Hepp (2006) offer cogent guidance on this issue, arguing that quantum effects are not part of the brain. The brain is simply too big, and while biology obeys quantum mechanics, it does not exhibit quantum effects. The biological features of the brain indicate that it is too large and has distances (millimeters) that are too long for quantum signals to remain coherent (Tegmark, 2000). The main argument of this book is that quantum computing is possibly the best computational platform for modeling the brain's neural signaling processes. The work is not proceeding from the assumption that there is something quantum-like taking place in the brain, but rather is inspired by the mathematical structure of quantum mechanics (Bruza *et al.*, 2015). The basic processes are necessary to enumerate as the building blocks of larger-scale behavior anyway (Churchland *et al.*, 1994).

## 1.6 Quantum Neuroscience and AdS/Brain

The current volume draws from contemporary progress in neuroscience and physics to ultimately propose AdS/Brain as a multiscalar theory of neural signaling that might be implemented with quantum computing. The advent of quantum computing is a concrete testament to the understanding of quantum mechanics and may facilitate the quest to further clarify the mysterious inner workings of the brain. One critique might be that it is too early for this work given the lack of human *in vivo* whole-brain activity data, and the developmental stage of quantum computing. However, the rate of data acquisition from connectomics projects and the specialized expertise of neuroscientists suggest that this is exactly the time for qualitatively new methods to address the challenges of the brain, to obtain a full model of neural signaling behavior. Further, quantum computing is part of the national competitiveness narrative for many countries and has substantial financial resources invested.

Computation methods are needed that are not just faster (server racks) or process data in parallel (supercomputing) but that run differently, more in line with quantum mechanical reality. There is an opportunity to define the computational neuroscience analysis techniques that will succeed in the areas of spiking neural networks, neural field theories, tensor networks and quantum kernel learning, photonic quantum networks for smart network computing, and quantum state teleportation with high-dimensional entangled qudits. A computational environment is needed with multiple levels of three-dimensional image representation and their behavioral manipulation through nonlinear dynamical models. It is clear that a deeper theoretical and experimental arsenal is necessary for the next eras of neuroscience and that quantum computing might help to open a new chapter in studying the brain.

## References

Aaronson, S. & Arkhipov, A. (2013). The computational complexity of linear optics. *Theor. Comput.* 9(4):143–252.

Aaronson, S. & Chen, L. (2016). Complexity-theoretic foundations of quantum supremacy experiments. arXiv:1612.05903.

Abbott, L.F., Bock, D.D., Callaway, E.M. *et al.* (2020). The mind of a mouse. *Cell.* 182(6):1372–76.

Acin, A. Bloch, I., Buhrman, H. *et al.* (2018). The quantum technologies roadmap: A European community view. *New. J. Phys.* 20(8):080201.

Aishwarya, S., Abeer, V., Sathish, B.B. & Subramanya, K.N. (2020). Quantum computational techniques for prediction of cognitive state of human mind from EEG signals. *J. Quantum. Comput.* 2(4):157–70.

Alagic, G., Alperin-Sheriff, J., Apon, D. *et al.* (2019). Status report on the first round of the NIST post-quantum cryptography standardization process. NISTIR 8240.

Alcazar, J., Leyton-Ortega, V. & Perdomo-Ortiz, A. (2020). Classical versus quantum models in machine learning: Insights from a finance application. *Machine Learning: Sci. Tech.* 1(3):035003.

Amari, S. (1977). Dynamics of pattern formation in lateral-inhibition type neural fields. *Biol. Cybern.* 27:77–87.

Arute, F., Arya, K., Babbush, R. *et al.* (2019). Quantum supremacy using a programmable superconducting processor. *Nature*. 574:505–10.

Baaquie, B.E. (2004). *Quantum Finance: Path Integrals and Hamiltonians for Options and Interest Rates*. Cambridge: Cambridge University Press.

Ball, P. (2020). Physicists in China challenge Google's "quantum advantage". *Nature*. 588:380.

Bassett, D.S. & Gazzaniga, M.S. (2011). Understanding complexity in the human brain. *Trends Cogn. Sci.* 15:200–9.

Biamonte, J., Wittek, P., Pancotti, N. *et al.* (2017). Quantum machine learning. *Nature*. 549(195):195–202.

Boixo, S., Isakov, S.V., Smelyanskiy, V.N. *et al.* (2018). Characterizing quantum supremacy in near-term devices. *Nat. Phys.* 14:595–600.

Bouland A., van Dam, W., Joorati, H. *et al.* (2020). Prospects and challenges of quantum finance. arXiv:2011.06492v1.

Breakspear, M. (2017). Dynamic models of large-scale brain activity. *Nat. Neurosci.* 20:340–52.

Bromley, T.R., Arrazola, J.M., Jahangiri, S. *et al.* (2020). Applications of near-term photonic quantum computers: Software and algorithms. *Quantum Sci. Technol.* 5(3):034010.

Bruza, P.D., Wang, Z. & Busemeyer, J.B. (2015). Quantum cognition: A new theoretical approach to psychology. *Trends Cogn. Sci.* 19:383–93.

Carminati, F. (2018). Quantum thinking required. *Cern Courier*. 58(9):5.

Chatterjee, R. & Yu, T. (2017). Generalized coherent states, reproducing kernels, and quantum support vector machines. *Quantum Inf & Computation.* 17(15–16):1292–1306.

Chern, S.-S. & Simons, J. (1974). Characteristic forms and geometric invariants. *Ann. Math.* Second Series. 99(1):48–69.

Churchland, P.S., Ramachandran, V.S. & Sejnowski T.J. (1994). A critique of pure vision. In *Large-Scale Neuronal Theories of the Brain*. Eds. Koch, C. & Davis J.L. Cambridge: The MIT Press, pp. 23–60.

Cirac, J.I. (2021). Quantum computing and simulation: Where we stand and what awaits us. *Nanophotonics*. 10(1):453–56.

Coombes, S., Lai, Y.M., Sayli, M. & Thul, R. (2018). Networks of piecewise linear neural mass models. *Eur. J. Appl. Math.* 29(5):869–90.

Costello, K. & Rimol, M. (2020). *Gartner Forecasts Worldwide Public Cloud End-User Spending to Grow 18% in 2021*. Gartner, Inc. https://www.gartner.com/en/newsroom/press-releases/2020-11-17-gartner-forecasts-worldwide-public-cloud-end-user-spending-to-grow-18-percent-in-2021.

Davis, J.B. & Hands, D.W., Eds. (2016). *Reflexivity and Economics: George Soros's Theory of Reflexivity and the Methodology of Economic Science.* New York: Routledge.

Feldman, M. (2018). Blue Brain project installs HPE supercomputer. *TOP500.* https://www.top500.org/news/blue-brain-project-installs-hpe-supercomputer/.

Feynman, R.P. (1985). Quantum mechanical computers. *Found Phys.* 16(6):507–31.

Feynman, R.P., Leighton, R.B. & Sands, M. (2005). *The Feynman Lectures on Physics: The Definitive and Extended Edition.* 2nd Edition. New York: Addison Wesley.

Flamini, F., Spagnolo, N. & Sciarrino, F. (2018). Photonic quantum information processing: A review. *Rep. Prog. Phys.* 82(1):016001.

Gao, R., Asano, S.M., Upadhyayula, S. *et al.* (2019). Cortical column and whole-brain imaging with molecular contrast and nanoscale resolution. *Science.* 363(6424):eaau8302.

Grumbling, E. & Horowitz, M. (2019). *Quantum Computing: Progress and Prospects.* Washington DC: US National Academies of Sciences.

Hamilton, K.E., Dumitrescu, E.F. & Pooser, R.C. (2019). Generative model benchmarks for superconducting qubits. *Phys. Rev. A.* 99(6):062323.

Han, X. & Hartnoll, S.A. (2020). Deep quantum geometry of matrices. *Phys. Rev. X.* 10(1):011069.

Harris, S. & Kendon, V.M. (2010). Quantum-assisted biomolecular modeling. *Phil. Trans. R. Soc.* 368(1924):3581–92.

Harrow, A.W., Hassidim, A. & Lloyd, S. (2009). Quantum algorithm for linear systems of equations. *Phys. Rev. Lett.* 103(15):150502.

Haven, E.E. (2002). A discussion on embedding the Black-Scholes option pricing model in a quantum physics setting. *Phys. A: Stat. Mech. Appl.* 304(3–4): 507–24.

Igarashi, J., Yamaura, H. & Yamazaki, T. (2019). Large-scale simulation of a layered cortical sheet of spiking network model using a tile partitioning method. *Front Neuroinform.* 13(71):1–15.

Jurcevic, P., Javadi-Abhari, A., Bishop, L.S. *et al.* (2020). Demonstration of quantum volume 64 on a superconducting quantum computing system. arXiv: 2008.08571v2.

Kendon, V.M., Nemoto, K. & Munro, W.J. (2010). Quantum analogue computing. *Phil. Trans. R. Soc.* 368(1924):3609–20.

Kiani, B.T., Villanyi, A. & Lloyd, S. (2020). Quantum medical imaging algorithms. arXiv:2004.02036.

Kitaev, A.Y. (1995). Quantum measurements and the Abelian Stabilizer Problem. arXiv:9511026.

Koch, C. & Hepp, K. (2006). Quantum mechanics in the brain. *Nature*. 440(30):611–2.

Komar, P., Kessler, E.M., Bishof, M. *et al.* (2014). A quantum network of clocks. *Nat. Phys*. 10(8):582.

LeCun, Y., Bengio, Y. & Hinton, G. (2015). Deep learning. *Nature*. 521 (7553):436–44.

Lee, R.S.T. (2020). *Quantum Finance: Intelligent Forecast and Trading Systems*. Singapore: Springer.

Leyton-Ortega, V., Perdomo-Ortiz, A. & Perdomo, O. (2019). Robust implementation of generative modeling with parametrized quantum circuits. arXiv: 1901.08047.

Li, C., Xu, Y., Tang, J. & Liu, W. (2019). Quantum blockchain: A decentralized, encrypted and distributed database based on quantum mechanics. *J. Quantum Comput*. 1(2):49–63.

Lichtman, J.W., Pfister, H. & Shavit, N. (2014). The big data challenges of connectomics. *Nat. Neurosci*. 17(11):1448–54.

Lloyd, S., de Palma, G. & Gokler, C. (2020). Quantum algorithm for nonlinear differential equations. arXiv:2011.06571v2.

Lynn, C.W. & Bassett, D.S. (2019). The physics of brain network structure, function and control. *Nat. Rev. Phys*. 1:318–32.

Markram, H. (2006). The blue brain project. *Nat. Rev. Neurosci*. 7:153–60.

Martin, A., Candelas, B., Rodriguez-Rozas, A. *et al.* (2019). Towards pricing financial derivatives with an IBM quantum computer. arXiv:1904.05803.

Martins, N.R.B., Angelica, A., Chakravarthy, K. *et al.* (2019). Human brain/cloud interface. *Front Neurosci*. 13(112):1–23.

Montero, M. (2017). Quantum and random walks as universal generators of probability distributions. *Phys. Rev. A*. 95(6):062326.

Motta, A., Schurr, M., Staffler, B. & Helmstaedter, M. (2019). Big data in nanoscale connectomics, and the greed for training labels. *Curr. Opin. Neurobiol*. 55:180–87.

Nielsen, M.A. & Chuang, I.L. (2010). *Quantum Computation and Quantum Information*. 10th-anniversary Edition. Cambridge: Cambridge University Press.

NSF. Quantum information and computation for chemistry. *NSF Workshop Report* 2016.

Nunez, P.L. (1974). The brain wave equation: A model for the EEG. *Math. Biosci*. 21:279–97.

Nunez, P.L., Srinivasan, R. & Fields, R.D. (2015). EEG functional connectivity, axon delays and white matter disease. *Clin. Neurophysiol*. 126(1):110–20.

Orus, R., Mugel, S. & Lizaso, E. (2019). Quantum computing for finance: Overview and prospects. *Rev. Phys.* 4:100028.

Otterbach, J.S., Manenti, R., Alidoust, N. *et al.* (2017). Unsupervised machine learning on a hybrid quantum computer. arXiv:1712.05771.

P&S Intelligence. (2020). Quantum computing market is poised to surpass $64,988.3 million by 2030: P&S Intelligence (Prescient & Strategic Intelligence Private Limited). Press Release. https://www.globenewswire.com/news-release/2020/02/10/1982087/0/en/Quantum-Computing-Market-is-Poised-to-Surpass-64-988-3-Million-By-2030-P-S-Intelligence.html.

Panetta, K. (2019). The CIO's guide to quantum computing. Gartner, Inc.

Pednault, E., Gunnels, J., Maslov, D. & Gambetta, J. (2019). On "quantum supremacy". *IBM.* https://www.ibm.com/blogs/research/2019/10/on-quantum-supremacy. Accessed March 15, 2021.

Pennisi, E. (2001). The human genome. *Science.* 291(5507):1177–80.

Potts, J.D. (2000). *The New Evolutionary Microeconomics: Complexity, Competence and Adaptive Behavior.* Cheltenham, UK: Edward Elgar Publishing.

Preskill, J. (2018). Quantum computing in the NISQ era and beyond. *Quantum.* 2:79.

Preskill, J. (2021). Quantum computing 40 years later. arXiv:2106.10522.

Rajan, D. & Visser, M. (2019). Quantum blockchain using entanglement in time. *Quantum Rep.* 1(2):1–9.

Reinsel, D. (2020). IDC's Global DataSphere Forecast shows continued steady growth in the creation and consumption of data. *IDC Report: Worldwide Global DataSphere Forecast, 2020–2024: The COVID-19 Data Bump and the Future of Data Growth* (Doc #US44797920).

Schumacher, B. (1995). Quantum coding. *Phys. Rev. A.* 51(4):2738–47.

Sejnowski, T.J. (2020). The unreasonable effectiveness of deep learning in artificial intelligence. *Proc. Natl. Acad. Sci.* 117(48):30033–8.

Shor, P.W. (1997). Polynomial-time algorithms for prime factorization and discrete logarithms on a quantum computer. *SIAM J. Comput.* 26(5): 1484–1509.

Sparrow, C., Martin-Lopez, E., Maraviglia, N. *et al.* (2018). Simulating the vibrational quantum dynamics of molecules using photonics. *Nature.* 557 (7707):660–67.

Stamatopoulos, N., Egger, D.J., Sun, Y. *et al.* (2020). Option pricing using quantum computers. *Quantum.* 4:291.

Sterratt, D., Graham, B., Gillies, A. & Willshaw, D. (2011). *Principles of Computational Modelling in Neuroscience.* Cambridge: Cambridge University Press.

Suzuki, Y., Uno, S., Raymond, R. *et al.* (2020). Amplitude estimation without phase estimation. *Quantum Inf. Proc.* 19:75.

Swan, M. (2016). Blockchain temporality: Smart contract time specifiability with blocktime. In *Rule Technologies. Research, Tools, and Applications. 10th International Symposium, RuleML 2016, Stony Brook, NY, USA, July 6–9, 2016. Proceedings*, pp. 184–96.

Swan, M. (2020). Black hole zero-knowledge proofs. *FQXi Undecidability, Uncomputability, and Unpredictability Essay Contest Entry*. https://fqxi.org/community/forum/topic/3442.

Swan, M., dos Santos, R.P. & Witte, F. (2020). *Quantum Computing: Physics, Blockchains, and Deep Learning Smart Networks*. London: World Scientific.

Taha, S.M.R. & Taha, Z.K. (2018). EEG signals classification based on autoregressive and inherently quantum recurrent neural network. *Int. J. Comput. Appl. Technol.* 58(4):340.

Tegmark, M. (2000). The importance of quantum decoherence in brain processes. *Phys. Rev. E.* 61(4):4194.

Treiblmaier, H., Swan, M., de Filippi, P. *et al.* (2021). What's next in blockchain research? An identification of key topics using a multidisciplinary perspective. *ACM SIGMIS Database: The DATABASE for Adv. Inf. Syst.* 52(1):27–52.

van Albada, S.J., Rowley, A.G. & Senk, J. (2018). Performance comparison of the digital neuromorphic hardware SpiNNaker and the neural network simulation software NEST for a full-scale cortical microcircuit model. *Front Neurosci.* 12:291.

Vescovi, R.F.C., Cardoso, M.B. & Miqueles, E.X. (2017). Radiography registration for mosaic tomography. *J. Synchrotron Radiat.* 24:686–94.

Vidal, G. (2008). Class of quantum many-body states that can be efficiently simulated. *Phys. Rev. Lett.* 101(11):110501.

Villalonga, B., Lyakh, D., Boixo, S. *et al.* (2020). Establishing the quantum supremacy frontier with a 281 Pflop/s simulation. *Quantum Sci. Technol.* 5:3.

von Bartheld, C.S., Bahney, J. & Herculano-Houzel, S. (2016). The search for true numbers of neurons and glial cells in the human brain: A review of 150 years of cell counting. *J. Comp. Neurol.* 524(18):3865–95.

Wang, J., Paesani, S., Ding, Y. *et al.* (2018). Multidimensional quantum entanglement with large-scale integrated optics. *Science*. 360:285–91.

Wang, Y., Li, Q., Liu, L. *et al.* (2019a). TeraVR empowers precise reconstruction of complete 3-D neuronal morphology in the whole brain. *Nat. Comm.* 10:3474.

Wang, Y.E., Wei, G.-Y., Brooks, D. (2019b). Benchmarking TPU, GPU, and CPU platforms for deep learning. arXiv:1907.10701.

West, H. (2021). Enterprise IT Infrastructure Survey, 1Q21: Insights on end-user 2021 IT compute infrastructure priorities and adoption of quantum computing. IDC Report #US47687021.

Woerner, S. & Egger, D.J. (2019). Quantum risk analysis. *NPJ Quantum Information*. 5:15.

Yin, W., Brittain, D., Borseth, J. *et al.* (2019). A petascale automated imaging pipeline for mapping neuronal circuits with high-throughput transmission electron microscopy. bioRxiv:791889.

Zhang, T., Dahlsten, O. & Vedral, V. (2020). Different instances of time as different quantum modes: Quantum states across space-time for continuous variables. *New J. Phys*. 22(023029):1–19.

Zheng, Z., Lauritzen, J.S., Perlman, E. *et al.* (2018). A complete electron microscopy volume of the brain of adult *Drosophila melanogaster*. *Cell*. 174: 730–43.e22.

Zhong, H.-S., Wang, H., Deng, Y.-H. *et al.* (2020). Quantum computational advantage using photons. *Science*. 370(6523):1460–63.

Zhu, D., Linke, N.M., Benedetti, M. *et al.* (2019). Training of quantum circuits on a hybrid quantum computer. *Sci. Adv*. 5(10):eaaw9918.

# Part 1

# Foundations

# Chapter 2

# Neural Signaling Basics

*In addition to secretory machines, nerve terminals are computational units*

— Sudhof (2004, p. 510)

**Abstract**

Chemical synapses are the brain's neural signaling processes between axon, presynaptic terminal, synaptic cleft, postsynaptic density, and dendritic spiking potentials from dendrite to soma (at the scale tiers of network, neuron, synapse, and molecule). Electrical signals from the action potential are converted to chemical signals in the presynaptic terminal, cross the synaptic cleft as neurotransmitters, are received at dendritic arbors, and are then reconverted to electrical signals as dendritic spikes. Synaptic integration is the process by which the brain integrates thousands of dendritic spikes and other incoming signals.

## 2.1 Scale Levels in the Brain

The human brain is a small 1.2–1.4 kg organ (Bigos *et al.*, 2015, p. 157) containing 86 billion neurons and 242 trillion synapses (Martins *et al.*, 2019, p. 4) and 85 billion glial cells (von Bartheld *et al.*, 2016). The brain transfers vast amounts of information between areas and rewires its connections as necessary with synaptic plasticity. Neurons in the cortex are arranged in layers, creating a complex communications network of neuronal connections or cortical circuits (Farhy-Tselnicker & Allen, 2018). The outermost gray matter of the cortex is a local area network (with mainly local connections) and the innermost white matter is a long-distance network (within itself) (Laughlin & Sejnowski, 2003).

The three elements involved in neural signaling are the sending neuron, the synapse, and the receiving neuron's dendritic arbors. The sending neuron's action potential is an electrical signal that is converted to a neurotransmitter-based chemical signal, sent across the synaptic cleft, and then reconverted to an electrical signal by the receiving neuron's dendrites. Protein complexes at the ends of the neurons transport calcium ions and molecules in and out of the cells. The relevant scales for neural signaling are those of the neuron, synapse, signaling pathway, and ion channel identified, respectively, as 100 $\mu$m, 1 $\mu$m, 1 nm, and 1 pm (Table 2.1) (Sterratt *et al.*, 2011). A related proposal similarly identifies the three levels of the neuron, synapse, and molecule, at 100 $\mu$m, 1 $\mu$m, and 1 Angstrom ($10^{-10}$) (Sejnowski, 2020, p. 30037). In quantum mechanics, atoms are on the order of nanometers ($10^{-9}$), and ions and photons are at the subatomic scale of picometers ($10^{-12}$). The scale pairings can be modeled as bulk-boundary relationships with the AdS/CFT correspondence in the AdS/Brain theory.

Since they are larger in scale and have more readily detectable electrical activity, action potential spikes from neurons have been the first and most studied aspect of neural signaling. The chemical operations of synapses are less well known, and the molecular propagation into dendritic arbors even less so. In computational neuroscience modeling (such as with the industry workhorse NEURON), neuronal and synaptic activity can be accommodated in a relatively straightforward manner with ordinary

Table 2.1. Neural signaling scale tiers.

| No. | Scale | Number | Size | Size (m) | NEURON | Microscopy |
|---|---|---|---|---|---|---|
| 1 | Neuron | 86 bn | 100 $\mu$m | $10^{-4}$ | ODE | EM |
| 2 | Synapse | 242 tn | 1 $\mu$m | $10^{-6}$ | ODE | EM/Light field |
| 3 | Signaling pathway | Unk | 1 nm | $10^{-9}$ | PDE | Light sheet |
| 4 | Ion channel | Unk | 1 pm | $10^{-12}$ | PDE | Light sheet |

differential equations (ODEs), but dendritic activities require more complicated partial differential equations (PDEs). In connectomics microscopy, single-neuron resolution is standard (Wang *et al.*, 2019), and single-molecule resolution for dendritic arbor analysis (detecting synaptic proteins at dendritic spines) is emerging (Gao *et al.*, 2019).

### 2.1.1 *Relative size of neural entities*

Understanding neural operations require thinking in various numeric scales. The standard units employed are the micron ($\mu$m, a millionth of a meter, $1 \times 10^{-6}$ meter) and the nanometer (a billionth of a meter, $1 \times 10^{-9}$ meter). One micron is 1,000 nm. As a heuristic, the diameter of a human hair is ~100 microns or 100,000 nm (the range is 17–181 microns) (Ley, 1999). A red blood cell is 7,000 nm and the smallest capillaries are 3,000 nm (Freitas, 2012, p. 69). Neurons are larger, having a 10,000–25,000 nm cell body (soma) and a 3,000–18,000 nm nucleus (Chudler, 2009).

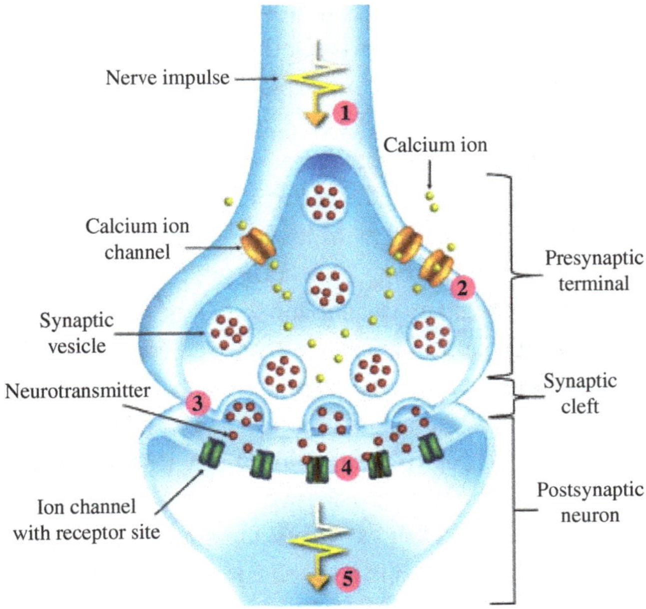


Figure 2.1. Neural signaling.

*Source*: Okinawa Institute of Science and Technology.

Presynaptic terminal research has studied in detail the calyx of Held (in the auditory pathway) in rats. The pathway forms a large nerve terminal 15,000 nm in diameter and makes about 500–600 synaptic contacts with the postsynaptic cell (Sudhof, 2004, p. 511). The presynaptic terminal has active zones on the synaptic cleft 50–100 nm wide and vesicles with an average radius of 20 nm (although stored in larger vesicles with a radius of 50–200 nm) (*Ibid.*, pp. 512, 523). The synaptic cleft between neurons is very small, 20–50 nm (Scimemi & Beato, 2009, p. 290), and glial cells are separated from each other by only 2 nm (Figure 2.1).

On the receiving neuron, the postsynaptic density is usually found at the tip of dendritic spines. Dendritic spines are long membrane protrusions on dendrites that receive the majority of synaptic inputs and are about 500–2,000 nm in length (Kim & Sheng, 2009, R723). The head of the dendritic spine or postsynaptic density is often a disk-like shape with an average diameter of 360 nm (range 200–800 nm) and a thickness of 40 nm (30–50 nm) (*Ibid.*). A similar estimate of the postsynaptic density is a diameter of 250–500 nm and a thickness of 50–100 nm (Meyer *et al.*, 2014). The postsynaptic density is positioned directly opposite the presynaptic active zone to receive the release of neurotransmitters.

In terms of glia, microglial cells are about the same size as neurons, 15,000–30,000 nm (Kettenmann & Verkhratsky, 2011), and astrocytes are even larger, 40,000–50,000 nm, with long branches wrapping around the neurons in their territory (Parent, 1996) (Table 2.2).

The postsynaptic density is an apparatus in a protein-dense area attached to the postsynaptic membrane stretched out in dendritic spines. Located across from specific active zones in the presynaptic terminal, the postsynaptic density orchestrates signal reception, becoming enlarged in the process and contributing to synaptic plasticity (the long-term potentiation or depression of synapses). The size of the postsynaptic density is dynamic and expands and shrinks during the signaling process. The signaling of many different proteins is implicated in the process. For example, Sonic hedgehog (Shh) signaling has an expansionary effect on the presynaptic terminals of both glutamatergic and GABAergic synapses in adult hippocampal neurons (Mitchell *et al.*, 2012, p. 4208). Glutamate

Table 2.2. Circulatory system entities and neural cells.

| Entity | Size (Microns) | Size (nm) |
|---|---|---|
| Human hair | 100 | 100,000 |
| Red blood cell | 7 | 7,000 |
| Smallest capillaries | 3 | 3,000 |
| Neuron cell body (soma) | 10–25 | 10,000–25,000 |
| Neuron cell body nucleus | 3–18 | 3,000–18,000 |
| Presynaptic terminal | 15 | 15,000 |
| Presynaptic terminal active zones | — | 50–100 |
| Synaptic cleft | — | 20–50 |
| Dendritic spine | 0.5–2 | 500–2,000 |
| Postsynaptic density (dendritic head) | — | 360 × 40 |
| Glial cells: Astrocytes | 40–50 | 40,000–50,000 |
| Glial cells: Microglial cells | 15–30 | 15,000–30,000 |

(excitatory action) and GABA (*gamma*-Aminobutyric acid) (inhibitory action) are the two most common neurotransmitters in the brain, comprising 90% of neurotransmitter activity.

The structural setup of the synapse facilitates the targeting of signals. The active zone (50–100 nm) on the sending presynaptic terminal is much smaller than the receiving postsynaptic density (360 nm or 250–500 nm), which effectively creates a large goalpost through which to receive incoming neurotransmitters. Further, the areas enlarge during signaling to additionally enhance signal reception.

## 2.2 Neural Signaling Overview

A neuron is an electrically excitable cell that communicates with other cells by sending a signal called an action potential across specialized connections called synapses. Each neuron is comprised of a cell body (soma), a long thin axon insulated by a myelin sheath for outbound signaling, and multiple dendrites for receiving inbound signals. Glial cells are non-neuronal cells that insulate neurons from each other, supply nutrients, and facilitate signaling.

Neurons have two main processes, sending and receiving signals. To send a signal, an axon transmits information from the neuron to neighboring neurons. To receive a signal, a neuron's dendrites interpret incoming information sent by the axons of other neurons. The signaling activity of neurons is both electrical and chemical. The axons of neurons produce and transmit electrical pulses called action potentials which travel along the axon like a wave. The action potential is a short electrical pulse that is 0.1 V in amplitude and lasts for one millisecond (Nicholls *et al.*, 2012, p. 14). The action potential is sent along the axon to the axon terminals in the synaptic nerve endings, from which the axon contacts the dendrites of other neurons. Synapses (from the Greek word for conjunction) consist of active zones on the edge of the presynaptic terminal on the outbound neuron, the postsynaptic density on the dendrites of the receiving neuron, and a ~20 nm gap between them (synaptic cleft).

The electrical current responsible for the propagation of the action potential along the axons cannot go across the synaptic cleft. A signal conversion is made so that the transmission across the gap between one neuron's axon and another's dendrites is accomplished by chemical messengers called neurotransmitters. Various chemical neurotransmitters are stored in vesicles (spherical bags) in the synaptic terminal at the nerve ending to be available for release across the synaptic junction.

At the presynaptic terminal (the bouton or bulbous area at the end of the neuron), the arrival of an electrical action potential causes voltage-gated calcium channels in the terminal wall to open and disgorge calcium into the terminal bulb. The calcium triggers synaptic vesicles located in the terminal to release their neurotransmitter contents into the synaptic cleft. In less than a millisecond, neurotransmitter diffuses across the gap and activates receptors in the membrane of the postsynaptic density (dendrites) in the receiving neuron, and also activates adjacent astrocyte processes. Astrocytes (glial cells) are present around the synaptic cleft to facilitate signaling and recycle neurotransmitters from the synaptic cleft back into synaptic vesicles (Shepherd, 1974).

Although each neuron has only one axon (which ends in multiple axon terminals for sending signals), it has multiple dendrites for receiving signals. On average, there may be about 2,800 synaptic connections to other neurons (Martins *et al.*, 2019). Other estimates are higher: That each neuron may have an average of 7,000 synaptic connections to other neurons (Finger, 1994), or 10,000 (Koch, 1999). Another analysis points out that although each neuron may have about 7,000 axon terminals from other neurons, redundancy suggests an effective connectivity to only 80 other neurons, mostly nearest neighbors (Cowan *et al.*, 2016, p. 2). Specialized cells such as the Purkinje cells in the cerebellum have over 1,000 dendritic branches, each with thousands of synaptic connections to other neurons (Mel, 2016). Synapses can be either excitatory or inhibitory, which serves to reinforce or dampen the signal that comes from the axon.

### 2.2.1 *Electrical-to-chemical interconnects*

Just as global telecommunications networks convert signals from electric to optical to electric for more expedient transmission across the intermediate portion of the network, the brain, likewise, converts signals from electric to chemical to electric. The neuron has an elaborate process for converting signals between the electrical and chemical regimes for efficient transfer (Table 2.3). A neuron receives signals via dendrite and soma (for example, from visual or motor stimulus), and sends them as an electrical action potential down the axon. The action potential is converted from an electrical to chemical signal in the presynaptic terminal and crosses the synaptic cleft as a chemical signal. In the postsynaptic density of the dendritic spine head, the chemical signal is processed and reconverted to an electrical signal to pass on to the soma of the receiving neuron. Whereas the general form of neural signaling is through chemical synapses as described, there are also exclusively electrical synapses

Table 2.3. Neural signal processing.

| No. | Location | Activity | Signal |
|---|---|---|---|
| 1 | Sending neuron axon | Action potential | Electric |
| 2 | Presynaptic terminal | Signal conversion | Electric-to-chemical |
| 3 | Synaptic cleft | Signal transmission | Chemical |
| 4 | Postsynaptic density | Signal reception | Chemical-to-electric |
| 5 | Dendritic arbors | Synaptic integration | Electric |

Table 2.4. Energy budget for signaling in the brain.

| No. | Brain Function | Energy (%) |
|---|---|---|
| 1 | Action potentials | 47 |
| 2 | Postsynaptic potentials | 34 |
| 3 | Resting potentials | 13 |
| 4 | Presynaptic calcium ($Ca^{2+}$) | 3 |
| 5 | Glutamate recycling | 3 |

*Source*: Attwell and Laughlin (2001, p. 1140).

(excitable cells which allow ions to pass directly from one cell to another) that are used in high-stakes rapid-signaling applications such as in the heart and escape reflexes.

### 2.2.2 *Neural signaling energy budget*

It is no mystery that creating electric energy potentials might use up a lot of the brain's estimated energy budget, but receiving signals (postsynaptic receptor potentials) uses up a full third, too, as dendrites produce and send action potentials (dendritic spikes) themselves (Table 2.4). Attwell and Laughlin (2001) estimate the energy expenditure of different aspects of information processing of the brain. Most demanding are action potentials and postsynaptic potentials (47% and 34% of the total energy signaling budget). Then are neuronal and glial resting potentials (13%), presynaptic calcium entry and neurotransmitter recycling (each 3%), and least demanding are calcium transients in spines and vesicle recycling (<1%).

## 2.3 Sending Neuron (Presynaptic Terminal)

Neurons communicate with each other at specialized contact points called synapses. Presynaptic neurons store neurotransmitters within presynaptic vesicles at the nerve terminal. During synaptic transmission, presynaptic vesicles fuse with the plasma membrane, releasing their neurotransmitter contents into the synaptic cleft to activate postsynaptic receptors on receiving dendrites. Neurotransmitter release is a multistage process which requires the priming of synaptic vesicles into a readily-releasable pool of vesicles. When an action potential (an electrical signal traveling along the neuron's axon) invades a nerve terminal, it promotes an influx of calcium ions ($Ca^{2+}$) that proceed to trigger the fusion of primed vesicles with the membrane's active zone, thereby causing neurotransmitter release.

The so-called "calcium hypothesis" describes how neurotransmitter release from presynaptic vesicles is triggered by elevations in the calcium ion ($Ca^{2+}$) concentration in the presynaptic terminal (Katz & Miledi, 1965). The three main steps in the presynaptic signaling cascade are $Ca^{2+}$ influx through voltage-gated calcium channels, buffered $Ca^{2+}$ diffusion from the channels to releasable vesicles, and activation of the $Ca^{2+}$ sensor for release (Meinrenken *et al.*, 2003, p. 665). An action potential arrives and there is a $Ca^{2+}$ influx (through a voltage-gated channel in the presynaptic terminal wall). $Ca^{2+}$ enters the terminal through three subtypes of calcium channels (P/Q-type, N-type, and R-type channels, with 50%, 25%, and 25% contributions, respectively) (*Ibid.*, p. 668). There may be, on average, at least ten open channels per $mm^2$ membrane (*Ibid.*).

Once the $Ca^{2+}$ influx in the presynaptic terminal is received as a result of the action potential, a number of steps of protein interaction-related steps are triggered in the terminal or bouton (the enlarged nerve ending at the end of the axon). Synaptotagmins are a family of membrane-trafficking proteins that function as calcium sensors in the regulation of neurotransmitter release.

Synaptotagmins serve as $Ca^{2+}$ sensors for release and also inhibit the spontaneous fusion of synaptic vesicles in the absence of an action potential. Synaptotagmins are implicated in early and late vesicle docking with the presynaptic (fusion) membrane. Two synaptotagmins (synaptotagmins 1 and synaptotagmins 7), mediate fast and slow neurotransmitter release, respectively, and maintain a readily-releasable pool of vesicles (Bacaj *et al.*, 2015).

The $Ca^{2+}$ sensor synaptotagmins form an interface with the SNARE complex. The SNARE complex consists of three proteins (synaptobrevin, syntaxin, and SNAP-25) and the synaptotagmins $Ca^{2+}$ sensor. The SNARE complex brings the synaptic vesicle and plasma membranes into juxtaposition and provides the energy for membrane fusion. Whereas synaptotagmins orchestrate the neurotransmitter-filled vesicles, the coordination with the SNARE complex binds the vesicle membrane to the plasma membrane and proceeds with exocytosis (in which the vesicles expel their contents into the synaptic cleft). Synaptotagmin displaces the protein complexin from the SNARE complex in the presence of calcium as one of the last steps in exocytosis. Calcium-bound synaptotagmin binds to the SNARE complex, causing the fusion clamp effect of complexin to be released, which allows vesicle fusion to occur and exocytosis to proceed (Sudhof, 2013).

Over 1,000 proteins function in the presynaptic nerve terminal, and hundreds are thought to participate in exocytosis (Sudhof, 2004, p. 510). The Munc13 and Munc18 proteins, for example, contribute to calcium sensitivity, and Munc13 is also related to the regulation of SNARE complex assembly (Lai *et al.*, 2017). Experimental evidence highlights the three-dimensional structure of the presynaptic terminal, finding that synaptic vesicles are tightly interconnected in the axonal bouton, and preferentially connected to active zones (Siksou *et al.*, 2007).

Other research indicates that presynaptic inhibition is more complicated and autonomous than had been thought (Jullie *et al.*, 2020). This is due to MOR (mu-type) opioid receptors in the GPCR (G protein-coupled receptor) family being diffusely distributed and laterally mobile across the axon surface, and recycling locally as a separate behavior from the synaptic vesicle cycle.

## 2.4 Receiving Neuron (Postsynaptic Density)

Neurotransmitters released at the presynaptic terminal are either excitatory or inhibitory. Whereas excitatory neurotransmitters depolarize the postsynaptic cell, inhibitory neurotransmitters hyperpolarize the postsynaptic cell. The inhibitory neurotransmitter often mitigates the effects of an excitatory neurotransmitter. The depolarization of the excitatory neurotransmitters is called an excitatory postsynaptic potential (EPSP), and the hyperpolarization of the inhibitory neurotransmitter is called inhibitory postsynaptic potential (IPSP).

The postsynaptic density is a dense protein-rich complex on the postsynaptic membrane that receives neurotransmitter signals, mostly via specialized protrusions called dendritic spines. Electron microscopy identifies the postsynaptic density as an electron-dense thickening of the postsynaptic membrane of excitatory synapses (Kim & Sheng, 2009). Excitatory synapses occur mainly on dendritic spines, whereas inhibitory synapses are typically formed on the shaft of dendritic arbors (Sheng & Kim, 2011). Postsynaptic densities are located across from the active zone of the presynaptic terminal of the sending neuron that releases excitatory neurotransmitters (mainly glutamate). Inhibitory synapses do not have a prominent postsynaptic density. The postsynaptic density comprises many different protein complexes and the space underneath it is occupied by actin filaments, the major cytoskeletal component of dendritic spines.

About 90% of excitatory synapses terminate on the dendritic spines of the receiving neuron. There are about 1–10 spines per micron length (1,000 nm) of dendrite (Sheng & Hoogenraad, 2007). Spine shapes are labeled as mushroom (60% of all spines in the adult cortex), stubby (20–25%), thin (10–20%), filopodia (2–15%), or branched (*Ibid.*). The postsynaptic density also serves as a signaling apparatus (including by compartmentalizing calcium) and is implicated in synaptic plasticity (Suzuki *et al.*, 2018). The size and shape of the postsynaptic density can change dynamically, and also the dendritic spines in response to long-term potentiation and long-term depression (Martins *et al.*, 2016).

The most numerous volume of molecules received at the dendritic synapse is calcium ions (Cugno *et al.*, 2019, p. 2), which geometrically are absorbed into a lattice structure (Suzuki *et al.*, 2018). Of the many different classes of postsynaptic density proteins identified by mass spectrometry, about half are related to structural form and the other half to function. Functional proteins include kinases (11%), GTPases (8%), metabolism (7%), translation (6%), mitochondria (6%), and membrane trafficking (5%). Structural proteins include cytoskeleton-actin (12%), cell adhesion (7%), receptors and channels (6%), and scaffolds (6%) (Sheng & Kim, 2011, p. 3). The most abundant postsynaptic density proteins are those from the CamKII (Calmodulin-dependent protein kinase type II) family, a GTPase-activating protein (SynGAP), and a scaffold protein PSD-95 (postsynaptic density 95) (Kim & Sheng, 2009, R724).

## 2.5 Synaptic (Dendritic) Spike Integration

Neurotransmitters are disgorged from the active zone on the edge of the presynaptic terminal and cross the 20-nm wide synaptic cleft directly into the postsynaptic density across the channel on the receiving neuron. Processing the signaling information, the dendrites in the postsynaptic density may convert the chemical signals back into electrical signals for onward transmission. The chemical-to-electric conversion is performed with the same membrane polarization and depolarization mechanisms that are used to generate the electrical signal of the axon's action potential. Dendritic membrane depolarization is triggered by incoming (afferent) chemicals (neurotransmitters), which are received at many locations on the dendrite. Dendrites have high densities of calcium channels, and calcium entry into the cell causes prolonged membrane depolarization and increased action potentials. The initiation of dendritic spikes is facilitated by the high input impedance of small-diameter branches, which allows a relatively small number of co-activated synapses on the same branch to produce a large local EPSP, and thus evoke a dendritic spike. The dendrites thus generate small local action potentials (dendritic spikes) and send them upstream in an information processing sequence in which they may be further aggregated and eventually lead to the neuron's cell body (soma) and axon to possibly trigger an outgoing action potential from that neuron.

Synaptic integration (or dendritic integration) is the neuron's information processing activity of amalgamating individually received molecular signals on dendrites into a global action. The majority of synaptic input neurons receive is made onto their dendrites, and so the morphology and membrane properties of dendrites play a key role in signal transformation. In particular, the structure of the dendritic tree and the position of synapses on the dendrites influence synaptic summation in different ways. Dendritic geometry is an active research topic. One project modeled the dendritic shape as elliptical spheroids and found that the curvature of the geometry gives rise to pseudoharmonic functions that can be used to predict the locations of maximum and minimum concentrations along the spine heads (Cugno *et al.*, 2019). In the basic setting, three elements are involved in the synaptic integration of incoming signals. There is the amplitude of the unitary postsynaptic potential, the manner in which non-simultaneous unitary events add in time (temporal summation), and the addition of unitary events occurring simultaneously in separate regions of the dendritic arbor (spatial summation) (Magee, 2000).

There is active dendritic integration at many intermediary steps along the way from the dendrite to the cell body (soma), not merely passive signal transmission (Williams & Atkinson, 2008). Dendritic spikes are generated in many regions of the dendritic tree. Dendrites do not merely forward signals to the neuron's cell body and axon, but process signals along the way. The number of dendritic integration compartments is defined by the electrical geometry of the neuron together with the dendritic distribution of voltage-activated ion channels. Dendritic synaptic inputs are integrated locally in the dendritic tree, leading to the generation of dendritic spikes as an intermediary processing signal. Synaptic input is integrated not only at the level of the axon, but also within the dendritic tree. The brain is the original smart network, with local intelligence built into its processing all the way from the dendrite to the cell body.

An intricate brain processing logic appears to be at work as a large number of incoming signals are received, but not necessarily transferred to the neuron's soma. For example, empirical dendritic recordings indicate that barrages of excitatory synaptic input generated distally (far away) in the dendritic tree of cortical pyramidal neurons do not sum to form a coherent signal, and rather are heavily attenuated and provide a weak drive for action potential firing (Williams & Atkinson, 2008, R1045). The implication is that some degree of intelligence is added by dendritic integration and spiking activity in order to transmit signals.

Spatial (near and far) and temporal properties (fast and slow) are implicated in dendritic signal transfer and amalgamation (and also signal amplitude and kinetics). Dendrite potentials closest to the soma (basal, proximal) are more heavily weighted than those that are farther away (distal, apical (apex of dendrite)). The closer to the cell body, the higher the signal amplitude. The most heavily transferred signals are fast signals from nearby dendrites, but even these are only transferred to the soma with 20–25% efficiency (Henze *et al.*, 1996, p. 341). Slow signals from farther away dendrites are efficiently transferred to the soma, which suggests a modulatory role on the resting potential of the cell. In other cases in which there is a joint signal from both closer and farther away dendrites (when nearby wave activity is superimposed on farther away activity), the neuron has a higher probability of firing an action potential. Further, the amplitude and kinetics of the electrical signal can vary as a function of position within the dendrite and signal frequency, adding even more complexity to the "neural algebra" by which incoming signals are aggregated.

Dendrites track not only how many incoming signals they receive but also how many neurons are involved in sending them, in both space and time. Dendritic spikes are more likely to occur when dendrites receive a coherent activation simultaneously from a number of presynaptic neurons, as opposed to when a presynaptic neuron fires alone (Losonczy *et al.*, 2008). Also, dendritic spikes have different levels, weak and strong, modulated by activity-dependent dendritic voltage-activated ion channels, as a sort of learning rule (*Ibid.*). Fast and slow times are implicated in two different ways. One is that fast and slow times are used in that local fast signals, and distant slow signals, are more likely to be transmitted to the soma. Another is that fast and slow times are used for fast network processing at the edge and slower processing at the core.

### 2.5.1 *Excitatory and inhibitory postsynaptic potentials*

The dendritic spiking and integration activity discussed so far applies mainly to excitatory signals. Excitatory synapses occur mainly on the tiny protrusions called dendritic spines. In contrast, inhibitory synapses are more hidden and typically form on the shaft of dendrites. Excitatory synapses differ from inhibitory synapses in their location and shape and in the type of neurotransmitter receptors they have and the processing activity they conduct. More is known about excitatory synapses as they have a distinctive structure and greater abundance. Signals from both excitatory and inhibitory synapses, though, consist of far-off (distal) and nearby (proximate) signals that are aggregated for upstream transmission. Dendrite potentials (signals) are aggregated into excitatory postsynaptic potentials (EPSPs) or inhibitory postsynaptic potentials (IPSPs). Synaptic computation is performed in dendritic trees when excitatory and inhibitory synapses are activated in specific spatial and temporal patterns.

Whereas excitatory potentials have a stimulatory impact, inhibitory potentials exert a blocking influence. At the soma and axon, inhibitory synaptic potentials have the ability to block action potential generation, and in the dendrites, the ability to block dendritic spike generation and propagation (Spruston *et al.*, 2016, pp. 36–7). By preventing dendritic spike generation, inhibitory synapses on individual dendritic branches act as gatekeepers that control whether or not a dendritic spike is generated.

### 2.5.2 *Dendritic pathologies*

Many pathologies are associated with improperly functioning dendritic arbors. Stress-related pathologies such as posttraumatic stress disorder (PTSD) are implicated in that chronic stress reduces arbor complexity and dendritic length (McKittrick *et al.*, 2000). Chronic stress-induced changes in behavior are often further attributed to changes in the hippocampus and targeted with pharmaceutical intervention. In addition, mutations in postsynaptic density proteins are associated with autism spectrum disorders, obsessive-compulsive disorder, and other neuropsychiatric illnesses (Sheng & Kim, 2011, p. 12).

Reduced levels of postsynaptic density proteins in the brain are a hallmark of Alzheimer's disease, possibly related to the substantial synapse loss that is a precursor to this neurodegenerative disorder. Seizure is also implicated as an abnormal brain state. Electrical activity in the brain is usually nonsynchronous, but neurons that fire in an excessive and synchronized manner can lead to seizures (Angus-Leppan, 2014). The mechanism of action is that ion channel mutations may confer a long-lasting depolarized resting state to neurons that then leads to hyperexcitability. The long-lasting depolarization is due to an influx of calcium ions from outside of the cell which triggers the extended opening of sodium channels and repetitive action potentials.

### 2.5.3 *Dendritic integration filtering*

There is even more complication and nuance to dendritic integration than discussed earlier. Central to dendritic integration is the idea that dendrites behave like electrical filters, reducing the amplitude of synaptic potentials as they travel from the dendritic site of generation to the cell body (Rall, 1995). The time course of EPSPs at the soma is slowed due to the filtering properties of the dendritic membrane between the synapse and the soma. The neuron responds more slowly to inputs received at distal dendrites than at proximal dendrites. Synaptic potentials generated in distal dendrites may attenuate over 100-fold by the time they reach the soma, suggesting that such synapses will be less efficient than more proximal synapses.

Two additional factors mitigate the disparity between proximal and distal synapses. First, the attenuation of synaptic *charge* is much less than the attenuation of fast synaptic *voltage* changes. Second, at least some synapses may scale their conductance to compensate for dendritic distance (Spruston *et al.*, 2016, p. 17). On the one hand, synaptic voltage, through EPSP attenuation and temporal filtering, depends not only on the distance of the synapse from the soma but also on the EPSP time course, with faster EPSPs attenuated and filtered more than slower EPSPs. On the other hand, the attenuation of synaptic charge depends only on distance from the soma and not on the time course of the charge entry at the synapse. Notably, the treatment of voltage and charge behaviors may be quite different in passive dendrites and active dendrites.

Filtering or other mechanisms may be at work in a new class of graded dendritic action potentials that have been discovered. Studying human pyramidal neurons, Gidon *et al.* (2020) identified some calcium-mediated dendritic action potentials whose waveform and effects on neuronal output have not been described previously. In contrast to typical all-or-none action potentials, these potentials appear to be graded in the sense of having maximal amplitudes for threshold-level stimuli but dampened amplitudes for stronger stimuli.

### 2.5.4 *Computational neuroscience and biophysical modeling*

The complexities of dendritic behavior are still emerging and eclipse the ability of contemporary modeling techniques. The opportunity for quantum computing is immediately clear in possibly providing a natural three-dimensional environment similar to the dendrite's own. This could improve on the simple three-dimensional cone models that have been proposed (Henze *et al.*, 1996). Meanwhile, computational neuroscience software applications such as NEURON, GENESIS, BRIAN, and NEST are the main options for modeling the complexities of dendritic behavior. However, although these platforms (particularly, NEURON and GENESIS) offer intricate single neuron models, a fuller simulation of brain network behavior is difficult, even with multicompartment models (Tikidji-Hamburyan *et al.*, 2017). Neuronal morphology is simplified into a point representation of the soma, and linear summations at the soma of the excitatory and inhibitory synaptic currents originating from dendrites. The point neuron framework does not incorporate the complete picture of the spatiotemporal aspects of dendritic integration. One proposed solution is an overlay to the existing point neuron model in NEURON, in the form of a synaptic integration current that captures a greater range of dendritic effects including the dendritic filtering effect (that far-off signals are attenuated) (Li *et al.*, 2019).

## 2.6 Neural Signaling and Quantum Computing

The obvious low-hanging fruit application for quantum neuroscience is synaptic integration. The problem is complex and three-dimensional and requires diffusion equation modeling with PDEs (to capture the effects of nonlinear calcium signaling). Although the electrical signaling behavior of the action potential being transmitted along the neuron's axon is somewhat well understood, having a predictive model of dendrite behavior is much more challenging. Pyramidal human dendritic arbors appear to perform extremely sophisticated logic operations. Further, dendritic behavior involves chemical signaling comprising complicated protein cascades at the subatomic scale. Current synaptic modeling software approaches include dendritic trees to some extent, but not full synaptic integration (Poirazi & Papoutsi, 2020). The underlying biology is still being characterized. Thus, synaptic integration modeling and microscopy imaging (electron microscopy, light field microscopy, and lattice light sheet expansion microscopy) might further inform each other as implemented in quantum neuroscience applications.

# References

Angus-Leppan, H. (2014). First seizures in adults. *Brit. Med. J.* 348:g2470.

Attwell, D. & Laughlin, S.B. (2001). An energy budget for signaling in the grey matter of the brain. *J. Cereb. Blood. Flow Metab.* 21:1133–45.

Bacaj, T., Wu, D., Burre, J. *et al.* (2015). Synaptotagmin-1 and -7 are redundantly essential for maintaining the capacity of the readily-releasable pool of synaptic vesicles. *PLoS Biol.* 13(10):e1002267.

Bigos, K.L., Hariri, A. & Weinberger, D. (2015). *Neuroimaging Genetics: Principles and Practices*. Oxford: Oxford University Press.

Chudler, E.H. (2009). Brain facts and figures. *Neuroscience for Kids*. https://faculty.washington.edu/chudler/facts.html#neuron.

Cowan, J.D., Neuman, J. & van Drongelen, W. (2016). Wilson–Cowan equations for neocortical dynamics. *J. Math. Neurosci.* 6(1):1–24.

Cugno, A., Bartol, T.M., Sejnowski, T.J. *et al.* (2019). Geometric principles of second messenger dynamics in dendritic spines. *Sci. Rep.* 9(1):11676.

Farhy-Tselnicker, I. & Allen, N.J. (2018). Astrocytes, neurons, synapses: A tripartite view on cortical circuit development. *Neural Dev.* 13(1):7.

Finger, S. (1994). *Origins of Neuroscience: A History of Explorations into Brain Function*. Oxford: Oxford University Press.

Freitas, R.A. Jr. (2012). Welcome to the future of medicine. Transhumanism and personal identity. In *The Transhumanist Reader*. Eds. More, M. & Vita-More, N. Oxford: Wiley-Blackwell, pp. 67–72.

Gao, R., Asano, S.M., Upadhyayula, S. *et al.* (2019). Cortical column and whole-brain imaging with molecular contrast and nanoscale resolution. *Science.* 363(6424)eaau8302.

Gidon, A., Zolnik, T.A., Fidzinski, P. *et al.* (2020). Dendritic action potentials and computation in human layer 2/3 cortical neurons. *Science.* 367(6743):83–7.

Henze, D.A., Cameron, W.E. & Barrioneuvo, G. (1996). Dendritic morphology and its effects on the amplitude and rise-time of synaptic signals in hippocampal CA3 pyramidal cells. *J. Comp. Neurol.* 369:331–44.

Jullie, D. Stoeber, M., Sibarita, J.B. *et al.* (2020). A discrete presynaptic vesicle cycle for neuromodulator receptors. *Neuron.* 105:663–77.

Katz, B. & Miledi, R. (1965). Effect of calcium on acetylcholine release from motor nerve terminals. *Proc. R Soc. Lond. B Biol. Sci.* 161:496–503.

Kettenmann, H. & Verkhratsky, A. (2011). Neuroglia: Living nerve glue. *Fortschr. Neurol. Psychiatr.* 79(10):588–97.

Kim, E. & Sheng, M. (2009). The postsynaptic density. *Curr. Biol.* 19(17): R723–24.

Koch, C. (1999). *Biophysics of Computation: Information Processing in Single Neurons*. Oxford: Oxford University Press.

Lai, Y., Choi, U.B., Leitz, J. *et al.* (2017). Molecular mechanisms of synaptic vesicle priming by Munc13 and Munc18. *Neuron*. 95:591–607.

Laughlin, S.B. & Sejnowski, T.J. (2003). Communication in neuronal networks. *Science*. 301(5641):1870–4.

Ley, B. (1999). Diameter of a human hair. *The Physics Factbook*. https://hypertextbook.com/facts/1999/BrianLey.shtml.

Li, S., Liu, N., Zhang, X. *et al.* (2019). Dendritic computations captured by an effective point neuron model. *Proc. Natl. Acad. Sci.* 116(30):15244–52.

Losonczy, A., Makara, J.K. & Magee, J.C. (2008). Compartmentalized dendritic plasticity and input feature storage in neurons. *Nature*. 452:436–41.

Magee, J.C. (2000). Dendritic integration of excitatory synaptic input. *Nat. Rev. Neurosci.* 1:181–90.

Martins, N.R.B., Angelica, A., Chakravarthy, K. *et al.* (2019). Human brain/cloud interface. *Front Neurosci.* 13(112):1–23.

Martins, N.R.B., Erlhagen, W. & Freitas, R.A. Jr. (2016). Human connectome mapping and monitoring using neuronanorobots. *J. Evol. Technol.* (26):1–25.

McKittrick, C.R., Magarinos, A.M., Blanchard, D.C., *et al.* (2000). Chronic social stress reduces dendritic arbors in CA3 of hippocampus and decreases binding to serotonin transporter sites. *Synapse*. 3685:942006.

Meinrenken, C.J., Borst, J.G.G. & Sakmann, B. (2003). Local routes revisited: The space and time dependence of the $Ca^{2+}$ signal for phasic transmitter release at the rat calyx of Held. The Hodgkin-Huxley-Katz Prize Lecture. *J. Physiol.* 547(3):665–89.

Mel, B.W. (2016). Towards a simplified model of an active dendritic tree. In *Dendrites*. Eds. Stuart, G., Spruston, N. & Hausser, M. Oxford: Oxford University Press, pp. 465–86.

Meyer, D. Bonhoeffer, T. & Scheuss, V. (2014). Balance and stability of synaptic structures during synaptic plasticity. *Neuron*. 82(2):430–43.

Mitchell, N., Petralia, R.S., Currier, D.G. *et al.* (2012). Sonic hedgehog regulates presynaptic terminal size, ultrastructure and function in hippocampal neurons. *J. Cell Sci.* 125:4207–13.

Nicholls, J.G., Martin, A.R., Fuchs, P.A. *et al.* (2012). *From Neuron to Brain*. 5th Edition. Sunderland, MA: Sinauer Associates, Inc.

Parent, A. (1996). *Carpenter's Human Neuroanatomy*. London: Williams & Wilkins.

Poirazi, P. & Papoutsi, A. (2020). Illuminating dendritic function with computational models. *Nat. Rev. Neurosci.* 21:303–21.

Rall, W. (1995). *The Theoretical Foundation of Dendritic Function: Selected Papers of Wilfrid Rall with Commentaries*. Cambridge: MIT Press.

Scimemi, A. & Beato, M. (2009). Determining the neurotransmitter concentration profile at active synapses. *Mol. Neurobiol.* 40:289–306.

Sejnowski, T.J. (2020). The unreasonable effectiveness of deep learning in artificial intelligence. *Proc. Natl. Acad. Sci*. 117(48):30033–38.

Sheng, M. & Hoogenraad, C.C. (2007). The postsynaptic architecture of excitatory synapses: A more quantitative view. *Annu. Rev. Biochem.* 76:823–47.

Sheng, M. & Kim, E. (2011). The postsynaptic organization of synapses. *Cold Spring Harb. Perspect. Biol.* 3(a005678):1–20.

Shepherd, G.M. (1974). *The Synaptic Organization of the Brain. An Introduction*. New York: Oxford University Press.

Siksou, L., Rostaing, P. & Lechaire, J.-P. (2007). Three-dimensional architecture of presynaptic terminal cytomatrix. *J. Neurosci*. 27(26):6868–77.

Spruston, N., Stuart, G. & Hausser, M. (2016). Principles of dendritic integration. *Dendrites*. 3rd Edition. Oxford: Oxford University Press, pp. 1–78.

Sterratt, D., Graham, B., Gillies, A. & Willshaw, D. (2011). *Prin. Comput. Model Neurosci*. Cambridge: Cambridge University Press.

Sudhof, T.C. (2004). The synaptic vesicle cycle. *Annu. Rev. Neurosci*. 27: 509–47.

Sudhof, T.C. (2013). Neurotransmitter release: The last millisecond in the life of a synaptic vesicle. *Neuron*. 80:675–90.

Suzuki, T., Kametani, K., Gui, W. & Li, W. (2018). Protein components of postsynaptic density lattice, a backbone structure for type I excitatory synapses. *J. Neurochem*. 144:390–407.

Tikidji-Hamburyan, R.A., Narayana, V., Bozkus, Z. *et al.* (2017). Software for brain network simulations: A comparative study. *Front Neuroinform*. 11(46): 1–16.

von Bartheld, C.S., Bahney, J. & Herculano-Houzel, S. (2016). The search for true numbers of neurons and glial cells in the human brain: A review of 150 years of cell counting. *J. Comp. Neurol.* 524(18):3865–95.

Wang, Y., Li, Q., Liu, L. *et al.* (2019). TeraVR empowers precise reconstruction of complete 3-D neuronal morphology in the whole brain. *Nat. Comm.* 10(3474):1–9.

Williams, S.R. & Atkinson, S.E. (2008). Dendritic synaptic integration in central neurons. *Curr. Biol.* 18(22):R1045–47.

# Chapter 3

# The AdS/Brain Correspondence

*The gauge/gravity duality is an equality between two theories. On one side we have a quantum field theory in d spacetime dimensions. On the other side we have a gravity theory on a d+1 dimensional spacetime*

— Maldacena (2014, p. 1)

**Abstract**

The AdS/CFT correspondence is a model of physical systems equating a complicated bulk volume to a boundary region with one less dimension. The model surpassed 20,000 journal citations in early 2021 and is applied in various areas of physics, information science, and neuroscience. A novel multi-tier AdS/Brain correspondence is proposed. AdS/DIY mathematics are elaborated with the four equations of the metric, operator, action, and Hamiltonian or Lagrangian.

## 3.1 The AdS/CFT Correspondence

The AdS/CFT correspondence (anti-de Sitter space/conformal field theory) is a solvable theory of quantum gravity proposed by Maldacena (1999). The work constitutes one of the most cited papers in any field (over 21,000 citations as of September 2021), including in all physics arXivs (Natsuume, 2016, p. 4). Although the correspondence is a conjecture that has not been mathematically proven, no serious inconsistencies appear to have arisen. The essence of the theory is that any physical system with a complicated bulk volume can be described by a boundary theory in one less dimension. This could be a room full of particles, a black hole, or a brain. The model formally states that there is an equivalence between a gravity theory (bulk) and a gauge theory (boundary). The theories can be related in part due to the fact that both operate on the basis of fields (gravitational fields and quantum fields) which can be mathematically related in matrix operations.

The AdS/CFT correspondence is also called the holographic correspondence or holographic duality (HD) because metaphorically, the boundary is a hologram in the sense of encoding a three-dimensional image on a two-dimensional surface. The holographic correspondence offers two views of the same physical system (boundary surface or bulk volume) and a mathematical formalism for solving in either direction (bulk-to-boundary or boundary-to-bulk). This book proposes the first instance, as far as the authors know, of using a multi-tier correspondence model (multiple graduated levels of bulk and boundary), in this case, to instantiate the scale tiers of the brain's neural signaling processes between axon, presynaptic terminal, synaptic cleft, postsynaptic density, and dendritic spiking potentials from dendrite to soma (at the scale tiers of network, neuron, synapse, and molecule). The resulting AdS/Brain theory is a composite theory of neural signaling that interprets the AdS/CFT correspondence in a matrix quantum mechanics formulation (a multiple matrix model for quantum mechanical systems (Han *et al.*, 2020)).

### 3.1.1 *Stating the AdS/CFT correspondence*

The AdS/CFT correspondence is a quantum field theory in $d$ spacetime dimensions that is equivalent to a gravity theory on a $d + 1$ dimensional spacetime (Maldacena, 2014, p. 1). An important target application of the correspondence is studying black hole solutions in various numbers of dimensions (*Ibid.*). As the $d$ and $d + 1$ format suggests, there can be different dimensional flavors of the correspondence. Most basic is $AdS_2$/CFT (two spatial dimensions in the bulk and one in the boundary).

The correspondence is initially stated in terms of $AdS_5/CFT_4$, namely, five bulk dimensions and four boundary dimensions (Table 3.1).

Table 3.1. The canonical AdS/CFT correspondence.

| Bulk | Boundary |
|---|---|
| 5D theory of quantum gravity ($AdS_5 \times S^5$) | 4D supersymmetric quantum gauge theory ($N = 4$ $SU(N)$ Yang–Mills theory) |
| Area of a minimal three-dimensional surface | Entanglement entropy of a boundary region |

The correspondence is the duality between a certain supersymmetric quantum gauge theory in four dimensions, $N = 4$ $SU(N)$ Yang–Mills theory, and a theory of quantum gravity, type IIB string theory, in a fluctuating spacetime that is an asymptotically five-dimensional AdS space times a spherical manifold, $AdS_5 \times S^5$ (the manifold "S" (as in $S^5$) is mostly ignored until computation begins). Yang–Mills theory is a gauge theory upon which the Standard Model of particle physics is based. The HD is simplest from the gravity point of view when the boundary quantum field theory is strongly coupled since in this limit, quantum gravity reduces to classical gravity in a weakly curved space.

AdS is a solution of classical gravity (of Einstein's equation with negative vacuum energy). The two theories have the same amount of degrees of freedom per unit volume and the same global symmetries. The theory draws from the holographic principle which says that the information stored in a spatial volume is encoded in its boundary area in $AdS_{d-1}$ (Susskind, 1995). The idea is to choose a bulk-boundary dimensional relationship relevant to the problem at hand, possibly beginning with the simple model of $AdS_2$/CFT and expanding into higher dimensionality. Although the AdS/CFT correspondence has long been conceived as a renormalization group method (Heemskerk & Polchinski, 2011), it is only recently with information-theoretic methods that an equation is available to perform this calculation explicitly (Harlow, 2017).

Following the correspondence itself, the second canonical proposal is the Ryu-Takayanagi formula for entanglement entropy (Ryu & Takayanagi, 2006). The formula says that the entanglement entropy of a region in the boundary is equivalent to the area of a bulk minimal surface. Entanglement entropy is a measure of the degree of quantum entanglement in a many-body quantum state. In the classical gravity limit of the bulk, the entanglement entropy of a region in the boundary quantum field theory is given by the area (in Planck units) of a minimal three-dimensional surface which hangs from the two-dimensional boundary region into the bulk as a geodesic (shortest length curve) (Swingle, 2012). The curve is a holographic screen in two senses: In one way, it projects bulk information onto the boundary, and, in another way, it hides other bulk information that is not revealed. Independent proofs have confirmed the Ryu-Takayanagi formula (Lewkowycz & Maldacena, 2013; Faulkner *et al.*, 2014). The entanglement entropy formula has been extended in the Hubeny-Rangamani-Takayanagi formula to accommodate covariance (measurement in a change of basis) (Hubeny *et al.*, 2007) and quantum formulations (Engelhardt & Wall, 2019).

## 3.2 AdS/CFT Correspondence Studies

### 3.2.1 *AdS/CFT hybrid approaches*

The AdS/CFT correspondence is implemented either directly as a tool in a content domain or via another tool aimed at a content domain, including itself as the content domain (in the study of HD). The AdS/CFT correspondence thus has various interpretations in other tools such as the Sachdev–Ye–Kitaev (SYK) model, tensor networks (TNs), and machine learning (ML) networks, as further directed to the study of a content domain. Current topics in HD include various dictionary mappings, bulk duals, bulk quantum mechanics, and theories of quantum gravity. A specific dictionary mapping on the research agenda, for example, is a complete gravity dual for the Ising model, since if such a dual exists, it seems likely to be complicated (Swingle, 2012; Harlow, 2017). AdS/CFT hybrid approaches are listed in Table 3.2.

### 3.2.2 *Duality lens*

The premise of the correspondence is that a duality lens can be applied to any physical system such that it can be understood either as a quantum field theory or as a gravity theory, using whichever side is more

Table 3.2. AdS/CFT hybrid approaches.

| No. | Approach | Result | Reference |
|---|---|---|---|
| 1 | AdS-SYK-HD | Bulk duals for cubic couplings | Gross and Rosenhaus (2017) |
| 2 | AdS-TN-HD | Entropy equals geodesics | Swingle (2012) |
| 3 | AdS-TN-HD | Exact holographic mapping | Qi (2013) |
| 4 | AdS-TN-HD | Expanded form of AdS/CFT | Hayden *et al.* (2016) |
| 5 | AdS-TN-QIT | Motzkin spin state walks | Alexander *et al.* (2018) |
| 6 | AdS-TN-QIT | Quantum error correction | Pastawski *et al.* (2015) |
| 7 | AdS-ML-QCD | QCD neural networks | Hashimoto (2019) |

Table 3.3. AdS/CFT correspondence directional duality.

| Direction | Domain | Known | Unknown |
|---|---|---|---|
| Boundary-to-bulk | Theoretical physics | Standard quantum field theory | Quantum gravity |
| Bulk-to-boundary | Condensed matter physics | Classical gravity | Unconventional materials quantum field theory |

convenient to compute. The directionality can be either way. Some systems are more complicated as formulated on the gravity side, and others from the quantum field theory perspective. This can be seen in two canonical problems to which the correspondence is applied. First, in the boundary-to-bulk direction, well-understood standard quantum field theories on the boundary are used to study the more complicated situation of quantum gravity and the emergence of gravity (and time and space) in the bulk. The duality view provides an indirect way to study gravity without the computational difficulty of studying gravity directly. Second, the bulk-to-boundary direction proves equally useful in other systems such as in condensed matter physics. Here, the quantum field theories by which unconventional materials behave are unknown, but can be interrogated through the bulk classical gravity that is well understood. Certain CFT states correspond to classical geometries in the bulk (Table 3.3).

## 3.3 Applied AdS/CFT

Many discipline-specific versions of the AdS/CFT correspondence have arisen as the theory continues to be applied to various fields. In theoretical physics, areas of study include quantum chromodynamics (QCD) and strongly coupled systems such as plasmas, condensed matter theory (CMT) and the SYK model, and chaotic thermal systems. The AdS/CFT correspondence sees application in neuroscience as a model for memory, a control tool for brain-cloud interfaces, and in the current work, as a multiscalar theory for neural signaling modeling. An early AdS/Brain proposal is the hypothesis of a nonlinear associative memory function in the human brain akin to the performance of a Fourier holograph (Willshaw *et al.*, 1969). In information science, the AdS/CFT correspondence is applied to TNs, quantum information theory (QIT), blockchain distributed ledgers, ML, and quantum ML (Table 3.4).

Table 3.4. Applied AdS/CFT correspondence studies.

| No. | AdS/CFT Correspondence Variation | | Reference |
|---|---|---|---|
| *Theoretical physics* | | | |
| 1 | AdS/CFT | AdS/conformal field theory | Maldacena (1999) |
| 2 | AdS/QCD | AdS/quantum chromodynamics | Natsuume (2016) |
| 3 | AdS/CMT | AdS/condensed matter theory | Hartnoll *et al.* (2018) |
| 4 | AdS/SYK | AdS/SYK model | Sachdev (2010) |
| 5 | AdS/Chaos | AdS/chaos (thermal systems) | Shenker and Stanford (2014) |
| 6 | AdS/Math | AdS/mathematics | Hazboun (2018) |
| *Neuroscience* | | | |
| 7 | AdS/Brain | AdS/neuroscience | Willshaw *et al.* (1969) |
| 8 | AdS/BCI | AdS/brain/cloud interface | Swan (2022) |
| *Information science* | | | |
| 9 | AdS/TN | AdS/tensor networks | Swingle (2012) |
| 10 | AdS/QIT | AdS/quantum information theory | Hayden *et al.* (2016) |
| 11 | AdS/DLT | AdS/blockchain technology | Kalinin and Berloff (2018) |
| 12 | AdS/ML | AdS/machine learning | Hashimoto *et al.* (2018b) |
| 13 | AdS/QML | AdS/quantum machine learning | Cottrell *et al.* (2019) |
| 14 | AdS/QSN | AdS/quantum smart networks | Swan *et al.* (2020) |

### 3.3.1 *AdS/QCD (quantum chromodynamics)*

The AdS/QCD correspondence is the research program to describe QCD (the quantum field theory of the strong force) in terms of a gravitational theory. In this formulation, QCD (strongly interacting particles) is the boundary, and a gravitational dual is the bulk. The strong force is difficult to test experimentally and the correspondence provides a means of investigating it more closely. The strong force pertains to quarks (matter particles) and gluons (force particles) which are bound together to comprise the protons and the neutrons in atomic nuclei. (In QCD, the fundamental degrees of freedom are quarks and gluons). Although the strong force is well understood, experiments are difficult because it is not possible to separate quarks and gluons as it is electrons in the standard setup of particle accelerator experiments. Other typical methods such as perturbation also do not work because the strong force is literally very strong. However, with the AdS/CFT correspondence, it is possible to study a strongly coupled gauge theory using the AdS spacetime bulk (Natsuume, 2016).

Quarks and gluons are normally confined inside protons and neutrons. However, at high enough temperatures, they become deconfined and form the quark-gluon plasma. Experimental evidence indicates that the quark-gluon plasma behaves like a fluid with low viscosity. Quark-gluon plasma viscosity is similar to that of black holes as predicted by the holographic correspondence. Viscosity is a measure of how quickly a thermal system returns to equilibrium after being perturbed. An example is throwing a pebble into a pond. Surface waves are generated but decay quickly, and the pond returns to a flat state. The pond has low viscosity and resets quickly. Black holes also have low viscosity and reset quickly.

When an object is dropped into a black hole, the shape of the black hole horizon momentarily becomes irregular, but the perturbation decays quickly and the black hole returns to its original symmetric shape. Viscosity can be computed by the dissipation rate of the perturbed state. In particular, the transport coefficients in the viscosity calculation measure how quickly the effect propagates. Quark-gluon plasmas have been found to have similar transport coefficients to those in other low viscosity systems such as black holes and hydrodynamic fluids. There are several proposals for a precise formula for computing the viscosity of the holographic bulk, for example, Gursoy *et al.* (2011) and Casalderrey-Solana *et al.* (2012). The upshot is that it is easy to perturb black hole spacetime with the holographic correspondence, whereas experimenting with quarks and gluons in real-life is very hard, and the two can be studied together through the duality relation of the correspondence.

Another team's AdS/QCD method takes a different approach. In this case, strong force empirical data are available, and the correspondence is used as a theoretical framework to compile and interpret the data (via a ML model). In one experiment, lattice QCD values (of a chiral condensate at finite-temperature) serve as input on the boundary and a thermal phase transition is the output of the bulk analysis (Hashimoto *et al.*, 2018a). In another experiment, meson mass spectra data are input on the boundary and a curved geometry formulation is the output of the bulk analysis (Akutagawa *et al.*, 2020) (Table 3.5).

### 3.3.2 *AdS/CMT (condensed matter theory)*

The AdS/CMT correspondence is the application of the AdS/CFT correspondence to problems in condensed matter physics. Unconventional materials have proven impervious to study with traditional methods, and the holographic correspondence offers a way to attack unsolvable quantum mechanical systems (exotic materials) with the bulk as a known gravity formalism. The main formulation of AdS/CMT is a bulk-to-boundary application of the correspondence. The bulk (Einstein's classical theory of gravity) is well understood and is used to evaluate the unknown quantum field theories of exotic materials on the boundary. The premise is that there is a holographic duality between black holes (bulk) and unconventional materials (boundary) (Sachdev, 2010). The assumption is that since

Table 3.5. Bulk-boundary: AdS/QCD (strong force).

| No. | Bulk | Boundary | Reference |
|---|---|---|---|
| 1 | AdS spacetime | Strongly coupled gauge theory | Natsuume (2016) |
| 2 | Thermal phase transition | Lattice chiral condensate | Hashimoto *et al.* (2018a) |
| 3 | Curved geometry | Meson mass spectra data | Akutagawa *et al.* (2020) |

black holes and unconventional materials have similar properties related to mass, temperature, and charge, they can be investigated with the duality lens of the correspondence.

An important application of the AdS/CMT correspondence is investigating high-temperature superconductors since they are not fully understood but could have an extremely transformative effect on future computational devices such as quantum computers. High-temperature superconductors are materials (such as cuprates, pnictides, and heavy fermions) that become superconducting (conducting electricity without resistivity) at relatively high temperatures (above 77 K (−196°C or −321°F)). "High-temperature" is a significant technical threshold as such materials do require bulky and expensive cryogenic freezing equipment (Flores-Livas *et al.*, 2020). In the AdS/CMT correspondence, high-temperature superconductors are the boundary. They constitute a CFT (boundary) in that the materials behave according to some unknown quantum field theory of interactions between the particles comprising the material, apparently governed by equations related to both the temperature and charge of the material. Classical gravity is the bulk, a well-understood computable theory. The method is to append a gravity bulk to the boundary field theory of the unconventional material to elicit its properties. Of particular interest is the conductivity (ability to conduct electricity) of the material as one of the first typical characterizations of materials, which is not possible with traditional methods (e.g. BCS (Bardeen–Cooper–Schrieffer) theory that applies to nonexotic superconducting materials (Bardeen *et al.*, 1957)).

The experimental analysis is as follows. The unconventional material organized per an unknown quantum field theory is appended to a bulk with a black hole behaving according to classical relativity. The two domains are linked together through the correspondence formalism. Then some electric current is applied to the boundary. Calculating the effect of applying the current to the exotic material is not possible because its properties are unknown. However, calculating the effect of applying the current is straightforward on the black hole side. When current or charge is applied to a black hole event horizon (boundary), some of the current falls into the black hole in the form of ripples in spacetime gravity. This makes the black hole larger, and the resulting growth can be measured as the entropy of the black hole with known formulas (from Bekenstein and

Hawking). Since entropy is the same as the loss of heat, via the correspondence, the loss of heat in the bulk is equal to the conductivity of the unconventional material (Hartnoll *et al.*, 2016).

Other methods do not allow the conductivity of the unconventional material to be calculated. However, with the AdS/CMT correspondence, black hole formulations can be used to describe dissipative processes that allow the investigation of unconventional materials. An important property in materials science is establishing a material's conductivity (ability to conduct electricity) and the converse, resistivity (ability to block the transmission of electricity). Articulating the properties of high-temperature superconductors, which have perfect conductivity (no loss), and how their operational deployment might proceed could have substantial use in constructing lossless computing systems. Some of the bulk-boundary relationships of AdS/CMT are outlined in Table 3.6.

### 3.3.3 *AdS/SYK (SYK model)*

The AdS/CMT correspondence is often applied with the SYK model (named after the authors, Sachdev & Ye, 1993; Kitaev, 2015), which is a solvable model of condensed matter systems with broad application in many fields of physics and beyond. More specifically, the SYK model is a model of quantum mechanical systems of Majorana fermions with all-to-all random interactions, that unlike many other models of strongly interacting quantum mechanical systems are readily solvable. Further, the SYK model is important as the minimal realization of the AdS/CFT correspondence (Sachdev, 2010).

AdS/SYK refers to the body of research that applies the correspondence through the SYK model. AdS/SYK is applied in both directions,

Table 3.6. Bulk-boundary: AdS/CMT (condensed matter).

| No. | Bulk | Boundary | Reference |
|---|---|---|---|
| 1 | Black hole gravity | Unconventional materials quantum field theory | Sachdev (2010) |
| 2 | Black hole entropy | Unconventional materials conductivity | Hartnoll *et al.* (2016) |

from bulk-to-boundary to facilitate the study of unknown quantum mechanical systems on the boundary via the well-understood bulk classical gravity, and from boundary-to-bulk to elaborate bulk duals (emergent bulk structure). For example, Gross and Rosenhaus (2017) examine the bulk dual of the SYK model as related to the cubic couplings of bulk interactions. Engelsoy *et al.* (2016) also investigate bulk duals, in particular through the dynamical time variable in the SYK model, to study black hole evaporation and the role of entropy, among other aspects. Garcia-Alvarez *et al.* (2017) propose the digital quantum simulation of a minimal AdS/CFT model in controllable quantum platforms using the SYK model as a protocol that reproduces a simplified low-dimensional model of quantum gravity in advanced quantum platforms as trapped ions and superconducting circuits.

### 3.3.4 *AdS/Chaos (thermal systems)*

AdS/Chaos refers to the application of the AdS/CFT correspondence to the study of chaotic systems. Chaos denotes the states of dynamical systems whose apparently random states of disorder and irregularity are in fact governed by deterministic laws that are highly sensitive to initial conditions. In theoretical physics, chaos is often synonymous with thermal systems (systems governed by heat), which often follow chaotic dynamics (a seemingly random evolution but one that can be described by laws). As in AdS/CMT, applying the correspondence in AdS/Chaos can provide a simplification for solving an otherwise intractable problem. Chaotic thermal systems are typically described by strongly interacting gauge theories, which cannot be easily computed. Chaos problems frequently entail solving classical general relativity problems, which suggests that they might be amenable to a gravity formulation via the holographic correspondence. The chaotic system is formulated with the correspondence in order to obtain computable coefficients for the timescale by which the strongly interacting thermal system will relax. Understanding how a chaotic system relaxes is a start toward characterizing the system.

Shenker and Stanford (2014) use the correspondence in the gauge-gravity formulation to explore bulk geometry. The experimental setup has highly entangled CFTs linked to black hole bulk geometry. A chaotic system is induced by acting on the bulk and the boundary with thermal-scale operators that are local at different times, such that perturbations create an intersecting network of shock waves. The resulting chaotic CFT dynamics and the associated fast information scrambling time are used to identify features of the resulting bulk geometries. The method is specifying the bulk and boundary regions, acting on both, and then finding out more about the bulk through the boundary.

In another example of AdS/Chaos, Maldacena *et al.* (2016) use holography to conjecture a bound on the growth rate of chaos in quantum thermal systems that have a large number of degrees of freedom. The usual mechanism for diagnosing chaotic systems, an out-of-time-order correlation function, is used (a quantum information operator that assesses temporal correlation). Long-time behavior that is sensitive to initial conditions in the CFT is connected to high-energy scattering processes in the bulk near the black hole horizon. A key finding is the claim that chaos can develop no faster than exponentially (per the influence of chaos on the out-of-time-order correlator). Analyzing an $AdS_5/CFT_4$ model ($N = 4$ Super Yang–Mills theory/$AdS_5$), Cotler *et al.* (2017) find that the late time behavior of horizon fluctuations in large AdS black holes is governed by random matrix dynamics that describe the fine-grained structure of energy levels in chaotic systems. Bulk-boundary representations of AdS/Chaos (thermal systems) applications appear in Table 3.7.

Table 3.7. Bulk-boundary: AdS/Chaos (thermal systems).

| No. | Bulk | Boundary | Reference |
|---|---|---|---|
| 1 | Black hole geometry | Highly entangled CFTs | Shenker and Stanford (2014) |
| 2 | High-energy scattering processes near the bulk black hole horizon | Long time behavior (sensitivity to initial conditions) in the CFT | Maldacena *et al.* (2016) |
| 3 | 5D AdS-Schwarzschild black hole metric | 4D super Yang–Mills theory | Cotler *et al.* (2017) |

### 3.3.5 *AdS/QIT (quantum information theory)*

*CFT: Quantum Field Theory -> Quantum Information State -> Qubits*

The AdS/QIT correspondence is the research program of interpreting the AdS/CFT correspondence in terms of QIT. The thought progression is that the boundary quantum field theory is described by quantum information states, which are represented by qubits. The correspondence is generally considered in the context of tangible physical systems such as a black hole or superconducting material. However, quantum computers are likewise physical systems and information-theoretical interpretation of the correspondence sees the boundary field theory as quantum states represented by qubits.

Information theory is concerned with the efficiency of information quantification, storage, and transmission. One problem of interest is determining the best information compression protocols for sending quantum states. AdS/QIT thus might operate a bulk-to-boundary analysis to find efficient information compression protocols for the boundary quantum states. AdS/QIT might go in the other direction as well, as a boundary-to-bulk analysis to interrogate bulk structures defined by boundary measures such as entropy.

One frequent application of the AdS/QIT correspondence is the relation between thermal density operators on the boundary and geometry in the bulk in the form of geodesic curves (the shortest path through the bulk's negatively curved AdS space). The boundary is density operators and the bulk is geometry (geodesic curves). Instead of using a traditional quantum mechanical entropy calculation (the sum over all minimal measurement bases) which is difficult to compute, a geometric calculation of entropy is applied via the correspondence. The shortest distance between two points on the boundary is the shortest length curve through the bulk. The shortest distance between two points on the boundary is interpreted as the number of qubits required to send a message (the quantum state) from one location to another. Entropy is a measure of the minimal number of qubits required to send a message. Hence, the question is posed in the boundary, namely, the most efficient compression of quantum state information (the number of qubits required to send the state), and solved in the bulk, by finding the shortest curve through the bulk geometry (Czech *et al.*, 2015).

Both the geometric and topological complexity of the bulk are a target of study (Raimond *et al.*, 2018). This is because different curves through the bulk have different meanings. Whereas the geodesic (the shortest curve) is equivalent to total entropy (the entropy of a boundary region), an arbitrary-length curve can be interpreted as conditional entropy (Czech *et al.*, 2015). There is also relative entropy (in the form of the Kullback–Leibler divergence) for computing how one probability distribution is different from another. These entropy measures are important for creating entanglement distillation in quantum information compression protocols (Horodecki *et al.*, 2007) (Table 3.8). Other work uses the measure of relative entropy in the boundary for a derivation of classical gravity in the bulk (Lashkari *et al.*, 2014).

### 3.3.6 *AdS/TN (tensor networks)*

AdS/TN is the idea of holographic TN, implementing the correspondence in the form of a TN. TNs factorize a high-order tensor into a network of low-order tensors. The structure of TNs is a hierarchical multilayered model that consolidates arbitrary microscale detail into increasingly fewer-node tiers in an overall apparatus that theoretically culminates in one macroscale kernel. TNs are an implementation of the renormalization group method in that the network structure preserves salient detail related to the individual scale tiers. In the blockchain world, TNs are similar to a Merkle tree, in which blocks of information are similarly rolled up in a hash-linked data structure into one cryptographic kernel (Merkle root) that calls the entirety of a data corpus.

A frequent implementation of AdS/TN is AdS/MERA. MERA (multiscale entanglement renormalization ansatz (guess)) is a tensor network structure designed to model quantum many-body systems by renormalizing

Table 3.8. Bulk-boundary: AdS/QIT (quantum information).

| No. | Bulk | Boundary | Reference |
|---|---|---|---|
| 1 | Geometric structure | Quantum states (qubits) | Hayden *et al.* (2016) |
| 2 | Geodesic (shortest curve) | Entanglement entropy | Swingle (2012) |
| 3 | Arbitrary length curve | Conditional entropy | Czech *et al.* (2015) |
| 4 | Einstein gravity derivation | Relative entropy | Lashkari *et al.* (2014) |

entanglement (Vidal, 2007). In a real-space renormalization procedure defined for quantum states, MERA represents a highly entangled many-body state (such as the ground state of a CFT) with a tensor network. MERA is constructed as a tensor network with alternating layers of disentanglers and isometries. The network structure has multiple input nodes and one output node; the system operates by coarse-graining up from microscopic system inputs to one (or few) macroscopic kernel(s). In each layer, unitary operators (disentanglers) remove local entanglement and isometries coarse grain the nodes into fewer representations in the next tier. The resulting network of unitary and isometric tensors encodes input such as ground state wavefunctions with the multilayered structure (Vidal, 2008). The alternating disentangler-isometry layers in MERA are similar to the alternating max pooling followed by convolutions and rectified linear unit (ReLU) activations in a neural network (LeCun *et al.*, 2015).

TNs provide a natural framework for interpreting the AdS/CFT correspondence. The tensor network input layer is the boundary and the rolled-up tiers point deeper into the bulk. The entropy of a boundary region is equal to the area of a corresponding bulk minimal surface per the Ryu–Takayanagi formula (2006). Swingle (2012) first suggested the tensor network interpretation of the AdS/CFT correspondence, by extending the Ryu–Takayanagi formulation to link the entropy of a boundary region to a bulk minimal curve (Table 3.9).

The work is demonstrated through a tensor network-based implementation of the Ising model. A key insight is running the tensor network

Table 3.9. Bulk-boundary: AdS/TN (tensor networks).

| No. | Bulk | Boundary | Reference |
|---|---|---|---|
| 1 | Geodesic | Entropy | Swingle (2012) |
| 2 | Qubit to protect | Protective ancilla | Pastawski *et al.* (2015) |
| 3 | Bulk entanglement wedge | Boundary region | Hayden *et al.* (2016) |
| 4 | Lattice: $d + 1$ Hilbert space | Lattice: Flat Hilbert space | Lee and Qi (2016) |
| 5 | Tile-based Motzkin walks | Motzkin spin-chain ground state | Alexander *et al.* (2018) |
| 6 | 2D ground states on a lattice | Gauged global symmetries | McMahon *et al.* (2020) |

backward. Whereas a tensor network has an endpoint, a black hole bulk does not. The coarse-grained final state in the tensor network completely factorizes (as the macroscale kernel), and then the renormalization process can be reversed to trace back through the network to calculate new aspects of the boundary starting from information already included in the entanglement roll-ups in the network. Calculating the entropy of a block of sites in the boundary is such a problem that lacks other tractable methods (concretized as obtaining the entropy of a block of sites in the Ising lattice model). Retracing back through the tensor network generates a curve of the minimum number of sites that must be passed through to obtain the boundary block entropy, thereby linking boundary region entropy to a bulk geodesic (the shortest path on a curved surface).

There are many other holographic tensor network implementations. Pastawski *et al.* (2015) build a tensor network with the correspondence using the bulk as an ancilla (ancillary bits) in the sense of having bulk logical degrees of freedom protect boundary physical degrees of freedom in a quantum error correction code structure (initially proposed by Almheiri *et al.* (2015)). Hayden *et al.* (2016) use holographic random TNs to propose an expanded model of the correspondence that applies to a wider range of spacetimes. Lee and Qi (2016) propose an exact holographic mapping method between the bulk and boundary Hilbert spaces of lattices and obtain analytic results for free fermion systems. Alexander *et al.* (2018) define exact holographic TNs for the Motzkin spin chain. The Motzkin model is a recently developed quantum mechanical model used to study quantum optimization problems as it is not constrained by the energy scaling profile typically associated with a CFT. McMahon *et al.* (2020) lift a traditional one-dimensional MERA implementation of critical ground states on a lattice to a two-dimensional bulk dual that allows a wider range of bulk-boundary operator mapping and in which horizon-like holographic screens emerge. Increasing the capacity of TNs to represent higher-dimensional systems is an ongoing research focus.

### 3.3.7 *AdS/ML (machine learning)*

The AdS/ML correspondence interprets the AdS/CFT correspondence as a neural network, with experimental data as the boundary and unknown quantum system structure as the bulk to be interrogated. It is a boundary-to-bulk analysis in which the known boundary is used to interrogate the unknown bulk. The premise is that the emergent neural network structure (as the network runs to produce an optimal solution) corresponds to emergent bulk structure that quantizes aspects of an unknown quantum system. Experimental data (boundary) is the input to ML networks (bulk). The emergent neural network structure (weights, layer depth) equates to the generation of the bulk metric, dilaton (hypothetical particle) profile, and other structural features of the bulk mechanics. The mapping between neural network parameters and the AdS/CFT correspondence appears in Table 3.10 (Hashimoto, 2019, p. 9).

In the standard deployment of AdS/ML, the first step is defining the boundary with training data (real-life data of quantum observables as training data for the neural network to learn). Supervised (discriminative) ML is used if the input data are labeled, and unsupervised (generative) learning of the input data are not annotated. The second step is interpreting the emergent network structure as the emergent bulk structure. The neural network weights (probabilities) are read as the bulk metric (an overall equation for the quantum system with space, time, curvature, volume, or other relevant parameters). The third step is using the bulk metric for the more complete description of specific aspects of interest in the quantum system such as scaling metrics, short-range and long-range correlations, and phase transition. Code is available for AdS/

Table 3.10. Mapping: AdS/ML (machine learning).

| No. | Deep Neural Network (Boltzmann Machine) | AdS/CFT Correspondence |
|---|---|---|
| 1 | Neural network architecture | Bulk spacetime geometry |
| 2 | Network depth | Emergent bulk radial direction |
| 3 | Network weights | Metric components |
| 4 | Hidden variables | Discretized fields in the bulk |
| 5 | Probability distribution given by the Boltzmann machine | Generating function of the QFT dual to the bulk gravity |
| 6 | Classical equations of motion | Fields propagating on spacetime |

Table 3.11. Bulk-boundary: AdS/ML (machine learning).

| No. | Bulk (Emergent Structure) | Boundary (Empirical Data) | Reference |
|---|---|---|---|
| 1 | Concrete bulk gravity metric and dilaton profile for AdS/QCD | QCD observables: Hadron spectra (rho and $a_2$ mesons) | 2020 |
| 2 | Consistent bulk geometry at various temperatures; black hole horizon | Lattice QCD data (finite-temperature chiral condensate) | 2021 |
| 3 | Bulk metric with finite-height IR wall (QCD thermal phase transition) | Lattice QCD data (finite-temperature chiral condensate) | 2018a |
| 4 | Bulk metric, mass, and quadratic coupling; gravitational model of a strongly correlated system | Magnetic response data for the strongly correlated material $Sm_{0.6}Sr_{0.4}MnO_3$ | 2018b |

*Sources*: Hashimoto *et al.* (2018a, Holographic QCD), Hashimoto *et al.* (2018b, AdS/CFT correspondence), Akutagawa *et al.* (2020, AdS/QCD), Hashimoto *et al.* (2021, Neural ODE).

ML (https://github.com/AkinoriTanaka-phys/DL_holographicQCD) and specific examples of the deployed method appear in Table 3.11.

## 3.4 AdS/DIY

The AdS/CFT correspondence can be applied practically in the notion of do-it-yourself AdS (AdS/DIY). The core concept is that any volumetric physical system can be described by a boundary theory in one less dimension, sort of like taking the derivative of a system to obtain the salient aspect. A basic example is a room, whose temperature and pressure are boundary theories in terms of being readily calculable averages of constituent bulk microstates.

To formulate the correspondence, first is defining the system and the two spaces, distinguishing a more complicated bulk region, and a more streamlined boundary in one less dimension. Second is choosing a relevant coordinate system and scale (units) for distance and curvature since lengths and energies will be measured in these units in the system. Third is defining the constituent elements and dynamics of the respective spaces. Fourth is defining a dictionary mapping between the two spaces that puts them into correspondence and describes how one domain can act upon the other. The correspondence might be defined on the basis of theories, states, operators, spatial structure, or other parameters (degrees of freedom) that have a correspondence between the two scale tiers of the system. Fifth is deploying the correspondence to solve problems from one side or the other, or asking a question in the boundary to return an answer from the bulk (or vice versa).

The two main dictionaries that describe the bulk-boundary mapping are the differentiate dictionary (Gubser *et al.*, 1998) and the extrapolate dictionary (Banks *et al.*, 1998). The differentiate dictionary makes use of the equivalence between the partition functions of the bulk and boundary theories, and the extrapolate dictionary relies on the fact that local CFT operators living in the boundary theory can be expressed as the limit of appropriately weighted bulk fields. Either of these dictionaries or a new mapping might be most relevant for the AdS/DIY operation.

### 3.4.1 *The AdS/CFT equations*

The AdS/CFT correspondence is a relationship between a quantum gravity theory and a quantum field theory. The basic statement of the correspondence is that any CFT in $d$-dimensional spacetime is equivalent to a quantum theory of gravity in $(d + 1)$ dimensional spacetime. Implementing the correspondence involves defining the bulk and the boundary and the equality relation between them.

The four kinds of equations that typically comprise the AdS/CFT correspondence are listed in Table 3.12. The most important is the metric, articulated as an equation in the form of ($ds$=), for the AdS space and the CFT. The *metric* (shortened from the metric tensor used in General Relativity) is the fundamental object of study and is used to define the space, time, distance, volume, curvature, and angles of any gravitational system, thereby providing a complete description of the geometric structure of the spacetime used in the formulation. Mathematically, the metric tensor is a function which takes as input a pair of tangent vectors at a point on a surface and produces a real number scalar. Dot products generalize vector properties in Euclidean space, and metric tensors are used similarly in AdS space to define the

Table 3.12. AdS/CFT correspondence equations.

| No. | Term | Description |
|---|---|---|
| 1 | Metrics (*ds*=) for the AdS space and the CFT | Specification of system space, time, curvature |
| 2 | Operators (*O*=) which act on observables | Functions acting on system observables |
| 3 | Local effective actions in AdS and CFT (*S*=) | Formulation of system energy and dynamics |
| 4 | Hamiltonian or Lagrangian (*H*=) or (*L*=) | Calculation of states of the dynamical system |

length of tangent vectors and the angle between them on a manifold. The metric tensor is integrated to give the length of curves on the manifold. A metric is defined for both the AdS and the CFT as the central equations of the correspondence.

The two respective spaces (AdS and CFT) have constituent elements upon which operators act to produce system observables. Any number of operators (*O*=) can be defined to act on the observable elements of the system. Then, bulk and boundary local effective actions (*S*=) are defined for the system. The action is an attribute of the dynamics that reflects kinetic and potential energy and which derives the equations of motion of the system. Finally, a Hamiltonian or Lagrangian is defined to enumerate and predict the different states of the dynamical system.

#### 3.4.1.1 *The AdS/CFT formalism*

The AdS/CFT relation postulates that the physics of an AdS spacetime can be described by a local quantum field theory on the boundary. Setting forth the correspondence involves first defining the two terms in field-theoretic language so that they can be equated, and then second, defining the equality relation between them. The first term to define is the AdS space of interest. AdS is a maximally symmetric spacetime with negative curvature. It is a solution to Einstein's equations with a negative cosmological constant. However, unlike the Einstein field equations of general relativity, the AdS/CFT equations are solvable. The second term to define is the CFT, which is constructed from the AdS formulation.

According to the AdS/CFT correspondence, the Hilbert spaces are identical, and all (physical or global) symmetries can be matched between the two theories. In particular, the spacetime symmetries or isometries of $AdS_{d+1}$ form the group $SO(2, d)$ and these act on the $CFT_d$ to create the conformal group. All states in both theories will be representations of this group (Kaplan, 2016, p. 11). More specifically, the isometries of AdS act on the boundary. Due to the symmetry relation, they send points on the boundary to other points on the boundary. This action is the action of the conformal group in $d$ dimensions, $SO(2, d)$. Thus, the quantum field theory is a CFT. Symmetry rescaling in the bulk translates into a dual representation on the boundary. This means that the boundary theory is scale invariant (Maldacena, 2014, p. 3). $SO(2, d)$ is the special orthogonal matrix operation (in the $2 \times d$ dimensions of the AdS) that is a linear transformation or rotation about the origin of a point in space that results in other measures or points in the space.

The AdS/CFT correspondence is formulated as a set of equations to implement the equality relation between the AdS bulk and the CFT boundary. The next step is specifying the spacetime of interest. Spacetimes might range between the most basic $AdS_2$/CFT (two dimensions of bulk space and one of boundary space) and Maldacena's initial $Ads_5/CFT_4$ specification (a five-dimensional theory of bulk quantum gravity equating to a four-dimensional supersymmetric quantum gauge theory ($N = 4$ Super Yang–Mills theory)). A familiar three-dimensional Euclidean space would have a metric ($ds$=) with three spatial terms, denoted X, Y, and Z (Natsuume, 2016, p. 89). An advanced formulation might have two time-like and three spatial dimensions in the AdS metric (Sokolowski, 2016, p. 3).

With the bulk-boundary space and time dimensions identified, next, a coordinate system for the model is defined. These are the global coordinates of the system. Applying the coordinates to the system, the AdS metric is then written in terms of the radius of curvature (Maldacena, 2014, p. 1; Harlow, 2017, p. 3). Then the metric for the CFT is specified based on populating the points in the CFT with the special orthogonal group matrix transformations governed by parameters of symmetry and dilation. Correlation functions (such as two-point correlation functions) and Green's functions are calculated in the CFT, as a means of further defining the CFT and providing standard formalisms to be used in the correspondence relation.

Finally, the equality of the two sides is articulated using field operators and a dictionary. The way the duality is deployed between the gravity theory (bulk) and the quantum field theory (boundary) is through field operators and a map. The map between the two theories might be a one-to-one map between individual operators. For example, in $AdS_5/CFT_4$, the map is between gauge invariant operators in the two domains (the $N = 4$ $SU(N)$ Super Yang–Mills boundary theory and the classical gravity fields in $AdS_5 \times S^5$ ($S^5$ is a manifold)). Overall, the map provides an explicit link between the two theories.

### 3.4.1.2 *Correspondence formulation example*

Harlow (2017) provides a useful demonstration of the correspondence. The same three steps apply, namely, defining the two terms and the relation between them. The two terms are defined as metrics (*ds*=). Harlow defines a metric for the AdS space (page 3), a metric for the CFT (page 6), and puts them into correspondence (page 8). Technically, the AdS space is an asymptotically AdS space (Henneaux and Teitelboim, 1985).

A metric (*ds*=) is defined for AdS space, a set of global coordinates is defined for the space, and the metric for AdS space is written in global coordinates. A metric (*ds*=) for the CFT is defined taking into account that conformal field theories are relativistic quantum field theories which have Poincaré symmetry and are invariant under dilations and special conformal transformations. The two metrics for AdS and CFT are equated by considering the map between the observables on the two sides. The idea is to establish a map between the observables by creating a dictionary that indicates how to view the duality as an isomorphism (one-to-one mapping) between the two Hilbert spaces. To implement the dictionary, local operators (*O*=) are defined to act on observables. The map from operators to states is implemented with path integrals.

The first line in the AdS/CFT dictionary (mapping between AdS and CFT) defines unitary operators which implement isomorphic symmetry groups between the AdS and CFT. This means that the spectrum of the Hamiltonian is the same in both AdS and CFT, and states decompose into the same irreducible representations of symmetry groups. The key point is that any operator on one side can be mapped to an operator on the other side. In the identity mapping, the Hamiltonians and the ground states of both are equal. With the dictionary in place, the next step is to define bulk and boundary local effective actions (*S*=).

With this basic setup of the AdS/CFT dictionary, a range of useful experiments can be carried out using correlation functions of local operators in the CFT. One typical experiment is a "scattering" investigation between the boundary and the bulk. The protocol is acting with boundary local operators, waiting for some time, and then measuring the boundary operators to obtain the corresponding formulation that comes out of the bulk. Black hole formation and evaporation can be examined this way. A more advanced AdS/CFT dictionary is needed to define operators in the CFT which represent bulk operators far from the boundary for investigations involving bulk reconstruction and the investigation of bulk structural emergence.

### 3.4.1.3 *Listing of AdS/CFT correspondence formulations*

For AdS/DIY, a survey of AdS/CFT correspondence literature delineating the mathematical formalisms appears in Table 3.13. First are the references for the initial statements of the correspondence. Next is Harlow and

Table 3.13. AdS/CFT correspondence mathematics.

| No. | Reference | Focus |
|---|---|---|
| *Early formulations of the correspondence* | | |
| 1 | Maldacena (1999, 2014) | Initial correspondence formulation: $AdS_5/CFT_4$ |
| 2 | Witten (1998) | Supergravity correlation functions in CFT |
| 3 | Klebanov and Witten (1999) | Symmetry breaking and the correspondence |
| *Standard formulations of the correspondence* | | |
| 4 | Harlow (2017, p. 3) | Expansive formulation for emergent bulk structure |
| 5 | Erdmenger (2018, p. 4) | Standard formulation with classical bulk gravity |
| *Additional formulations of the correspondence* | | |
| 6 | Zaanen *et al.* (2012, p. 11) | Formulation beginning from the CFT side |
| 7 | Kaplan (2016, p. 3) | Context of quantum field theories |
| 8 | Guo *et al.* (2016, p. 6) | Generating function of correlation functions |
| 9 | Zaffaroni (2000, p. 21) | Describes boundary CFT with a Lagrangian |

Erdmenger as two standard sources for the formalisms. Both include the basics. Harlow (2017) is good for boundary-to-bulk investigation of new topics such as quantum gravity theories and bulk quantum mechanics. Erdmenger (2018) is good for bulk-to-boundary investigations, using classical gravity to interrogate condensed matter situations such as the Kondo problem. The rest are formulations for various specific problems.

## References

Akutagawa, T., Hashimoto, K. & Sumimoto, T. (2020). Deep learning and AdS/QCD. *Phys. Rev. D.* 102(2):026020.

Alexander, R.N., Evenbly, G. & Klich, I. (2018). Exact holographic tensor networks for the Motzkin spin chain. arXiv:1806.09626v2.

Almheiri, A., Dong, X. & Harlow, D. (2015). Bulk locality and quantum error correction in AdS/CFT. *J. High Energ. Phys.* 1504:163.

Banks, T., Douglas, M.R., Horowitz, G.T. & Martinec, E. (1998). AdS dynamics from conformal field theory. hep-th/9808016.

Bardeen, J., Cooper, L.N. & Schrieffer, J.R. (1957). Microscopic theory of superconductivity. *Phys. Rev.* 106(1):162–4.

Casalderrey-Solana, J., Liu, H., Mateos, D. *et al.* (2012). Gauge/string duality, hot QCD and heavy ion collisions. arXiv:1101.0618. (An introductory text on AdS/QCD).

Cotler, J.S., Gur-Ari, G., Hanada, M. *et al.* (2017). Black holes and random matrices. *J. High Energ. Phys.* 1705:118.

Cottrell, W., Freivogel, B., Hofman, D.M. & Lokhande, S.F. (2019). How to build the thermofield double state. *J. High Energ. Phys.* 1902:58.

Czech, B., Hayden, P., Lashkari, N. & Swingle, B. (2015). The information theoretic interpretation of the length of a curve. *J. High Energ. Phys.* 1506:157.

Engelhardt, N. & Wall, A.C. (2019). Coarse-graining holographic black holes. *J. High Energ. Phys.* 1905:160.

Engelsoy, J., Mertens, T.G. & Verlinde, H. (2016). An investigation of $AdS_2$ backreaction and holography. *J. High Energ. Phys.* 1607:139.

Erdmenger, J. (2018). Introduction to gauge/gravity duality. In *Proceedings of Theoretical Advanced Study Institute Summer School 2017, "Physics at the Fundamental Frontier"*, Boulder, Colorado, USA, June 4–July 1, 2017. arXiv:1807.09872v1, PoS(TASI2017)001.

Faulkner, T., Guica, M., Hartman, T. *et al.* (2014). Gravitation from entanglement in holographic CFTs. *J. High Energ. Phys.* 1403:051.

Flores-Livas, J.A., Boeri, L., Sanna, A. *et al.* (2020). A perspective on conventional high-temperature superconductors at high pressure: Methods and materials. *Phys. Rep.* 856:1–78.

Garcia-Alvarez, L., Egusquiza, I.L., Lamata, L. *et al.* (2017). Digital quantum simulation of minimal AdS/CFT. *Phys. Rev. Lett.* 119(04):040501.

Gross, D.J. & Rosenhaus, V. (2017). The bulk dual of SYK: Cubic couplings. *J. High Energ. Phys.* 1705:92.

Gubser, S.S., Klebanov, I.R. & Polyakov, A.M. (1998). Gauge theory correlators from non-critical string theory. *Phys. Lett. B.* 428:105–14.

Guo, M., Niu, C., Tian, Y. & Zhang, H. (2016). Modave lectures on applied AdS/CFT with numerics. In *Proceedings, 11th Modave Summer School in Mathematical Physics*. arXiv:1601.00257v2, PoS Modave2015(2016)003.

Gursoy, U., Kiritsis, E., Mazzanti, L. *et al.* (2011). Holographic bulk viscosity: GPR vs EO. *Lect Notes Phys.* 828:79.

Han, X., Hartnoll, S.A. & Kruthoff, J. (2020). Bootstrapping matrix quantum mechanics. *Phys. Rev. Lett.* 125(04):041601.

Harlow, D. (2017). TASI lectures on the emergence of bulk physics in AdS/CFT. In *Proceedings of Theoretical Advanced Study Institute Summer School 2017, "Physics at the Fundamental Frontier"*, Boulder, Colorado, USA, June 4–July 1, 2017. arXiv:1802.01040, PoS(TASI2017)002.

Hartnoll, S.A., Lucas, A. & Sachdev, S. (2018). *Holographic Quantum Matter.* Cambridge: MIT Press.

Hartnoll, S.A., Ramirez, D.M. & Santos, J.E. (2016). Thermal conductivity at a disordered quantum critical point. *J. High Energ. Phys.* 1604:022.

Hashimoto, K., Sugishita, S., Tanaka, A. & Tomiya, A. (2018a). Deep learning and holographic QCD. *Phys. Rev. D.* 98(106014):1–15.

Hashimoto, K., Sugishita, S., Tanaka, A. & Tomiya, A. (2018b). Deep learning and the AdS/CFT correspondence. *Phys. Rev. D.* 98(046019):1–7.

Hashimoto, K. (2019). AdS/CFT as a deep Boltzmann machine. *Phys. Rev. D.* 99(106017):1–13.

Hashimoto, K., Hu, H.-Y. & You, Y.-Z. (2021). Neural ordinary differential equation and holographic quantum chromodynamics. *Mach Learn: Sci. Technol.* 2(03):035011.

Hayden, P., Nezami, S., Qi, X.-L. *et al.* (2016). Holographic duality from random tensor networks. *J. High Energ. Phys.* 11(9):1–57.

Hazboun, J.S. (2018). Constructing an explicit AdS/CFT correspondence with Cartan geometry. *Nucl. Phys.* B929:254–65.

Henneaux, M. & Teitelboim, C. (1985). Asymptotically anti-de Sitter spaces. *Commun. Math. Phys.* 98:391–424.

Heemskerk, I. & Polchinski, J. (2011). Holographic and Wilsonian renormalization groups. *J. High Energ. Phys.* 1106:031.

Horodecki, M., Oppenheim, J. & Winter, A. (2007). Quantum state merging and negative information. *Commun. Math. Phys.* 269(1):107–36.

Hubeny, V.E., Rangamani, M. & Takayanagi, T. (2007). A covariant holographic entanglement entropy proposal. *J. High Energ. Phys.* 0707:062.

Kalinin, K.P. & Berloff, N.G. (2018). Blockchain platform with proof-of-work based on analog Hamiltonian optimisers. arXiv:1802.10091v1.

Kaplan, J. (2016). Lectures on AdS/CFT from the bottom up. Johns Hopkins Lecture Course.

Kitaev, A. (2015). A simple model of quantum holography. KITP strings seminar and entanglement 2015 program. http://online.kitp.ucsb.edu/online/entangled15/. Accessed March 15, 2021.

Klebanov, I.R. & Witten, E. (1999). AdS/CFT correspondence and symmetry breaking. arXiv: 9905104v2.

Lashkari, N., McDermott, M.B. & van Raamsdonk, M. (2014). Gravitational dynamics from entanglement "thermodynamics". *J. High Energ. Phys.* 04(195).

LeCun, Y., Bengio, Y. & Hinton, G. (2015). Deep learning. *Nature.* 521 (7553):436–44.

Lee, C.H. & Qi, X.-L. (2016). Exact holographic mapping in free fermion systems. *Phys. Rev. B.* 93(03):035112.

Lewkowycz, A. & Maldacena, J. (2013). Generalized gravitational entropy. *J. High Energ. Phys.* 1308:090.

Maldacena, J.M. (1999). The large N limit of superconformal field theories and supergravity. *Intl. J. Theor. Phys.* 38(4):1113–33.

Maldacena, J. (2014). The gauge/gravity duality. In *Black Holes in Higher Dimensions*. Ed. G. Horowitz. Cambridge: Cambridge University Press.

Maldacena, J., Shenker, S.H. & Stanford, D. (2016). A bound on chaos. *J. High Energ. Phys.* 1608:106.

McMahon, N.A., Singh, S. & Brennen, G.K. (2020). A holographic duality from lifted tensor networks. *NPJ Quantum Info.* 6(36):1–13.

Natsuume, M. (2016). *AdS/CFT Duality User Guide*. London: Springer.

Pastawski, F., Yoshida, B., Harlow, D. & Preskill, J. (2015). Holographic quantum error-correcting codes: Toy models for the bulk/boundary correspondence. *J. High Energ. Phys.* 06(149):1–53.

Qi, X.L. (2013). Exact holographic mapping and emergent space-time geometry. arXiv:1309.6282.

Raimond, A., Erdmenger, J., Hinrichsen, H. *et al.* (2018). Topological complexity in AdS3/CFT2. arXiv:1710.01327v2.

Ryu, S. & Takayanagi, T. (2006). Aspects of holographic entanglement entropy. *J. High Energ. Phys.* 0608:045.

Sachdev, S. (2010). Strange metals and the AdS/CFT correspondence. *J. Stat. Mech.* 1011:P11022.

Sachdev, S. & Ye, J. (1993). Gapless spin-fluid ground state in a random quantum Heisenberg magnet. *Phys. Rev. Lett.* 70:3339–42.

Shenker, S.H. & Stanford, D. (2014). Multiple shocks. *J. High Energ. Phys.* 1412:046.

Sokolowski, L.M. (2016). The bizarre anti-de Sitter spacetime. arXiv:1611.01118v1.

Susskind, L. (1995). The world as a hologram. *J. Math. Phys.* 36(11):6377–96.

Swan, M. (2022). B/CI: Quantum computing, holographic control theory, and blockchain IPLD for the brain. In: *Nanomedical Brain/Cloud Interface: Explorations and Implications*. Ed. Boehm, F. Boca Raton FL: CRC Press.

Swan, M., dos Santos, R.P. & Witte, F. (2020). *Quantum Computing: Physics, Blockchains, and Deep Learning Smart Networks*. London: World Scientific.

Swingle, B. (2012). Entanglement renormalization and holography. *Phys. Rev. D.* 86(6):065007.

Vidal, G. (2007). Entanglement renormalization. *Phys. Rev. Lett.* 99(22):220405.

Vidal, G. (2008). Class of quantum many-body states that can be efficiently simulated. *Phys. Rev. Lett.* 101(11):110501.

Willshaw, D.J., Buneman, O.P. & Longuet-Higgins, H.C. (1969). Non-holographic associative memory. *Nature*. 222(5197):960–62.

Witten, E. (1998). Anti de Sitter space and holography. IASSNS-HEP-98-15.

Zaanen, J., Sun, Y.W., Liu, Y. & Schalm, K. (2012). The AdS/CMT manual for plumbers and electricians. Brussels Lecture Notes.

Zaffaroni, A. (2000). Introduction to the AdS/CFT correspondence. *Class Quant. Grav.* 17:3571–97.

# Chapter 4

# Tabletop Experiments

*[T]he technology for the control of complex quantum many-body systems is advancing rapidly, and we appear to be at the dawn of a new era in physics—the study of quantum gravity in the lab*

— Susskind and team. Brown *et al.* (2019, p. 2)

**Abstract**

This chapter describes a photonic particle accelerator-on-a-chip, quantum gravity testing with Rydberg atoms, a black hole on a superconducting chip solution, and quantum simulators of the Sachdev–Ye–Kitaev (SYK) model. The SYK model constitutes a minimal realization of the anti-de Sitter space/conformal field theory (AdS/CFT) correspondence. Due to information-theoretic formulations, foundational physics findings from black holes and the holographic correspondence can be applied in manageable tabletop experiments to study a variety of complex quantum systems including the brain.

## 4.1 Black Holes and Quantum Gravity in the Lab

A surprising development is the inventive experiments that are bringing large-scale phenomena such as particle accelerators, black holes, and quantum gravity into reach in the form of models that can be studied in the laboratory. A large part of this effort is facilitated by the anti-de Sitter space/conformal field theory (AdS/CFT) correspondence, which indicates how two different descriptions of the same underlying physical system are equivalent. The implication is that certain quantum mechanical systems are dynamically equivalent to black holes in quantum gravity, and therefore can be used as a means of studying them. Conversely, if a quantum mechanical system can be shown to have the same kind of dynamics as a black hole (such as fast information scrambling and chaotic behavior), it may qualify as a holographic dual. The upshot is that the experimental tools needed to study black holes are the same ones that physicists have already been developing to solve quantum computational problems. The insight is that both situations require storing a complex system of many particles and accurately controlling how they interact (which is also similar to the brain's activity in neural signaling).

## 4.2 Particle Accelerator on a Chip

One of the most tangible tabletop experiments with near-term benefits is the advent of a laser-driven particle accelerator that fits on a silicon chip (Sapra *et al.*, 2020). The accelerator-on-a-chip project led by Vuckovic at Stanford's Nanoscale and Quantum Photonics Laboratory presents the first experimental demonstration of a waveguide-integrated dielectric laser accelerator. The problem addressed is that the size and cost of conventional radio-frequency accelerators have limited the reach of traditional particle accelerators. Instead, creating a dielectric laser accelerator provides a compact and cost-effective solution to power accelerator nanostructures with visible or near-infrared pulsed lasers, and results in a $10^4$ reduction of scale (Wootton *et al.*, 2016). Earlier examples of dielectric laser accelerators used free-space lasers directly incident on the accelerating structures, but that still limited the scalability and integrability of the technology. Sapra *et al.*'s (2020) waveguide-integrated dielectric laser accelerator overcomes these problems and is able to achieve an initial energy of 83.4 keV over 30 $\mu$m, and peak acceleration gradients of 40.3 MeV/m.

Particle accelerators are measured in terms of the energy scale at which they operate, as to the number of electron volts marshaled (Table 4.1). The accelerator-on-a-chip initializes at 83.4 thousand electron volts and has a peak gradient of 40 million electron volts. To put this

Table 4.1. Accelerator energy scales (electron Volts).

| No. | Abbr. | Description | Size (eV) | Capacity Example |
|---|---|---|---|---|
| 1 | KeV | Kilo (thousand) electron volts | 1,000 | 83.4 keV (initial) |
| 2 | MeV | Mega (million) electron volts | 1,000,000 | 40.3 MeV (peak) |
| 3 | GeV | Giga (billion) electron volts | 1,000,000,000 | 9 GeV |
| 4 | TeV | Tera (trillion) electron volts | 1,000,000,000,000 | 7 TeV (14TeV) |

in context, the Stanford linear accelerator (SLAC) operates at 50 GeV (billion electron volts). The Large Hadron Collider (LHC), 9 km in diameter, currently operates at about 7 TeV (trillion electron volts) with a planned expansion to 14 TeV with the High-Luminosity Large Hadron Collider (HL-LHC) to open in 2026.

Chip-based accelerators provide an accessible lower-cost alternative to conventional radio-frequency-based electron accelerators with accelerators operating with optical and near-infrared sources. While the larger macroscale accelerators emphasize foundational theoretical physics experiments, chip-based accelerators could have a range of practical applications in targeted cancer therapies, compact imaging sources, and tabletop lasers. In principle, optical accelerators on a chip could replace traditional radio-frequency-based electron accelerators for many applications. Chip-based accelerators not only scale down the wavelength of the source but also all other components of the accelerator. The implication is that an accelerator that spans kilometers could one day fit inside a volume the size of a shoebox.

Also, although chip-based accelerator energies are currently lower than traditional macroscale accelerators, this could change. There are high losses in metals at optical frequencies, and so the elements that make up the accelerator-on-a-chip cannot simply be miniaturized but must be reinvented in appropriate material systems. A roadmap is proposed to reinvent the related components (dielectric material systems such as silicon, silicon dioxide, and silicon nitride).

Further, integrating the accelerator with photonic waveguides also represents a design challenge due to difficulties in accounting for scattering and reflections of the waveguide mode from sub-wavelength features.

Sapra *et al.* (2020) address this by using an inverse design approach to develop a waveguide-integrated dielectric laser accelerator on a 500 nm device layer silicon-on-insulator platform.

The chip-based particle accelerator uses lasers to accelerate electrons along an etched channel (channels are etched into silicon chips in the fabrication process). As electrons flow through the channel, laser light accelerates the particles to high speeds. The idea of using lasers in accelerators stretches back to the invention of the laser (late 1950s). Lasers produce electromagnetic waves with much shorter wavelengths than the microwaves used in a full-scale accelerator, which means they can accelerate electrons moving through a much smaller space. The device size can be extremely small. The electrons in the chip-based accelerator, for example, travel along a channel that is only 3 $\mu$m (3,000 nm) wide (about half the width of a 7 $\mu$m (7,000 nm) wide human red blood cell (Freitas, 2012, p. 69)). Although laser-driven devices can accelerate electrons in a much smaller space than full-scale accelerators, they require much greater precision to line up the laser and the electrons so that the light waves push the particles in the correct direction with as much energy as possible (Hughes *et al.*, 2018). Previous proof-of-concept prototypes required separate devices to generate the electrons, but the accelerator-on-a-chip integrates the components in one chip.

## 4.3 Quantum Gravity in the Lab

### 4.3.1 *Quantum gravity*

Quantum gravity in the lab refers to laboratory experiments designed to probe aspects of quantum gravity indirectly. A theory of quantum gravity is needed to solve contemporary puzzles about black holes, the Big Bang, and dark energy. Various theories of quantum gravity have been proposed, and what is new is the possibility of testing some of these theories in the laboratory. Traditional methods for studying quantum phenomena such as particle accelerators are not feasible for studying the much smaller scale of quantum gravity. A particle accelerator to generate the forces necessary to study quantum gravity at the $10^{-35}$ meters Planck-length scale would be the size of the entire Milky Way galaxy, and hence indirect methods are needed (Preskill, 2020).

Newtonian gravity (1687) was a substantial advance that unified the observed behavior of both terrestrial and celestial objects. The law states that bodies attract with a force that is directly proportional to the product of their masses and inversely proportional to the square of the distance between their centers (Newton, 1729, p. 392). Newtonian gravity continues to describe short-range gravity such as throwing a ball on Earth. However, other theories are needed to explain the intricacies of longer-range gravity in celestial motion. General relativity, Einstein's theory of gravitation (1915), proves such a formulation of gravity.

The two predominant theories in physics are general relativity and quantum mechanics. On the one hand, general relativity describes objects that are very large and very heavy such as planets. On the other hand, quantum mechanics describes objects that are very small and very light such as particles. A theory that incorporates aspects of both general relativity and quantum mechanics is needed to study objects that are very small and very heavy. These objects include black holes and the Big Bang and might enlighten an understanding of dark matter and dark energy. Dark energy contributes 68% of the total energy in the present-day observable universe, dark matter 27%, and ordinary (baryonic) matter 5% (Carroll, 2007, p. 46). The different theories of gravitation are listed in Table 4.2.

#### 4.3.1.1 *Justification for quantum gravity in the lab*

The central phenomenon studied in quantum gravity is the formation and eventual evaporation of black holes due to quantum effects. The AdS/CFT correspondence provides the theoretical and mathematical justification for indirect quantum gravity experiments. The holographic correspondence establishes an equivalence between two different formulations of the same physical system. Per the equivalence, a black hole's life cycle can be

Table 4.2. Gravitational theories.

| Newtonian Gravity | General Relativity |
|---|---|
| Human-scale objects (apples) | Very large and very heavy objects (planets) |
| Quantum Mechanics | Quantum Gravity |
| Very small and very light objects (particles) | Very small and very heavy objects (black holes) |

described in a completely different language that does not involve gravity at all. Instead, the holographic dual of gravity (the bulk theory) is a quantum system that consists of many particles strongly interacting with one another (the boundary theory). A goal of quantum gravity experiments in the laboratory is to continue to define the dictionary that translates between the bulk and boundary languages.

A key difficulty in the attempt to understand the quantum nature of spacetime and gravity has been the lack of experimental means. Gravity is a relatively weak force, and thus probing quantum gravity directly would mean going to experimentally infeasible energy scales. A consequence of the holographic principle, however, and its concrete realization in the AdS/CFT correspondence is that nongravitational systems with sufficient entanglement exhibit characteristics of quantum gravity. This suggests that it may be possible to use tabletop physics experiments to probe quantum gravity indirectly.

### 4.3.2 *Wormholes and holographic teleportation*

Brown *et al.* (2019) propose holographic teleportation protocols for quantum information transfer that can be readily executed in tabletop experiments with an outline for experimental realization in two platforms, Rydberg atom arrays, and trapped ions. The holographic teleportation protocols are quantum communication directions for how to transmit the quantum states and operators of a system. The teleportation protocols are holographic in that they exhibit behavior similar to that seen in black hole wormhole constructions. Information scrambled into one half of an entangled system unscrambles into the other half, after a weak coupling between the two halves. The work develops research in operator size growth and distribution in the context of information transmission.

#### 4.3.2.1 *Operator size and size winding distribution*

A key innovation of the research is an analysis of operator size distributions and growth, ideas that have been studied in connection to holography and many-body physics. The standard canon is that operators grow in size and complexity as a quantum system evolves in time, and because operator size can be computed, it can be used as a metric for determining other aspects of the system. New terms, teleportation-by-operator-size and winding-size-distributions, are introduced in this work to establish practical quantum communications protocols based on wormhole-like (holographic) physics. Teleportation-by-operator-size describes how information transmission couplings are sensitive to operator size. Winding-size-distributions (winding and unwinding the size of the distribution) refer to a wavefunction ansatz (guess) in which coefficients in the size basis acquire an imaginary phase that is linear in the size of the operators. The *winding* size distribution produces wormhole-like physics as opposed to the *conventional* size distribution, in which coefficients are uniformly summed over the square of the absolute value in the usual treatment of a quantum system.

#### 4.3.2.2 *Holographic teleportation protocols*

The research formalizes the holographic protocols (that instantiate the wormhole-like physics) with a state transfer protocol and an operator transfer protocol. A quantum circuit is outlined for each. A specific configuration is provided and the circuits can be created in a laboratory (Brown *et al.*, 2019, p. 4). The teleportation protocols and the quantum circuits are designed to exhibit the reoccurrence feature of information scrambling. Information scrambling is a process whereby initially simple information becomes so thoroughly mixed across the degrees of freedom of a system that it is inaccessible to local measurements. Here, a special property is the recoherence phenomenon of scrambling-unscrambling information in which information disappears and then reappears at distance focused into view. The information disappears (is scrambled) in one side of an entangled coupled system and then reappears in the other side of the system at some future moment in time. Teleportation refers to the transfer of information, not matter (analogous to a fax machine). Quantum teleportation uses preexisting entanglement between two states together with classical communication to send a quantum message.

### **4.3.3** ***Preparing the thermofield double state***

A thermofield double state is prepared. The thermofield double state is an entangled state between two copies of a quantum state. The reduced density matrix of each copy is thermal (allowing a physical understanding based on heat through the system's thermal properties). The thermofield double state serves as a "model organism" or "model state" in the sense of being a basic construction in quantum physics to probe different aspects of a system. Here, the thermofield double state is executed by preparing a special entangled state of two copies of the physical system, as the left and right systems. At infinite-temperature, the thermofield double state is a collection of (entangled) Bell pairs between the left and right systems. For general Hamiltonians and noninfinite-temperature, there is no known procedure to prepare the thermofield double state. However, there are approximate methods for systems of interest (such as the Sachdev–Ye–Kitaev (SYK) model and various spin chains) employed by this work.

The quantum circuits act on a $2n$-qubit state (just $2n$, not $2^n$). The qubits are divided into $n$ qubits on the left and $n$ qubits on the right (creating two copies of the system). The qubits are described by a Hamiltonian that is assumed to be scrambling (dissipating its quantum state information among the constituent parts of the system). Also, the system must be able to effectively evolve forward and backward in time with the system Hamiltonian. The left and right qubits are initially entangled in the "thermofield double" state (two copies of a system being entangled per thermal purification). The left and right systems are further partitioned into "message" qubits and "carrier" qubits.

The procedure consists of two phases, one for scrambling and one for unscrambling. To scramble the information, the left side of the system is used. The idea is to insert a message and scramble it on the left side of the system. The first step is evolving the left qubits "backward in time" by acting on them with the inverse of the time-evolution operator. The second step is inserting the message into the message subsystem (partition) of the left qubits at the earlier time. The third step is evolving the left system "forward in time" by acting on it with the time-evolution operator. The result is that the forward evolution rapidly scrambles the message among the left qubits. The left side of the system has a scrambled message in it.

The next phase is unscrambling the information and seeing what happens. The left and right sides of the system (which are entangled per the setup) are now coupled by acting on the qubits with a coupling operator.

The result is that each of the left carrier qubits is coupled to mirror image carrier qubits on the right. Then all $n$ of the right qubits (carrier and message) are evolved "forward in time" by acting on them with the time-evolution operator. At this stage, the recohering phenomenon occurs. The message, buried and scrambled on the left, reappears on the right. Since the left and right systems are coupled, it is possible to recover the message on the right. Interpreting the result in the context of black hole physics, the message has traveled across a wormhole, a wormhole through the bulk attached to two different boundary conformal field theories (constructed as the thermofield double left and right sides).

The point of the experiment is to investigate the information scrambling time of quantum systems. Scrambling time is important in terms of how much information can be sent and recovered with high fidelity, for example, in terrestrial quantum communications protocols. The scrambling time is the timescale for information to spread across the entire system. Due to entanglement, information recovery is possible. Since the two systems are entangled at the time of the original message, before it is scrambled, it is not a surprise that it is recovered. If the two systems were not entangled when the message was scrambled, the expectation would be that it would not be recovered on the other side. Even though the two sides need to be further coupled to recover the message on the right side, the key point is that the two sides were entangled at the time of the original message insertion.

Summarizing the experimental setup, the process is to first entangle the two sides of the system (left and right) by configuring a thermofield double state. Second is to evolve the left side of the system backward in time, insert a message, and evolve forward in time such that the message is scrambled. Third, the two sides of the system are further coupled and the original message pops out on the right side. This work uses out-of-time-order correlation (OTOC) functions to run the system evolution backward and forward. Another strategy for understanding the evolution of thermofield double states is machine learning. In an AdS/QML (quantum machine learning for the study of the holographic correspondence) application, machine learning is used to learn the operator mapping between the left and right system evolutions in the thermofield double state (Cottrell *et al.*, 2019).

#### 4.3.3.1 *Obtain wormhole-like physics with size winding*

A key experimental target in this research is understanding more about the information scrambling time in quantum systems with the practical objective of developing more efficient quantum communications protocols. Toward this goal, a salient innovation is the introduction of the size-winding distribution to enable greater fine-tuning of the quantum system than the traditional method of the conventional-size distribution. In the winding size distribution, an imaginary phase that is linear in the size of the operators is introduced into the coefficients, which allows greater manipulability than the conventional size distribution in which the coefficients are simply summed.

The result is that the size winding distribution gives a different ansatz (guess) for the operator wavefunction. The manipulability of the size winding distribution allows it to be applied as usual at the late time of the quantum system, after information scrambling is complete, and also at intermediate times, while information scrambling is still in process. Whereas the late-time size winding is necessarily damped because the scrambling process is complete, the intermediate-time size winding can be more granular or perfect because scrambling is still in process. Thus, there are two different forms of the size winding distribution, the dampened form deployed at the late time and the perfect form deployed at the intermediate times of the quantum system evolution (Table 4.3). The size winding feature means both size winding and size unwinding in the

Table 4.3. Operator growth and size winding.

| | Operator Growth Time | |
|---|---|---|
| | Late Time | Intermediate Time |
| Size winding | Damped size winding | Perfect size winding |
| # of qubits teleported | One qubit | Many qubits |
| Signal dependence | Weak signal dependence, high fidelity | Strong signal dependence, limited fidelity |
| Operator transfer | Weak operator transfer | Strong operator transfer |
| Geometrical wormhole | No signature | Strong signature |

*Source*: Adapted from Brown *et al*. (2019, p. 7).

wormhole system with the two different sides. Depending on the coupling, a signal can be transferred left to right in the system. The action of the coupling can unwind the distribution in one direction and wind it in the opposite direction (tuning one side of the system from the other).

If only considering late time, the result is that a single-qubit infinite-temperature large-time example does not correspond to geometrical motion through a semi-classical wormhole. Whereas only a single qubit can be teleported with high fidelity in the high-temperature limit, with the right encoding of information, many qubits can be sent at low temperature and intermediate time in a holographic system hosting a traversable wormhole. Hence, since the strong signature of a geometrical wormhole is indicated in the intermediate-time perfect size winding system configuration, the idea is to work toward the higher fidelity teleportation of many qubits. The overall benefit is that size winding implements the holographic correspondence by providing a clean mechanism for operator transfer that abstracts the complicated way that geometrical wormholes work in the bulk, to the more accessible level of the boundary theory. Further, since a system's scrambling time is determined by its geometry, the size winding analysis can be applied to study emergent bulk structure.

### 4.3.4 *Rydberg atoms and trapped ions*

The experimental setup of the holographic teleportation protocols to transfer information that is discussed in this work can be implemented in atomic physics laboratory settings. Although the AdS/CFT correspondence may have an infinite number of degrees of freedom, quantum systems in laboratory can be realized using a finite number of degrees of freedom. Four steps are as follows. First, a thermofield double state associated with the Hamiltonian is prepared. This means preparing a special entangled state of two copies of the physical system, the left, and right systems. At infinite-temperature, the thermofield double state comprises a collection of Bell pairs between left and right (or the appropriate fermionic version).

Second, the system is effectively evolved forward and backward in time with the system Hamiltonian. With a fully controlled fault-tolerant quantum computer, it would be more straightforward to implement backward time evolution than forward time evolution. However, implementing forward and backward time evolution in a specialized quantum simulator (QSim) requires specific capabilities. In the context of measurements of out-of-time-order correlators (OTOCs), various techniques have been developed to achieve this level of control, at least approximately.

Third, the weak left-right coupling of the system given by the velocity operator must be applied. The coupling must be applied suddenly, in between the other time-evolution segments of the circuit. Fourth, local control operations are applied to delete and insert qubits, perform local unitary operations, and make local measurements on a general basis. This requires some degree of individual qubit addressability, although in the simplest cases only a small number of qubits need to be targeted. With these capabilities, in principle, the holographic protocols for state transfer and operator transfer outlined in the research can be realized. Two such quantum hardware platforms are Rydberg atom arrays and trapped ions.

#### 4.3.4.1 *Rydberg atom arrays*

One of the most obvious platforms for implementing holographic teleportation protocols for information transfer is Rydberg atom arrays. Rydberg atom arrays are a useful experimental formulation that that involves atoms (often alkali metals) in a highly excited state (the Rydberg state). The excited state tiers are several orders of magnitude larger than the atomic ground state (i.e. the electron is far from the nucleus), have long decay periods, and indicate an exaggerated response to electric and magnetic fields. These properties make Rydberg atom arrays an experimental model that is easy to deploy for the study of strong interactions and other quantum phenomena.

In a test implementation of the holographic teleportation protocols, information is encoded in a pair of levels in 87Rb (a ground state and a Rydberg state) such that the effective Hamiltonian can be written in a spin-chain form (Bernien *et al.*, 2017). An infinite-temperature thermofield double state (i.e. Bell pairs) has been achieved using Rydberg atoms (Levine *et al.*, 2019). Approximate methods might be similarly applied for finite-temperatures. The needed left-right coupling is feasible in a

Rydberg system, and used to prepare the Bell states. The backward time evolution can be engineered in different ways. One possibility is to work in the blockade regime, in which effective dynamics take place in a constrained Hilbert space. The parameters can be reversed with echo pulse sequences as the mechanism for forward and backward time evolution.

An interesting system to consider is a Floquet version of the Rydberg Hamiltonian known as the kicked quantum Ising model. The kicked model is appealing because the infinite-temperature thermofield double state is easier to prepare and because it allows easier control of the system time evolution. Although experiments are restricted to infinite-temperature (due to heating), the model is interesting because it can enhance chaos and offer more exact backward and forward time evolution. For example, to study chaotic systems, the entanglement entropy of subsystems grows as rapidly as possible when starting from a product state (Bertini *et al.*, 2019). The hyperfine encoding for qubits (in the Floquet model as opposed to using the Rydberg level directly) is likewise useful for gate-like time dynamics (Levine *et al.*, 2019).

#### 4.3.4.2 *Trapped ions*

Rydberg atom arrays have a natural spatial structure to their interactions, but other systems can also be considered that support few-body but geometrically nonlocal interactions. One such system is an ion trap quantum processor (Wright *et al.*, 2019). By directing the vibrational modes of an ionic crystal, it is possible to engineer a rich pattern of all-to-all interactions. Such systems are interesting because they mimic the structure of the SYK model and other matrix models that exhibit low-energy dynamics governed by a simple gravitational effective theory. Analog or digital versions of the platform can be considered. A small-scale preparation of approximate thermofield double states on a digital ion trap quantum processor has been demonstrated (Zhu *et al.*, 2019).

## 4.4 Black Hole on a Chip

Pikulin and Franz (2017) propose the design for a superconducting chip to study black holes via the holographic correspondence. The work proceeds from the justification that the SYK model is a solvable boundary theory with which to study black holes (gravity) in the bulk (discussed in more detail in the next section). The SYK model is a calculable model of Majorana zero mode fermions with random infinite range interactions. Majorana fermions are a canonical model used to study strongly coupled matter particles (fermions). The work proposes one of the first physical implementations of the SYK model in a solid-state system (a superconducting chip), alongside other proposals to realize the SYK model in ultracold gases (Danshita *et al.*, 2017) and digital quantum simulations (Garcia-Alvarez *et al.*, 2017).

The research proposes using the Fu–Kane superconductor chip, a device designed specifically to study Majorana fermions (Fu & Kane, 2008). The superconductor chip orchestrates Majorana fermions into a two-dimensional state in a format that resembles a spinless superconductor, and that does not break time reversal symmetry. Junctions in the superconducting device provide a way to create, manipulate, and fuse Majorana bound states. The chip has three layers and a hole in the center. The bottom layer is a topological insulator such as Bismuth Selenium ($Bi_2Se_3$). The top layer is an ordinary superconductor, namely, Niobium (Nb with 41 electrons) or Lead (Pb with 82 electrons). Niobium is a superconductor of choice because it has a relatively high critical temperature (temperature at which it becomes superconducting) for a single element. The middle layer is a very thin interface between the insulator and the superconductor.

The chip structure is designed to host unpaired Majorana zero modes which create magnetic vortices in the shape of a lattice. Two-fermion interactions dominate, but four-fermion interactions are needed for the SYK model. To facilitate this, the interface superconductor is tuned to its neutrality point, at which the low-energy Hamiltonian is dominated by the four-fermion terms and a chiral symmetry suppresses the two-fermion terms. A further step is necessary to obtain the infinite range interactions that are also part of the SYK model. A hole is fabricated in the superconducting layer of the chip to pin the vortices. Effectively infinite-ranged interactions among the fermions are obtained by pinning the required number of Majorana zero modes to the same region of space. A superconducting phase is applied to induce the vortex pinning, binding the

Majorana zero modes to the hole. Pinning costs condensation energy, so the superconducting phase must be applied to pin the vortices because, otherwise, they prefer a lower-energy location such as a material impurity.

The superconducting device setup with the Majorana fermions pinned to the hole (threaded by magnetic flux quanta in the presence of disorder) allows the numerical calculation of the Majorana wavefunctions. Assuming that the constituent electrons interact via screened Coulomb potential, the four-fermion coupling constants between the Majorana zero modes can be calculated exactly. These are used as input data for the many-body Majorana Hamiltonian which is diagonalized numerically for $N$ up to 32. Other work likewise confirms numerical methods for the diagonalization of the SYK Hamiltonian for $N$ up to 32 on a desktop computer, and possibly $N$ up to 42 ($7 \times 6$ qubits in a two-dimensional lattice) on a supercomputer (Boixo *et al.*, 2018, p. 595). Quantum computing platforms might substantially expand the reach of such numerical analysis.

Several technical advances were necessary to make the method possible. One is the ability to tune the chemical potential in the chip to its neutrality point by applying the superconducting phase. Another is the controllable design feature of the size and shape of the hole in the superconducting chip. An irregular-shaped hole is required to obtain random trajectories in the zero mode wavefunctions (often termed "billiards" in chaos studies).

### 4.4.1 *Fast scramblers*

Black holes are fast scramblers (scrambling initial state information with maximum possible efficiency) and exhibit quantum chaos (seemingly random but deterministic ballistic-then-saturation growth eras). Therefore, one way to assess whether a quantum theory is a holographic dual of a black hole is to find that its dynamics exhibit fast scrambling and chaotic behavior. The standard way to check for scrambling is with OTOC functions. An OTOC allows the quantum chaotic behavior to be quantified. For black holes in Einstein gravity, scrambling is exponentially fast and the decay rate is given by the Lyapunov exponent. A corresponding calculation of the OTOC is expected for the SYK model in the large-$N$ limit. In the black hole on a chip setup, the system size is too small to show the expected Lyapunov exponent, but the OTOC decays rapidly to zero which is consistent with expected results.

## 4.5 QSims: The SYK Model and Beyond

### 4.5.1 *The SYK model*

QSims are another form of tabletop experiment that brings theoretical concepts into the practical setting. A key first-level objective in simulating quantum systems is implementing the SYK model as a known and solvable model of strongly interacting systems. The SYK model is also important because it is a simple model of a black hole and constitutes a minimal realization of the AdS/CFT duality. Thus, the SYK model is useful for exploring otherwise unreachable physics (black holes, strongly interacting systems, and high-temperature superconducting materials) in tabletop laboratory experiments.

In condensed matter physics and black hole physics, the SYK model is a mathematical framework proposed by Sachdev and Ye (1993) and expanded by Kitaev (2015). Definitionally, the SYK model is a model of strongly interacting quantum systems with random all-to-all couplings among $N$ Majorana fermions (a basic matter-based system) that is solvable in the large-$N$ limit. In mathematical implementation, the SYK model is a model of $Q$ spin-polarized fermions on $N$ sites, typically described by a Hamiltonian (the SYK Hamiltonian).

The SYK model is useful for studying a range of problems because it is solvable, and since many difficult quantum problems can be formulated in terms of the SYK model, including information scrambling problems, chaotic systems, black holes, and superconductors. For example, in the context of high-temperature superconductors (non-Fermi liquids with "strange metal" behavior), the SYK model is exactly solvable at large $N$ and exhibits an explicit non-Fermi liquid behavior with nonzero entropy density at vanishing temperature.

The SYK model shares important properties with black holes in that both are fast scrambling and maximally chaotic systems. A feature of the

SYK model is that for large $N$ and strong coupling, it is possible to sum the Feynman diagrams to obtain out-of-order-time correlation functions (among other properties). The results of this exercise suggest that the SYK model is maximally chaotic (having the same Lyapunov exponent as black holes in Einstein gravity). The property of being maximally chaotic, together with the emergence of an approximate conformal symmetry at low temperatures, indicates that the holographic dual of the SYK model is a theory of Einstein gravity (Polchinski & Rosenhaus, 2016).

The SYK model is a minimal configuration of the AdS/CFT correspondence and can be applied in either direction to calculate unknown aspects of a quantum system (Table 4.4). In the bulk-to-boundary application, the holographic SYK model can be used to calculate attributes of an unknown quantum field theory of an exotic superconducting material on the boundary from a known bulk theory of classical gravity, for example, to study non-Fermi liquids (high-temperature superconductors) (Luo *et al.*, 2019). In the boundary-to-bulk application, the holographic SYK model takes a known condensed matter field theory on the boundary to calculate an unknown bulk gravity, for example, beyond classical gravity toward a theory of quantum gravity (Gross & Rosenhaus, 2017).

There are two reasons why the SYK model is attractive to the study of quantum gravity. First, in the long-distance (IR) bulk, the SYK model is nearly conformally invariant (resistant to small conformal changes) and also nearly diffeomorphism invariant (even more strongly resistant to certain local changes). Second, the SYK model has the same Lyapunov exponent as a black hole. These two features suggest the existence of a gravitational dual in $AdS_2$ (the discrete model of the correspondence with a one-dimensional CFT and two-dimensional bulk). However, the nature of the bulk dual is largely unknown, except that it likely contains $AdS_2$ dilaton gravity (a simplified form of gravity based on a hypothetical

Table 4.4. Bulk-boundary: Holographic SYK model.

| No. | Direction | Known | Unknown |
|---|---|---|---|
| 1 | Boundary-to-bulk | Condensed matter field theory | Quantum gravity |
| 2 | Bulk-to-boundary | Classical gravity | Non-Fermi liquids |

particle (dilaton)) (Almheiri & Polchinski, 2015). The solvability of SYK at large $N$, in principle, provides the ability to derive the bulk specification directly. Gross and Rosenhaus (2017) provide a systematic construction of the bulk dual to the SYK model framed as a $0 + 1$ dimensional theory of a large number of Majorana fermions with random interaction. The program involves solving the SYK model at large $N$ (in the $1/N$ expansion), analyzing the two-, four-, and six-point functions of the fermions, and extracting the resulting operators to determine the mass of bulk fields and their cubic couplings. The resulting bulk structure of fields and couplings is a start toward a theory of quantum gravity and can be applied to a variety of bulk-boundary analysis problems.

### 4.5.2 *Tabletop platforms for quantum simulation*

A first group of tabletop platforms for quantum simulation involves simulating lattice gauge theories and the SYK model with ultracold atomic platforms and does not use quantum computing (Table 4.5). First is a proposal for modeling inaccessible high-energy physics problems (lattice gauge theories) with low-energy models such as ultracold atoms in an optical lattice (Zohar *et al.*, 2016). Second is a similar setup with ultracold

Table 4.5. Tabletop platforms: SYK model and beyond.

| No. | Description | What Is Modeled | Hardware Platform |
|---|---|---|---|
| *Nonquantum computing methods* | | | |
| 1 | High-energy system simulation | Lattice gauge theories | Ultracold atoms |
| 2 | SYK study of black holes | SYK | Ultracold gases |
| 3 | Black hole on a chip | SYK | Superconducting chip |
| *Quantum computing methods* | | | |
| 4 | SYK digital quantum simulation | SYK | Trapped ions, circuits |
| 5 | Error-corrected SYK model | SYK | Post-NISQ devices |
| 6 | Quantum gravity in the lab | SYK and wormholes | Rydberg, trapped ions |
| 7 | SYK experimental demonstration | SYK | 4-qubit NMR |
| 8 | Ryu-Takayanagi formula simulation | Entanglement entropy | 6-qubit NMR |
| 9 | Scrambling Hamiltonian, chaos | Information scrambling | Rydberg, trapped ions |

gases in an optical lattice to implement the SYK model (Danshita *et al.*, 2017). Third is the black hole on a chip project as a physical realization of the SYK model in a solid-state system (Pikulin & Franz, 2017).

A second group of tabletop platforms for quantum simulation relies on quantum computing setups, implementing various methods for simulating the SYK model and beyond. The fourth project is a protocol for the quantum digital simulation of the SYK model in either a trapped ion or superconducting circuit platform Garcia-Alvarez *et al.* (2017). Fifth is a quantum algorithm that features state preparation oracles and lower gate complexity and is conducive to post-NISQ device (error correction) implementation (Babbush *et al.*, 2019). NISQ (noisy intermediate-scale quantum) devices are currently available quantum computers that do not require error correction. Sixth is the proposal to study quantum gravity in the laboratory by creating quantum systems with wormhole-like behavior (Brown *et al.*, 2019).

Two projects employ nuclear magnetic resonance (NMR) quantum computing for real-life demonstrations. One is an SYK model with $N = 8$ Majorana fermions using a 4-qubit NMR QSim to study non-Fermi liquids (high-temperature superconductors) (Luo *et al.*, 2019). The team extends the work using a 6-qubit NMR QSim to calculate the Ryu–Takayanagi formula for bulk-boundary entanglement entropy as a key result of the AdS/CFT correspondence (Li *et al.*, 2019).

Finally, QSims are extending into new territory beyond SYK model implementations to establish other exactly solvable canonical models. For example, since black holes and the SYK model are known to be fast scramblers, it might be possible to write an information-theoretic simplification of this relationship. Such a simplification is proposed by rewriting the Hamiltonian (from the usual SYK Hamiltonian to a scrambling Hamiltonian) to more expediently calculate information scrambling (the spread of information across a system) in quantum systems (Belyansky *et al.*, 2020). Fast scrambling is a property of black holes, chaotic systems, and other quantum problems. The scrambling Hamiltonian can be realized experimentally with QSims such as the dressed (nonfree floating) Rydberg states of neutral atoms, cavity-QED (quantum electrodynamics) setups, coupled chains of superconducting qubits, and trapped ions. These and other projects are elaborated in greater detail in what follows.

### 4.5.3 *Simulation with ultracold gases*

#### 4.5.3.1 *Large-scale and small-scale physics*

One of the first quantum simulations proposals is to simulate high-energy physics with a low-energy, nonrelativistic, many-body system (ultracold atoms) (Zohar *et al.*, 2016). This is surprising as it would not seem that the two kinds of systems have much in common particularly given their scale differences. Understanding this in context, the Standard Model of particle physics is the theory that describes elementary particles and three of the four fundamental forces in the universe (electromagnetic, weak, and strong interactions), but not the gravitational force. The Standard Model has been tested extensively in the context of both large-scale and small-scale physics. An extraordinary range of experimental results from cosmological observations and particle accelerators has measured both high-energy scales up to $10^{12}$ eV (electron Volts) and low-energy scales down to $10^{-7}$ eV (a range of nineteen orders of magnitude) (Table 4.6).

Besides the energy scale, there are also other differences between large-scale and small-scale physical systems in the formal structure and the underlying physical principles that govern them. On the one hand, the physics of high-energy phenomena is relativistic, with dynamical structure and constrained symmetries (local gauge invariance and Lorentz invariance). On the other hand, low-energy systems such as ultracold atoms are nonrelativistic, with less dynamical structure (per conserved quantities) and also without constrained symmetry (systems manifest

Table 4.6. Physics: Nineteen orders of magnitude.

| System | Energy Scale | Structure | Physical Principles |
|---|---|---|---|
| High-energy physics (field theories) | $10^{12}$ eV | Relativistic | Dynamical structure, constrained symmetries: Local gauge invariance, Lorentz invariance |
| Low-energy systems (ultracold atoms) | $10^{-7}$ eV | Nonrelativistic | Causal spacetime, charge conservation, no local gauge invariance, no Lorentz invariance |

neither local gauge invariance nor Lorentz invariance). Among other effects, this leads to a causal spacetime structure and charge conservation laws (seen as long-range interactions in QED and quark confinement in QCD).

The point is that it is not obvious that the two domains could come together and that high-energy field theories might be simulated by the physics of ultra-low-energy systems. What is new is the possibility of configuring an atomic system there are ways to configure an atomic system to manifest both local gauge invariance and Lorentz invariance. Specifically, local gauge invariance can arise either as an effective, low-energy symmetry, or as an exact symmetry, following from the conservation laws in atomic interactions. Hence, Zohar *et al.* (2016) suggest that it is possible for high-energy physics to be simulated by low-energy, non-relativistic, many-body systems such as ultracold atoms.

### 4.5.3.2 *Ultracold atoms in optical lattices*

The team investigates quantum simulations of lattice gauge theories using ultracold atoms (via the Hamiltonian formulation of lattice gauge theories). A quantum simulation of abelian and nonabelian lattice gauge theories in $1 + 1$ and $2 + 1$ dimensions is constructed using ultracold atoms in optical lattices. The result is the possibility that QSims and cold atoms tabletop experiments could become standard for studying high-energy physics phenomena such as the confinement of dynamical quarks, phase transitions, and other strong force effects in quantum chromodynamics (QCD), which are inaccessible using other methods, both experimentally and computationally.

Three requirements are identified for simulating a gauge theory. First, the theory must contain both fermions and bosons. The fermions represent matter fields and the bosons represent gauge fields. Ultracold atoms are a good candidate for a simulation platform since bosonic and fermionic atoms are freely available in these systems. Second, ultimately, the theory must be Lorentz invariant (holding in any inertial frame). This might be problematic, but the lattice gauge theories can be simulated to obtain this symmetry in the continuum limit, which is manageable with the structure of optical lattices as the simulating systems. Third, the theory must have local gauge invariance, which is the symmetry responsible for gauge-matter interactions. This is the most problematic aspect since local gauge invariance is not a fundamental symmetry in cold atom systems. To achieve gauge invariant interactions which are not fundamental to ultracold atoms, two methods are applied to obtain effective symmetry and exact symmetry. The effective symmetry method imposes gauge invariance as a constraint in that the gauge invariance is constrained to be an emerging, low-energy symmetry. The exact symmetry method maps gauge invariance into a fundamental symmetry of the atoms, per the laws of conservation of hyperfine angular momentum in atomic collisions.

#### 4.5.3.3 *Black hole in a tabletop gas*

One of the first implementations of the SYK model was proposed by Danshita *et al.* (2017). The work uses an SYK-based model to produce black hole-like conditions in an experimental setting with ultracold gases for the potential study of quantum gravity. The work relies on the idea that quantum gravity can be studied in optical-lattice systems loaded with ultracold gases by using the holographic principle. The SYK model is considered as a specific example, as it consists of spin-polarized fermions with all-to-all random connectivity, and its low-temperature state has been conjectured to be dual to an $AdS_2$ black hole as the quantum gravitational system (Sachdev, 2010). The work introduces a variant of the SYK model (that is equivalent to the original SYK model in the large-$N$ limit) and can, in principle, be created by confining ultracold fermionic atoms into optical lattices and coupling two atoms with molecular states via photo-association lasers (Table 4.7).

The SYK model is represented as a model of $Q$ spin-polarized fermions on $N$ sites given by a Hamiltonian. Calculating the physical

Table 4.7. Bulk-boundary: Black hole in a gas.

| No. | Bulk | Boundary | Reference |
|---|---|---|---|
| 1 | $AdS_2$ black hole | SYK Model: Spin-polarized fermions with an all-to-all random connectivity | Sachdev (2010) |
| 2 | Quantum gravitational system | Optical-lattice systems loaded with ultracold gases | Danshita *et al.* (2017) |

observables of the system is possible by measuring the OTOC functions and the single-particle Green's function, which characterize the properties of the black hole, by the use of a control qubit consisting of an atom in a double well. The proposal is incomplete due to practical difficulties in realizing the model with then-current experimental technology (including related to the fact that particles on lattice systems tend to move the most dominantly in nearest-neighbor interactions). However, the importance of the proposal is in articulating some of the first steps toward the experimental realization of the SYK model, and hence laboratory systems dual to black holes.

### 4.5.4 *Simulation with quantum computing*

#### 4.5.4.1 *SYK simulation with ion traps and circuits*

Transitioning quantum simulation efforts onto the quantum computing platform, one of the first efforts is defining a protocol for the digital quantum simulation of the SYK model (Garcia-Alvarez *et al.*, 2017). The aim is to reproduce a simplified low-dimensional model of quantum gravity in available quantum platforms such as trapped ions and superconducting circuits. The proposal calls for simulating the AdS/CFT correspondence with the simplest quenched-disorder SYK model (an SYK model with a quenched-disorder Hamiltonian). Both Majorana fermions and complex fermions can be studied, by solving the model for Majorana fermions at finite $N$, or for complex fermions in the large-$N$ limit. The quantum algorithm can be implemented with ion traps or superconducting circuits. Either platform can implement the quantum algorithm design based on the multiqubit Molmer-Sorensen gate (which implements the exponentials of tensor products of Pauli matrices). A method is also given for probing nonequilibrium dynamics with OTOC functions and information scrambling.

In the same area of research, Babbush *et al.* (2019) suggest a more scalable algorithm for the simulation of the SYK model with quantum platforms. Gate complexity is reduced by using a new method for encoding the Hamiltonian with state preparation oracles and random quantum circuits. The algorithm anticipates post-NISQ devices by being conducive to application with known error-correcting codes (surface codes) and possibly accommodating larger-scale ($N > 100$) SYK model quantum simulations (a size thought to be intractable on NISQ devices).

#### 4.5.4.2 *Demonstrations with NMR QSims*

Some of the earliest real-life demonstrations of tabletop SYK model implementations are achieved with the NMR platform. A generalized SYK model with $N = 8$ Majorana fermions using a 4-qubit NMR QSim is realized by Luo *et al.* (2019). The NMR platform is selected as it is one of the most fully controllable quantum systems. Well-characterized qubits can be produced with long decoherence times, and there is fine control over the nuclear spins through radio-frequency fields. This enables the ability to simulate the dynamics of a generalized SYK model. The aim of the research is using the SYK model to study non-Fermi liquids (such as high-temperature superconductors). So far, the quantum simulation of non-Fermi-liquid states in strongly interacting systems has not been possible.

The experimental realization of the SYK model is challenging because it is difficult to simulate the Hamiltonian which has strong randomness and fully nonlocal fermion interactions. How to initialize the simulated system into specific states at different temperatures and measure the related dynamical properties is also unclear. A QSim with individual and high-fidelity controllability is key, and ideally, the simulation process should be easy to manipulate digitally.

The SYK model describes a strongly interacting quantum system with random all-to-all couplings among $N$ Majorana fermions. At large $N$, the model is exactly solvable and exhibits an explicit non-Fermi liquid behavior with a nonzero entropy density at vanishing temperature. Non-Fermi liquids ("strange metals" or anomalous matter phases) are systems in which Fermi liquid behavior breaks down, meaning systems that deviate from resistivity at low temperatures, which suggests that more exotic physics is taking place. In condensed matter physics, one of the most well-known (yet poorly understood) non-Fermi liquids is the "strange metal" phase of high-temperature superconductors (such as in cuprates (high-temperature ceramic superconductors) with optimal doping). In these systems, the resistivity scales linearly with the temperature for a large range of their behavior. The strange metal phase can be viewed as the parent state of high-temperature superconductors, in contrast to the role of the Fermi liquid in ordinary superconductors. Non-Fermi liquids are a research frontier and other work has constructed non-Fermi liquid states based on SYK physics, with potential application to condensed matter systems (Patel *et al.*, 2018). QSims for the SYK model could greatly extend research in this area.

The quantum simulation of the SYK model is demonstrated on a nuclear-spin-chain simulator. The observed results include the fermion pairing instability of the non-Fermi liquid state and the chaotic-nonchaotic transition at simulated temperatures, as predicted in previous theories. The experiment highlights the first steps toward the quantum simulation of non-Fermi-liquid states in strongly interacting systems. As the realization of the SYK model in practice, the results provide a new direction in the investigation of other key features of non-Fermi liquid states, as well as quantum chaotic systems and the AdS/CFT duality.

A further aspect of the work is the use of machine learning for system control. Such ML/Quantum Simulation applications, the application of machine learning to quantum simulation, could become a standard digital toolkit method. The scalability of control techniques is an obstacle when performing higher-dimensional digital quantum simulations. Earlier work from the team proposes a method that utilizes the power of quantum processors together with machine learning techniques to enhance quantum control (Lu *et al.*, 2017). Specifically, this is in the form of a quantum processor optimizing its own control sequence by using measurement-based feedback control. The method is efficient in the sense that it requires polynomial time for optimization with the number of qubits. Improvement of control fidelities has been demonstrated on a 12-qubit system. The machine learning control method can be scaled up to many qubit systems, and thus might underpin future quantum simulation tasks involving SYK models of greater complexity as well as other models.

#### 4.5.4.3 *Ryu–Takayanagi entanglement entropy simulation*

Extending the work to quantum gravity-type problems, the team announces the simulation of entanglement entropy using a 6-qubit NMR QSim (Li *et al.*, 2019). A key result of the AdS/CFT correspondence, the

Ryu-Takayanagi formula for bulk-boundary entanglement entropy, is demonstrated by measuring relevant entanglement entropies on a perfect tensor state. The fidelity of the experimentally prepared 6-qubit state is 85.0% via full state tomography and reaches 93.7% if the signal-decay due to decoherence is taken into account. The experiment could serve as a core module in the simulation of more complex tensor network states to examine the holographic correspondence. As one of the early experimental attempts to study AdS/CFT via quantum information processing, the work could open up new directions for investigating quantum gravity phenomena on QSims. The research is an example of AdS/TN/QSim: AdS with tensor networks implemented on a quantum simulator.

#### 4.5.4.4 *Scrambling Hamiltonian*

Extending this research trajectory, Belyansky *et al.* (2020) propose a simpler-than-SYK model as a generic technology to generate Hamiltonians for the characterization and study of a quantum system's dynamics. The underlying need is to establish a greater range of exactly solvable models for quantum problems. The premise is that it is now possible to simulate fast scrambling using QSims without having to rely on the SYK setup (with its nontrivial SYK Hamiltonian) and that a simplified model can be used. Fast scrambling (the spread of quantum information across a system) is a signature of black holes, chaotic systems, and other complex quantum many-body problems of interest. The idea is that although complicated quantum systems (such as high-temperature superconductors) can be formulated as an SYK problem (solvable with some effort), instead they might be cast as an information scrambling problem (more easily solvable). Whereas the SYK model sees condensed matter systems (through the holographic correspondence) as having black hole-like properties (solvable), the fast-scrambling model sees quantum systems (including condensed matter systems) as having information-theoretic properties (more easily solvable). The advance is one of quantum information theory.

More specifically, scrambling refers to the spread of an initially local quantum information over the many-body degrees of freedom of the entire system, rendering it inaccessible to local measurements. Scrambling is also related to the Heisenberg dynamics of local operators and can be probed via the squared commutator of two local, commuting, unitary, and Hermitian operators. One operator grows so fast that it eventually fails to commute with the other. The formalism produces two exactly solvable models. One comprises a random circuit with Haar random local unitaries and a global interaction, and the other is a classical model of globally coupled nonlinear oscillators. Numerical analysis provides further evidence of the relationship by studying the time evolution of an OTOC and the entanglement entropy in spin chains of intermediate sizes.

The streamlined scrambling Hamiltonian can be realized experimentally in a variety of state-of-the-art QSims. The most natural setup is with the Rydberg dressing (holding in place) of neutral atoms. The spin can be encoded in two ground states with one ground state dressed to two Rydberg states such that one of the Rydberg states leads to all-to-all interactions and the other produces nearest-neighbor interactions. Other similar spin models can be implemented with cavity-QED setups, using photon-mediated all-to-all interactions of the Heisenberg form together with nearest-neighbor interactions achieved by Rydberg dressing one of the ground states. The resulting Hamiltonian differs on the basis of the local interactions but leads to qualitatively similar information scrambling. Other possibilities include a chain of coupled superconducting qubits (with all-to-all flip-flop interactions mediated via a common bus) and trapped ions.

## References

Almheiri, A. & Polchinski, J. (2015). Models of $AdS_2$ backreaction and holography. *J. High Energ. Phys.* 1511:014.

Babbush, R., Berry, D.W. & Neven, H. (2019). Quantum simulation of the Sachdev-Ye-Kitaev model by asymmetric qubitization. arXiv:1806.02793v2.

Belyansky, R., Bienias, P., Kharko, Y.A. *et al.* (2020). A minimal model for fast scrambling. *Phys. Rev. Lett.* 125(13):130601.

Bernien, H., Schwartz, S., Keesling, A. *et al.* (2017). Probing many-body dynamics on a 51-atom quantum simulator. *Nature.* 551:579–84.

Bertini, B., Kos, P. & Prosen, T. (2019). Entanglement spreading in a minimal model of maximal many-body quantum chaos. *Phys. Rev. X.* 9(2):021033.

Boixo, S., Isakov, S.V., Smelyanskiy, V.N. *et al.* (2018). Characterizing quantum supremacy in near-term devices. *Nat. Phys.* 14:595–600.

Brown, A.R., Gharibyan, H., Leichenauer, S. *et al.* (2019). Quantum gravity in the lab: Teleportation by size and traversable wormholes. aXiv:1911.06314v1.

Carroll, S. (2007). *Dark Matter, Dark Energy: The Dark Side of the Universe.* Pasadena, CA: The Teaching Company.

Cottrell, W., Freivogel, B., Hofman, D.M. & Lokhande, S.F. (2019). How to build the thermofield double state. *J. High Energ. Phys.* 1902:058.

Danshita, I., Hanada, M. & Tezuka, M. (2017). Creating and probing the Sachdev-Ye-Kitaev model with ultracold gases: Towards experimental studies of quantum gravity. *Prog. Theor. Exp. Phys.* 17(83):083I01.

Freitas, R.A. Jr. (2012). Welcome to the future of medicine. Transhumanism and personal identity. In *The Transhumanist Reader.* Eds. More, M. & Vita-More, N. Oxford: Wiley-Blackwell, pp. 67–72.

Fu, L. & Kane, C.L. (2008). Superconducting proximity effect and Majorana fermions at the surface of a topological insulator. *Phys. Rev. Lett.* 100(9): 096407.

Garcia-Alvarez, L., Egusquiza, I.L., Lamata, L. *et al.* (2017). Digital quantum simulation of minimal AdS/CFT. *Phys. Rev. Lett.* 119(4):040501.

Gross, D.J. & Rosenhaus, V. (2017). The bulk dual of SYK: Cubic couplings. *J. High Energ. Phys.* 1705:092.

Hughes, T.W. *et al.* (2018). On-chip laser-power delivery system for dielectric laser accelerators. *Phys. Rev. Appl.* 9(5):054017.

Kitaev, A. (2015). A simple model of quantum holography. KITP strings seminar and entanglement 2015 program. http://online.kitp.ucsb.edu/online/entangled15/. Accessed March 15, 2021.

Levine, H., Keesling, A., Semeghini, G. *et al.* (2019). Parallel implementation of high-fidelity multiqubit gates with neutral atoms. *Phys. Rev. Lett.* 123(17): 170503.

Li, K., Han, M., Qu, D., *et al.* (2019). Measuring holographic entanglement entropy on a quantum simulator. *NPJ Quantum Inf.* 5(30):1–6.

Lu, D., Li., K., Li, J. *et al.* (2017). Enhancing quantum control by bootstrapping a quantum processor of 12 qubits. *NPJ Quantum Inf.* 3(45):1–7.

Luo, Z., You, Y.-Z., Li, J. *et al.* (2019). Quantum simulation of the non-Fermi-liquid state of Sachdev-Ye-Kitaev model. arXiv:1712.06458v2.

Newton, I. (1729, 1687). In [experimental] philosophy particular propositions are inferred from the phenomena and afterwards rendered general by induction. *Principia.* Book 3. *General Scholium. Trans. A. Motte.* Vol 2. p. 392.

Patel, A.A., McGreevy, J., Arovas, D.P. & Sachdev, S. (2018). Magnetotransport in a model of a disordered strange metal. *Phys. Rev. X.* 8(2):021049.

Pikulin, D.I. & Franz, M. (2017). Black hole on a chip: Proposal for a physical realization of the Sachdev-Ye-Kitaev model in a solid-state system. *Phys. Rev. X.* 7(3):031006.

Polchinski, J. & Rosenhaus, V. (2016). The spectrum in the Sachdev-Ye-Kitaev model. *J. High Energ. Phys.* 1604:001.

Preskill, J. (2020). Spotting quantum black holes in the lab. *Quanta.* https://www.quantamagazine.org/john-preskill-quantum-computing-may-help-us-study-quantum-gravity-20200715/.

Sachdev, S. & Ye, J. (1993). Gapless spin-fluid ground state in a random quantum Heisenberg magnet. *Phys. Rev. Lett.* 70:3339–42.

Sachdev, S. (2010). Strange metals and the AdS/CFT correspondence. *J. Stat. Mech.* 1011:P11022.

Sapra, N.V., Yang, K.Y., Vercruysse, D. *et al.* (2020). On-chip integrated laser-driven particle accelerator. *Science.* 367(6473):79–83.

Wootton, K., McNeur, J. & Leedle, K. (2016). Dielectric laser accelerators: Designs, experiments, and applications. In *Reviews of Accelerator Science and Technology: Vol. 9: Technology and Applications of Advanced Accelerator Concepts*. London: World Scientific, pp. 105–26.

Wright, K., Beck, K.M., Debnath, S. *et al.* (2019). Benchmarking an 11-qubit quantum computer. arXiv:1903.08181.

Zhu, D., Johri, S., Linke, N.M. *et al.* (2019). Variational generation of thermofield double states and critical ground states with a quantum computer. arXiv: 1906.02699.

Zohar, E., Cirac, J.I. & Reznik, B. (2016). Quantum simulations of lattice gauge theories using ultracold atoms in optical lattices. *Rep. Prog. Phys.* 79(1):014401.

# Chapter 5

# Neuronal Gauge Theory

*It is only slightly overstating the case to say that physics is the study of symmetry*

— Nobel Physicist, Anderson (1972, p. 394)

**Abstract**

This chapter studies symmetry, the property that systems look the same from different points of view (whether a face, a cube, or the laws of nature), and symmetry breaking (phase transition). A neuronal gauge theory interprets the brain as a multiscalar system with a global symmetry (invariant property). In the process of neural signaling, the global symmetry is maintained by the application of gauge fields with energy minimization as the gauge-invariant property of the brain system.

## 5.1 Concept of the Neuronal Gauge Theory

The laws of nature originate in symmetries, and much of foundational physics is based in symmetries and symmetry breaking. For example, the understanding of symmetry breaking in superconductivity helped to facilitate the quantum computational advance of the Josephson junction (to manage quantum interference and make use of quantum tunneling) (Anderson, 1972, p. 396). Likewise, an enumeration of relevant symmetry breaking behavior in living things (such as the brain) might be crucial to understanding these domains (*Ibid.*, p. 395).

The concept of the neuronal gauge theory for modeling the brain is proposed by the Friston laboratory (Sengupta *et al.*, 2016). The work is an application of previous research regarding the free energy principle which argues that any self-organizing system that is at equilibrium with its environment must be minimizing its free energy (Friston *et al.*, 2006). The free energy principle takes the form of a predictive mechanism about the steady state and the free energy needed to maintain an organism, and is thought to be greatly conserved across types of organisms. Energy minimization is a model widely used in fields ranging from materials analysis to deep learning. Typically, the problem is framed as the analysis of how a dynamic system finds the shortest path to the lowest-energy configuration of the system. A notable model for energy minimization computations is the spin glass (a disordered ferromagnet), and in the sense that both systems minimize energy, the brain is like a spin glass.

These ideas are developed in the proposal for a neuronal gauge theory in which the gauge invariance (nonchanging property of a system) is the principle of variational free energy minimization (Sengupta *et al.*, 2016). A gauge theory is a theory specifying that certain global properties of a physical system do not change as a result of local transformations (changes). For example, a ball can be tossed around a room and have different locations (local transformations), while the laws of gravitation (global symmetries) always hold. The gauge invariance is the laws of gravity as an overall system property. Many powerful theories in physics are described by gauge invariance or system dynamics that are invariant under certain kinds of local transformations. The brain as a system presumably remains invariant under different kinds of local transformations, and might be explained by a neuronal gauge theory. In the specific neuronal gauge theory proposed by Sengupta *et al.* (2016), the overarching principle that does not change (gauge invariance) is free energy minimization and the local transformations are the stimulus received by system elements such as stochastic fluctuations in the brain due to thermal energy, ion channel chattering, and irregular synaptic input from other neurons (Table 5.1).

Table 5.1. Neuronal gauge theory.

| | Local Transformation | Global Invariance |
|---|---|---|
| A ball in a room | Different locations | Laws of gravitation |
| Neuronal gauge theory | System element stimulus | Free energy minimization |

The problem domain is the specification of the bulk properties of the brain. The aim of the neuronal gauge theory is to serve as a general principle for neuronal dynamics that holds at various timescales (for example, evolutionary, developmental, and perceptual timescales). The gauge theory as posed centers around an energy minimization principle arguing that energy minimization extends to any biological system (whether neuron, brain, or body) as the operation of an organism resolving uncertainty about its external milieu, either by changing its internal states or its relationship to the environment.

The empirical demands of neuroimaging and optogenetics have forced the need to characterize the relationship between the activity of neurons and their system-level behavior. These technical innovations call for theories that describe neuronal interactions and reveal the underlying principles of the brain. A gauge-theoretic formalism in neuroscience might provide a quantitative framework for modeling neural activity and also show that neuronal dynamics across scales (from single neurons to population activity) can be described by the same principle.

### 5.1.1 *Gauge theory*

A gauge theory formalism is naturally suggested as a physics-based approach to the brain as a physical system. A central organizing principle of the universe and physical systems in general is thought to be gauge theories which describe overarching properties (symmetries) that are invariant irrespective of scale. Gauge theories arose to understand classical electromagnetism and general relativity together in the context of the gauge symmetries that appear in the relativistic quantum mechanics of electrons (quantum electrodynamics). Electrons are controlled by both spin and charge, which necessitates a formulation such as a gauge theory (with symmetry-type principles) to explain their behavior (Griffiths, 1995, p. 175). Such gauge theories are widely applied in condensed matter physics, high energy physics, and other fields.

General relativity, electromagnetism, and quantum field theory can be consolidated within the framework of gauge theory (O'Raifeartaigh & Straumann, 2000). The AdS/CFT correspondence likewise formulates gravity as being equal to gauge theory in one less dimension (Maldacena, 1998). Gauge-theoretic formalisms highlight the fact that both general relativity and quantum mechanics are based on fields (gravitational fields and quantum fields) which can be analyzed together mathematically as matrices. The centrality of gauge theory as a physical theory of the universe and its possibility of uniting large-scale and small-scale systems (such as general relativity and quantum mechanics) suggests the utility of gauge-theoretic approaches to neural dynamics.

#### 5.1.1.1 *The principle of variational free energy*

Neuronal gauge theories might be specified on the basis of various properties of invariance. For Sengupta *et al.* (2016), the variational free energy principle is a good candidate as a central invariance principle. Minimizing variational free energy indicates that every aspect of the brain (from neuronal signaling to synaptic connection strengths, as well as higher-order behavior) can be described as a process that minimizes variational free energy. Variational free energy is a measure of the approximate amount energy available in a system. In the neural context, variational free energy is a measure of the probability of receiving certain sensory inputs and stimulus, based on the brain's indirect model of how these inputs are caused (Friston *et al.*, 2006). The "variational" aspect of variational free energy is due to its derivation from variational calculus. Variational calculus is using small changes in functions to find minima and maxima such as geodesics (the shortest length curve connecting two points), and features heavily in information theory.

In the simplest formulation, variational free energy reduces to prediction error in the same way that estimating the parameters of a statistical model can be reduced to minimizing the sum of squared error. Variational free energy's statistical model therefore suggests a machine learning implementation (which is also based on error minimization). When physical laws such as Hamilton's principle of least action are applied to variational free energy, the resulting behavior is statistical inference, giving the brain (or any self-organizing system) the characteristics of a system trying to estimate or infer the causes of its sensory exchanges with the world.

Minimizing variational free energy is a statistical data analysis technique, often used in Bayesian (iteratively updating) models. If the brain were shown to minimize variational free energy, it might be considered more formally as a Bayesian (self-updating) system. Such evidence could support the Bayesian brain hypothesis (that the brain updates itself in an ongoing manner) (Knill & Pouget, 2004). A Bayesian inference model of the brain, based on formulating the free energy principle as a neuronal gauge theory, might lead to new inference schemes for analyzing neuroscience data. Such methods might provide new ways for inferring the underlying structure in empirical data.

The aim of a neuronal gauge theory is to understand complex neural dynamics in simpler yet formal terms. For example, gauge theories are used to model complex weather patterns such as the Coriolis effect (curvilinear motion in a rotating frame of reference). A similar method could be applied to understanding the effects of inbound neural signals on postsynaptic responses as a necessary consequence of much simpler invariances or symmetries. In the Bayesian brain model, neuronal activity encodes representations (Bayesian beliefs) and the Lagrangian (variational free energy) is a probability distribution function. The gauge-theoretic perspective allows the specification of a structure of patterns or responses that is independent of the usual noise of stochastic fluctuations from thermal energy, ion channels, and synaptic communication. These latter are the local transformations and free energy minimization is the gauge invariance (unchanging property).

### 5.1.1.2 *Symmetry, gauge invariance, and the Lagrangian*

Symmetry, gauge invariance, and the Lagrangian are related ideas in physics. Symmetry and gauge invariance are used as synonyms and mean the unchanging overall system parameters in the face of small local changes.

The Lagrangian is a mathematical function describing the system's dynamics across local and global states that remain unchanged.

In everyday use, symmetry means balance, proportion, and evenness. In mathematics, symmetry has a more precise definition, and refers to an object that is invariant under some transformations including translation, reflection, rotation, or scaling. The two meanings are not at odds in that they both point to aspects of an object or system that are consistent or unchanging. Symmetry is a statement that something looks the same from different points of view, which could be a face, a cube, or the laws of nature (Weinberg, 1980) (Table 5.2).

Symmetry may be further classified as global or local. Symmetry is global if a system or theory is invariant under a transformation identically performed at every point in the spacetime in which the physical processes occur. Local symmetry is a stronger constraint and serves as a cornerstone of gauge theories. A local symmetry's group parameters are spacetime-independent whereas a global symmetry's group parameters are spacetime-dependent. In addition to being a property of objects, symmetry may be observed with respect to the passage of time, as a spatial relationship, through geometric transformations, through other kinds of functional transformations. Symmetry is also observed as a feature of abstract objects including theoretic models, language, and music. In physics, symmetry is synonymous with invariance (lack of change) under transformation. The concept has become one of the most powerful tools of theoretical physics, as it has become evident that practically all laws of nature originate in symmetries.

Symmetry, gauge invariance, and the Lagrangian are considered together in the overall frame of gauge theories. The terms symmetry and gauge invariance are used synonymously in physics. Symmetry (invariance) and gauge invariance are used to refer to the system property of a nonchanging Lagrangian (system dynamics function) under a group of

Table 5.2. Symmetry definition.

| No. | Use | Interpretation | Meaning |
|---|---|---|---|
| 1 | Everyday | Balance | Looking the same from different points of view |
| 2 | Physics | Invariance | |

local transformations. The Lagrangian is a system dynamics function, a function that describes the state of a dynamic system in terms of position coordinates and time derivatives, and potential energy and kinetic energy, and is invariant under local transformations. The overall frame is that of a gauge theory which is a field theory in which the Lagrangian (state of a dynamic system) does not change (is invariant) under local transformations (that are mathematically described by certain Lie groups). The Lie group is a widely used algebraic formulation of a continuous group in which spaces are combined, allowing all points in a space to be multiplied and divided.

The concept of gauge refers to a system being organized in discrete tiers. An analogy can be drawn to the twelve-gauge shotgun, which only accommodates bullets in its size tier. Similarly in physics, a gauge is a mathematical formalism that regulates scale tiers (as redundant degrees of freedom) in the system description, with the Lagrangian. A system may have various degrees of freedom, meaning parameters, the number of independent parameters required to characterize a system. The same system parameters (degrees of freedom) may be relevant to a system description at multiple tiers (for example, location is a reoccurring parameter). Analyzing a system as to which properties remain invariant across scale tiers requires some sort of renormalization to streamline redundant degrees of freedom, which is the operation of a gauge theory. Summarizing, the gauge theory is a field theory which the Lagrangian (system dynamics) does not change (is invariant) under local transformations. Definitions related to this cluster of terms are as follows:

- *Gauge*: A formalism rendering systems in discrete scale tiers.
- *Gauge bosons*: Force particles that are the quanta of gauge fields.
- *Gauge field*: A (vector) field generated by the Lie algebra that describes the gauge theory. Gauge fields are included in the Lagrangian to ensure its invariance under the local group transformations (gauge invariance).
- *Gauge group (symmetry group)*: Lie group (algebraic formulation) formed by all possible gauge transformations.
- *Gauge invariance*: Unchanging global property of a system. The system property of a nonchanging Lagrangian (system dynamics function) under local transformations.

- *Gauge theory*: A field theory in which the Lagrangian (state of a dynamic system) does not change (is invariant) under local transformations from certain Lie groups.
- *Gauge transformation*: Transformations between possible gauges (levels, degrees of freedom) in a system.
- *Lagrangian*: System dynamics function: a function that describes the state of a dynamical system in terms of position coordinates and time derivatives, and potential energy and kinetic energy, and is invariant under local transformations.
- *Lie group*: A continuous group combining regions of space by allowing all points in a space to be multiplied and divided.
- *Symmetry*: Balanced (everyday), invariance (physics); property of looking the same from different points of view (for example, a face, a cube, or the laws of nature).
- *Symmetry group*: (see gauge group).

## 5.2 Details of the Neuronal Gauge Theory

Gauge theories originate in physics but can be applied to many other fields, including biology to analyze cell structure, morphogenesis, and embryonic development. For example, a gauge-theoretic treatment has been used to study the self-organization of dendritic spines (Kiebel & Friston, 2011). Sengupta *et al.* (2016) posit a gauge theory for the central nervous system more generally to describe overall brain function. A gauge theory is a field theory, and the proposal for the brain-wide gauge-field theory is partially motivated by empirical evidence that visual perception is a field-based phenomenon (Zeki, 2005).

In a gauge theory, the Lagrangian (overall system dynamics) is invariant under continuous symmetry transformations. A gauge theory of the brain would therefore require a Lagrangian plus three elements, a system with symmetry, local forces applied to the system, and a gauge field(s) to compensate for the perturbations that are introduced by the local forces. In the neuronal gauge theory, the system with symmetry (invariant aspects across tiers) is the nervous system. The local forces or local transformations are sensory stimuli received by brain elements. The gauge fields are part of the brain environment and apply continuous forces to act on the brain elements to produce local perturbations that counteract the effect of the local force stimulus. The gauge theory is a mechanism that acts to constantly rebalance the system such that symmetry (gauge invariance) is maintained. The four aspects of interpreting the brain in a gauge-theoretic format are listed in Table 5.3. These include first having a system with conserved symmetry, second, there being local forces in the system, third having the structural aspect of gauge fields in the system, and finally, having a Lagrangian equation to describe the system's dynamics.

Simplifying, in the "ball in a room" example, local transformations are the location of the ball in the room and the system property that is invariant is the law of gravity. In the neuronal gauge theory, the local transformations are the stimulus from local forces received by the brain elements and the system property that is invariant is the Lagrangian (system dynamics). The Lagrangian is the focal object of analysis because it must maintain the gauge invariance of the system. A Lagrangian can be defined on the basis of the variational free energy minimization principle. Such a free energy Lagrangian has been specified previously to measure of aspects of functional brain architecture including hierarchical organization and the asymmetries between forward and backward connections in cortical hierarchies. By formal analogy with Lagrangian mechanics, the free energy of the system can be written as a function of time (Friston, 2008, p. 6), thus providing a description of neuronal dynamics.

## 5.2.1 *Rebalancing global symmetry*

The neuronal gauge theory sees a system immersed in its environment as an extended hierarchy. The gauge theory can be applied at various nested

Table 5.3. Neuronal gauge theory: Four elements.

| Element | Generic Gauge Theory | Neuronal Gauge Theory |
|---|---|---|
| Symmetry | System with conserved symmetry | Central nervous system |
| Local transformations | Local forces acting on the system | Sensory stimuli |
| Gauge field | Zone of invariance to local transformations | Counter-compensation for local perturbations |
| Lagrangian | System dynamics function | Free energy Lagrangian |

levels. At every scale tier (gauge), the Lagrangian is disturbed by local transformations (changes in forward or bottom-up sensory input), and compensatory adjustments must be made to keep the Lagrangian invariant (via backward or top-down messages) (Sengupta *et al.*, 2016, p. 7). Variational free energy reduces to prediction error in the statistical implementation (the same way that estimating the parameters of a statistical model can be reduced to minimizing the sum of squared error). In the variational free energy minimization context, the bottom-up or forward adjustment messages convey the prediction error from a lower hierarchical level to a higher level, and the backward or top-down messages are predictions of statistics in the level below. The predictions are produced to explain away prediction errors in the lower levels.

The gauge field is the enforcement mechanism of the Lagrangian in maintaining global symmetry (formalized by Lie algebra terms in the Lagrangian). The gauge field incorporates the prediction errors and other system information, and is applied to preserve global symmetry despite the perturbing action of local forces. The local forces are prediction errors that serve to increase variational free energy, thereby activating the gauge fields to reduce or minimize such growth in free energy, and explain away or eliminate the importance of the local transformations in the global symmetry calculation. The gauge fields are based on the fact that variational free energy is a scalar quantity determined by probability measures. The gauge theory is the rebalancing mechanism that preserves system symmetry (gauge invariance). In the free energy model, the consequence of the nervous system maintaining its Lagrangian is that energy (prediction error) is minimized across all scale tiers. This suggests that the complexities of multiscalar neural behavior might be modeled with a neuronal gauge theory.

#### 5.2.1.1 *Information-theoretic interpretation*

Central to the neuronal gauge theory is the multi-tier rebalancing of local transformations per overall gauge principles. Gauge theories have an information-theoretic interpretation through information geometry and entropy. The neuronal gauge theory argument is that macroscale brain emergence is a force that manifests from the curvature of information geometry in the same way that gravity is manifested when the spacetime continuum is curved by massive planetary bodies. Macroscale emergence in the brain can be seen in the apparatus of a gauge theory interpreted by information geometry and entropy.

Sengupta *et al.*'s (2016) method is a free energy based interpretation of the information geometry and mean-field approximation approach developed by Amari (1995) and others (which also configures neural field theories). The probability measures executed in the neuronal gauge theory produce not a flat, but a curved (Riemannian) landscape. Such negative curvature has a hyperbolic geometry. Traversing a curved manifold requires a distance measure that corresponds to the distance between two statistical distributions. In differential geometry, the distance measure is often provided by the Fisher information metric, an approximation of the local geometry of a probability distribution which quantifies the amount of information that a random variable carries about an unknown parameter. The Fisher information represents the curvature of the relative entropy (Kullback–Leibler divergence). Distance in the curved geometry corresponds to the relative entropy of traveling from one point on the manifold to another. The shortest-length curve or geodesic is a central formulation in information geometry (Amari, 1995, p. 15), as well as general relativity and the AdS/CFT correspondence. The AdS/Information Geometry interpretation appears in Table 5.4.

The neuronal gauge theory uses a free energy based model developed by Jordan *et al.* (1998). The proposal is a variational Fokker–Planck method with a Langevin (stochastic time evolution) equation whose ensemble density minimizes variational free energy. Fokker–Planck equations describe time-dependent dynamics, specifically the time evolution of the probability density function of particle velocity under the influence of drag forces equivalent to the convection-diffusion equation in Brownian motion. Here, the Fokker–Plank energy minimization approach provides the information-geometric manifold coordinates that are used to apply the

Table 5.4. AdS/Information Geometry.

| Bulk | Boundary | Mathematical Formulation |
|---|---|---|
| Geodesic | Neural signal | Fisher information, Kullback–Leibler divergence |

gauge field. The gauge field is formulated as a Levi-Civita connection (covariant derivative), an operation on the tangent bundle that differentiates vector fields. The gauge field is formalized as a vector field comprised of independent coordinates on the manifold base, and compares two points or distributions. The gauge field (Levi-Civita connection) is applied to enact the local forces that form the neuronal dynamics in the neuronal gauge theory.

#### 5.2.1.2 *Implications*

The concept of the neuronal gauge theory is presented as an apparatus with a compensatory mechanism (gauge fields) to maintain the invariance of a global symmetry across all scale levels of a system. The Lagrangian is the formula describing the system dynamics and the implicit mechanism used to rebalance the local forces to maintain gauge invariance. Free energy minimization is proposed as one candidate for a gauge-invariant property in the brain, but there could be others. From the information-geometric perspective, the invariance preservation mechanism entails finding the shortest path on a curved manifold (geodesic). The gauge theory model could be implemented for further investigation on any variety of classical and quantum computational systems including machine learning platforms, neural networks, tensor networks, spiking neural networks, and photonic platforms.

Two of the key benefits of the neuronal gauge theory are having a method for finding the shortest path on curved manifolds (concretized with coordinates) and having an entropy-based formulation. A considerable challenge in neural modeling is the map-territory problem, namely, transforming the physical space the neural realities to the phase space of the model (Golubitsky & Stewart, 2003). The modeling process can disconnect variables and result in coordinate transformation issues (for example, in EEG and fMRI analysis, scale changes can be lost when instantiating the three-dimensional cortex as a representation in a plane) (Cocchi *et al.*, 2017). The neuronal gauge theory contributes a schema of concretized coordinates for the curved manifold analysis. Further, the natural structure of the gauge theory allows a symmetry property in phase space to be translated into a symmetry property in the physical space.

The benefit of articulating the symmetries of a dynamical system with a gauge theory is that one dynamical system can be more readily mapped to another by aligning the higher-order properties. Symmetry is an ongoing topic in quantum computing algorithm design. For example, one effort formalizes the connection between the quantum symmetry properties of the Quantum Approximate Optimization Algorithm (QAOA) and the underlying symmetries of the objective function to be optimized (Shaydulin *et al.*, 2020).

### 5.2.2 *Diffeomorphism invariance*

Gauge theories are a fundamental tool that might aid in the understanding of the brain and also continue to contribute to theoretical physics. Although gauge theories have helped to bring general relativity and quantum mechanics closer together in the picture of both having fields (gravitational fields and quantum fields) that can be computed with matrices, there is more work to be done. On the one hand, general relativity is a geometrical theory of gravity in which the effects of gravity are due to the curvature of space and time. On the other hand, fundamental particle interactions are described as quantum field theories that are invariant under gauge transformations. To unify gravity with particle theories, one proposed strategy is to rewrite general relativity more formally as a gauge theory. Gravity (general relativity) is already considered to be a gauge theory in some respects because it is diffeomorphism invariant.

Diffeomorphism invariance refers to a system that is invariant to diffeomorphism (manifold changes). A diffeomorphism is a mapping between two smooth manifolds. A diffeomorphism invariant system is one that does not change with certain kinds of mappings between smooth (differentiable) manifolds. The gauge symmetry in general relativity can be identified as being invariant under diffeomorphism (manifold) transformations. However, the nature of this symmetry, how it is implemented, and how it behaves as a gauge transformation is unknown. Spontaneous symmetry breaking and the Higgs mechanism (by which particles acquire mass) are important in particle physics gauge theories, and these same formulations might likewise contribute to a gravity gauge theory that is diffeomorphism invariant (Chung, 2008).

Table 5.5. The Standard Model of particle physics.

| No. | Fundamental Force or Theory | Symmetry |
|---|---|---|
| 1 | Electromagnetic force | U(1) |
| 2 | Weak force | SU(2) |
| 3 | Strong force (Quantum Chromodynamics (QCD)) | SU(3) |
| Standard Model: Unified symmetry group | | SU(3) × SU(2) × U(1) |

### 5.2.3 *Symmetry and Yang–Mills theory*

Symmetry is implicated in the current understanding of the Standard Model of particle physics developed from Yang–Mills theory. The Yang–Mills theory is a gauge theory based on a special unitary group SU($n$) described by Lie algebra (Yang & Mills, 1954). The behavior of elementary particles is described using nonabelian Lie groups. The Yang–Mills theory is at the heart of the unification of the electromagnetic force and weak forces (i.e. U(1) × SU(2)) together with quantum chromodynamics, the theory of the strong force (based on SU(3)) (Jaffe & Witten, 2006). This results in the unified symmetry group of the Standard Model (Table 5.5). The Lie group often plays the role of symmetry (invariance) in physical systems, indicating the overall system properties that remain unchanged in the face of local transformations.

## References

Amari, S. (1995). Information geometry of the EM and EM algorithms for neural networks. *Neural Netw.* 8(9):1379–408.

Anderson, P.W. (1972). More is different. *Science.* 177(4047):393–96.

Chung, J.P. (2008). Diffeomorphism invariance in general relativity. *Honors Theses.* Colby College. Paper 53.

Cocchi, L., Gollo, L.L., Zalesky, A. & Breakspear, M. (2017). Criticality in the brain: A synthesis of neurobiology, models and cognition. *Prog. Neurobiol.* 158:132–52.

Friston, K. (2008). Hierarchical models in the brain. *PLoS Comput. Biol.* 4(11):e1000211.

Friston, K., Kilner, J. & Harrison, L. (2006). A free energy principle for the brain. *J. Physiol. Paris.* 100:70–87.

Griffiths, D.J. (1995). *Introduction to Quantum Mechanics.* Upper Saddle River, NJ: Prentice Hall.

Golubitsky, M. & Stewart, I. (2003). *The Symmetry Perspective: From Equilibrium to Chaos in Phase Space and Physical Space*. Berlin: Birkhauser.

Jaffe, A. & Witten, E. (2006). Quantum Yang-Mills theory. In *Millennium Prize Problems*. Providence RI: American Mathematical Society, pp. 129–52.

Jordan, R., Kinderlehrer, D. & Otto, F. (1998). The variational formulation of the Fokker-Planck equation. *SIAM J. Math. Anal.* 29(1):1–17.

Kiebel, S.J. & Friston, K.J. (2011). Free energy and dendritic self-organization. *Front. Syst. Neurosci.* 5(80):1–13.

Knill, D.C. & Pouget, A. (2004). The Bayesian brain: The role of uncertainty in neural coding and computation. *Trends Neurosci.* 27(12):712–9.

Maldacena, J. (1998). The large N limit of superconformal field theories and supergravity. *Adv. Theor. Math. Phys.* 2:231–52.

O'Raifeartaigh, L. & Straumann, N. (2000). Gauge theory: Historical origins and some modern developments. *Rev. Mod. Phys.* 72(1):1–23.

Sengupta, B., Tozzi, A., Cooray, G.K. *et al.* (2016). Towards a neuronal gauge theory. *PLoS Biol.* 14(3):e1002400.

Shaydulin, R., Hadfield, S., Hogg, T. & Safro, I. (2020). Classical symmetries and QAOA. arXiv:2012.04713v1.

Weinberg, S. (1980). Conceptual foundations of the unified theory of weak and electromagnetic interactions. *Science*. 210(4475):1212–8.

Yang, C.N. & Mills, R. (1954). Conservation of isotopic spin and isotopic gauge invariance. *Phys. Rev*. 96(1):191–5.

Zeki, S. (2005). The Ferrier Lecture 1995 behind the seen: The functional specialization of the brain in space and time. *Philos. Trans. R. Soc. Lond. B. Biol. Sci*. 360(1458):1145–83.

# Part 2

# Substrate

# Chapter 6

# Quantum Information Theory

*It from bit … all things physical are information-theoretic in origin*

— Wheeler (1990, p. 356)

**Abstract**

This chapter describes information-theoretic formulations as a control lever for quantum mechanical processes such as quantum computing. Entropy is a key measure of the interconnectedness of subsystems within a system and can be manipulated in the information compression and quantum teleportation of the state information between locations. Quantum walks and out-of-time-order correlation (OTOC) functions manage forward and backward time evolution in quantum systems.

## 6.1 Quantum Information

Wheeler's quote points to the idea that information is the key to understanding reality. The intuition is that in order to truly comprehend reality, which involves unifying general relativity and quantum mechanics, it is necessary to develop a deeper understanding of the behavior of information, particularly in quantum systems. Hence, the field of quantum information has arisen as the discipline of thinking about information in many different kinds of quantum mechanical situations such as qubits, harmonic oscillators, and fermion systems. The quote update for the quantum computing era is "it from qubit", or more appropriately, "it from qudit" (multistate unit of quantum information).

### 6.1.1 *Entropy and quantum information*

The first topic to be clarified is what is meant by information. The usual definition of information is facts provided or learned about something that resolves uncertainty. Etymologically, information comes from the verb to "in form", to give a form or an idea to something. In this way, information can be seen as a coalescing of order out of disorder, the rendering of salience out of randomness. Physicist Davies (1992, p. 16) suggests that the real question is why there is any order at all "given the limitless variety of ways in which matter and energy can arrange themselves".

Conceptually, information theory can be seen as a way of organizing and quantifying the correlations observed in real-life phenomena (how interrelated subsystems of a system are). The methods of information theory provide concrete functions and quantities to evaluate correlations, including entropy, mutual information, channel capacity, and error correction. Entropy plays this kind of role in statistical mechanics, namely, quantifying the underlying relationships in complex systems, and the same concept extends to quantum systems.

#### 6.1.1.1 *Classical information theory*

Information theory arose in the context of efficient signal processing in communications. Shannon was interested in the fundamental limitations of signal processing and data compression. He proposed information-theoretic entropy as a measure of the minimum number of bits needed to communicate a message produced by a statistical source (Shannon, 1948). Hence, classical information theory is often understood as the study of the quantification, storage, and communication of information. Information is taken to be an ordered sequence of symbols from an alphabet. Horodecki *et al.* (2007) articulate three building blocks that comprise classical information theory. These are entropy (the information content of something or the minimum number of bits needed to communicate a message), mutual information (the knowledge held in common between entities), and conditional entropy (the total entropy minus partial entropy as the additional amount information that must be sent to relay a message).

Bennett and Shor (1998, p. 2724) suggest that quantum information theory is the natural completion of classical information theory: "At a more fundamental level, it has become clear that an information theory based on quantum principles extends and completes classical information theory, somewhat as complex numbers extend and complete the reals".

Quantum information theory has to do with the same topics of information generation, storage, and transmission in quantum networks for quantum communication and quantum computing. In the broadest sense, quantum information theory is formulating quantum mechanics from an information-theoretic perspective (Nielsen & Chuang, 2010). The term "quantum information" specifically denotes the information of the state of a quantum system. It can be given formally (by the technical von Neumann entropy measure) or informally (by the general computational status of a system). In practice, quantum information theory is the counterpart of classical information theory. Relevant topics in quantum information theory include quantum information encoding, error correction, channel capacity, entanglement, and quantum cryptography. A lexicon of terms appears in Table 6.1.

### 6.1.1.2 *Entropy*

Entropy is a widely used term in various contexts, always meaning about the same thing, namely, the number of different ways a system can be arranged. Entropy refers to a desk becoming messy, stirring milk into

Table 6.1. Lexicon: Classical and quantum information.

| Term | Definition |
|---|---|
| Classical information | Facts that give form to something (in-form) |
| Quantum information | State information of a quantum system |
| Classical information theory | Quantification, storage, and sending of information |
| Quantum information theory | Information-theoretic version of quantum physics |

coffee, a black hole evaporating, or sending a message across the quantum internet. The more different ways the system can be organized (microstates), the higher the entropy, and the more information that is required to send the full details of the system to another location. Entropy arose in the context of studying thermodynamics and heat dissipation, and was formulated as statistical mechanical entropy by Boltzmann (2011, 1896) and in the modern formulation by Gibbs (1902). von Neumann applied the Gibbs entropy to quantum mechanics to take the minimum over all measurement bases of the system (1932).

Shannon used entropy in information-theoretic terms to describe the information bits required to encode, compress, and transmit messages (1948). In these situations, entropy is a quantitative measure of the number of possible microscopic configurations (microstates) of a system that are consistent with its macroscopic quantities such as volume, pressure, and temperature. There is no practical distinction between thermodynamic entropy and information-theoretic entropy (Harlow, 2017). Both von Neumann entropy and Shannon entropy have the operational interpretation of the number of bits (qubits) required to transmit the system state information (relevant microscopic degrees of freedom) from one location to another. Rényi (1961) entropy is another form of entropy often used in quantum information theory as a composite of four other entropy measures (Shannon, Hartley, collision, and minimum entropy).

The AdS/CFT correspondence has sponsored further advance in entropy formulations. The Ryu and Takayanagi (2006) formula relates the bulk and the boundary regions through entanglement entropy. Entanglement entropy is a measure of the information content (entanglement) between two quantum subsystems. The Ryu–Takayanagi formula states that the boundary entanglement entropy is equal to the area of a corresponding minimal surface in the bulk. This can be seen as the entanglement entropy of a region in the boundary being given by the area of a minimal three-dimensional surface which hangs from the two-dimensional boundary region into the bulk as a geodesic (shortest length curve) (Swingle, 2012). An additional advance is the geometric formulation of quantum mechanical entropy. Despite the von Neumann formula, minimizing over all measurement bases in a strongly interacting quantum mechanical system is cumbersome and sometimes intractable. Instead,

Czech *et al.* (2015) extend the geodesic-based geometrical formulation to quantum mechanical entropy. Using the holographic correspondence, the idea is to evaluate entropy with geometry, through the geometrical quantity of the shortest length curve through the bulk that corresponds to a boundary region.

## 6.1.2 *Superposition, entanglement, and interference*

The SEI properties (superposition, entanglement, and interference) are the central attributes of quantum mechanical objects that are relevant to quantum computing (Swan *et al.*, 2020, p. 48). Superposition is the property that an unobserved particle exists in all possible states simultaneously, but once measured, collapses to just one state. Entanglement is the property of particles being connected such that their states are related, even when separated by a large distance. Interference is the property of waves reinforcing or canceling each other out (cohering or decohering), which is important for measuring wave amplitudes in many-particle systems.

### 6.1.2.1 *Superposition and interference*

The superposition and interference properties of quantum mechanics are demonstrated by the canonical double-slit experiment (Nielsen & Chuang, 2010). In the first setup of the experiment, there is just one slit. A laser is shone through the slit and illuminates a screen in the distance. The resulting pattern is a curve with a peak in the middle and weaker peaks further out on the screen in diminishing size. If the slit is narrowed, the width of the peak broadens, and in the limit of an infinitely thin slit, there is an infinite-width peak. In the second setup of the experiment, there are two slits. In this case, the wave front hits both slits with little waves coming out from each slit that interfere with each another. The pattern on the screen shows multiple peaks with interference which is not surprising as they indicate the expected behavior of classical wave formations.

The third setup of the experiment considers the quantum mechanical scale. The laser is turned down to emit only one photon at a time. The emitted light is composed of one individual photon. Thus, it seems that the photon could only take the path through the upper slit or the lower slit.

However, when performing a measurement and looking at the screen, the result is the same pattern as that of the two-slit experiment with multiple peaks and interference. In order to generate such an interference pattern, the photon would need to pass through both slits. Since there is only one photon, not the photon but something related to it must be two places at once. This idea is called superposition, that a quantum object simultaneously exists in what would seem to be two mutually exclusive domains from a classical perspective (Lee, 2020, p. 7).

#### 6.1.2.2 *Two-state qubit systems and quantum computing*

In information-theoretic terms, the quantum double-slit experiment is a qubit system (a two-state system) (Bennett & DiVincenzo, 2000). The coinage of the term "qubit" is credited to Schumacher (1995). The two states can be labeled as zero and one. If the photon is passing through the upper slit, it is a zero, and through the lower slit, it is a one. Since quantum mechanics allows both states to occur at the same time, superposition is modeled mathematically as a linear combination of the two possibilities. The principle of superposition is that multiple incompatible classical realities can coexist simultaneously.

There are many different ways to make a two-state qubit system for the purpose of quantum computing. Most qubit systems use binary state properties that can be labeled in a quantum object (atom, ion, photon) related to energy, spin, or other physical properties. The simplest atom, for example, is the hydrogen atom (with one proton and one electron). To make a qubit system, the lowest energy state (the ground state) is labeled zero, and the first excited state is labeled one. The qubit states (one and zero) are literal translations of the real-life physical properties of the quantum object. A quantum computer is a physical system.

A basic approach to quantum computing is applying energy to the hydrogen atom qubit system to create states that are between the zero and the one (Rieffel & Polak, 2014, p. 13). These are not states in which the electron is halfway between the zero orbit and the one orbit, but states in which there is some amplitude (probability, which appears as a coefficient) associated with the zero orbit and some amplitude associated with the one orbit, that coexist. Superconducting circuits are another platform for quantum computing, ideally realized by the semiconductor industry. In a superconducting circuit, the two-state qubit system is typically constructed such that the current flowing one way in a Josephson junction circuit is a zero, and the current flowing the other way is a one. Another semiconductor-related method is quantum dots which are a microfabricated structure in which there is a potential well, and the electron prefers to be in one location or the other. Whether the electron is in the left or the right well is encoded as the zero or the one. The presence or absence of a charge is another standard form of qubit system, as is binary polarization in optical systems.

#### 6.1.2.3 *Entanglement and Bell pairs*

Entanglement is the property of particles being connected such that their states are related, even if they are separated by a large distance. Entanglement is produced when a pair of quantum objects such as photons interacts physically. For example, a laser beam fired through a certain type of crystal can cause individual photons to be split into pairs of entangled photons. The photons can be separated by a large distance, hundreds of miles or more. When observed, one photon takes on one state (spin-up, for example). The entangled photon, though now far away, immediately takes on the opposite state (spin-down).

A qubit exists in a superposition of two states until collapsing to one of them when measured. By analogy to a coin flip, a qubit exists in the state of Heads and Tails at the same time. The probability of being in Heads and the probability of being in Tails sum to one. If two qubits are entangled, it means that if one ends up in Heads, the other is in Tails. Both qubits do not need to be measured, because if one is measured, the other's state is known automatically due to their being entangled. The entanglement relationship ends when one side is measured. Qubits may participate in high-dimensional entanglement schemes by being simultaneously entangled according to one or more attributes such as spin, polarization, and angular momentum, in a dense juggernaut of quantum computational information (Erhard *et al.*, 2020). For each attribute, there are two values, and if one qubit is measured in "spin up", the other is correspondingly in "spin down".

Entangled particles are called Bell pairs (after Bell's theorem). Einstein objected to the idea of such "spooky action at a distance" since faster-than-light-travel is not possible. That is true, but entanglement is also true. Particles that are in physical proximity, entangled, and then separated remain entangled, and when one half of the pair is measured, the other immediately collapses to the opposite value (Weihs *et al.*, 1998). Quantum entanglement has been demonstrated numerous times and is exploited as a standard feature in quantum communication.

## 6.2 Quantum Toolbox

### 6.2.1 *Quantum teleportation*

Quantum entanglement is harnessed is in quantum teleportation. Quantum teleportation is a technique for sending quantum information from one location to another, for example, between two parties, A and B. This is possible if A and B share an entangled Bell pair and have a classical communications channel available to them. The idea of quantum teleportation is sending information, not matter, more like a fax machine than a means of transportation (as science fiction suggests). In quantum teleportation, the state of a particle or quantum system is transmitted from one physical location to another. It is analogous to sending a fax in that only information is sent and the final product relies on some sort of feedstock being present at the receiving location to generate the state.

In an experimental setup, A and B might teleport the state of a photon from A across some distance to B (Nielsen & Chuang, 2010, p. 26). First, A packages up the information describing the quantum state of the photon in the form of a qubit. Then A and B use an existing Bell pair, or create a new Bell pair with an entangled state between two new photons, to initiate the teleportation. They separate the Bell pair photons so each has one qubit of the entangled Bell pair. Next, A interacts the qubit state with A's half of the entangled Bell pair, and then measures the two qubits, obtaining one of four possible classical results (00, 01, 10, 11). A sends this information to B using a classical channel. Depending on A's message, B performs one of four pre-specified operations on B's half of the entangled pair to recover the original state. Through entanglement, in the form of the entangled pair, A and B are able to transfer the quantum state information of the original photon from one location to another. Notably, quantum teleportation is secure because the Bell pair has information shared exclusively between themselves and no other particles. This property might be used to provide a high level of information security in quantum communication and computation. A further extension is blind quantum computing, protocols in which one party cannot access a quantum computer, and another party facilitates the computation with the input, output, and task remaining hidden (Childs, 2005), in a sort of quantum zero-knowledge proof technology method.

### 6.2.2 *Quantum error correction*

Quantum error correction is becoming more prominent in considering the potential future applications that extend beyond NISQ devices to universal fault-tolerant quantum computing, including as motivated by real-life applications in quantum finance. Fault tolerance means preventing a few errors from escalating to many. Various quantum error correction techniques are used to protect quantum information (i.e. quantum states) from environmental noise. Such noise arises in quantum communication as quantum states pass through noisy channels, and in quantum computation as quantum states are transformed through a sequence of computational steps and exposed to environmental decoherence (Brun, 2019). Classical error correction methods such as making redundant copies or checking information integrity before transmission are not possible in quantum systems since information cannot be copied or inspected (per the no-cloning and no-measurement principles of quantum mechanics). Quantum error correction therefore relies on entanglement instead of redundancy. The quantum state to be protected is entangled with a larger group of states from which it can be corrected indirectly (one qubit might be entangled with a 9-qubit ancilla of extra qubits, for example).

The basic errors that occur are a bit flip, a sign flip (the sign of the phase), or both. Basic error correcting codes are applied to diagnose the error, and correspond to the usual Pauli matrices for manipulating qubits in the X, Y, and Z dimensions of a Hilbert space. The error is expressed as a superposition of basis operations given by the Pauli matrices. If there is an error, the same Pauli operator is applied to act again on the corrupted qubit to reverse the effect of the error. The unitary correction returns the state to the initial state without measuring the qubit directly.

The basic form of the quantum error correcting code (QECC) is the stabilizer code, as the quantum version of linear codes used in classical systems (Brown, 2020). In the application of stabilizer codes, the quantum information to be protected is stored in a larger quantum state (ancilla) that is accessible through QECCs. The QECCs are a subspace of the larger Hilbert space of the protective ancilla. The code subspace is the eigenspace of a set of commuting Pauli operators (called stabilizer generators) acting on the qubits. A stabilizer code is defined by three parameters: The number of underlying physical qubits to be protected, the number of logical qubits in the protective ancilla, and the minimum distance of the code (the smallest number of simultaneous qubit errors that can be tolerated) (Swan *et al.*, 2020, p. 325). A stabilizer code acts to correct any damaged information in this schema, and can be applied within other analytical frameworks; MERA tensor network-based stabilizer codes, for example (Kim & Kastoryano, 2017).

Stabilizer codes are the general method for protecting static quantum information from noise, for example, in quantum communications networks. However, the dynamical process of quantum computing itself also introduces errors since information is not only stored but also processed. For universal quantum computing, fault-tolerant error correction is needed to prevent a few errors from escalating during the quantum computation process. Topology-based stabilizer codes (the toric code and the surface code) are proposed as the primary method for fault-tolerant error correction. Particle movement and its correction are interpreted in the structure of lattice topologies. Toric codes are stabilizer codes defined on a two-dimensional lattice with periodic boundary conditions (which gives them the shape of a torus), with stabilizer operators on the spins around each vertex and plaquette (face) (Kitaev, 1997). Surface codes are a more generic formulation of topology-based stabilizer codes, which are also defined on two-dimensional spin lattices, and take various shapes, but are not necessarily toroidal.

Other fault-tolerant stabilizer codes are also proposed related to Majorana fermion braiding and color codes (gauge color fixing).

In particular, color codes are a family of topological quantum error-correcting codes that use less computationally demanding gauge-fixing instead of magic state distillation to execute non-Clifford gates (Brown *et al.*, 2016). "Color" coding refers to the minimal number of colors needed to code a system so that each cell touches no other cell of the same color (states on a map is a canonical color-coding problem). Color coding has a more compact encoding but requires more elaborate hardware (Litinski, 2019, p. 28). Further, the ability to conduct "lattice surgery" by choosing different decoders, including with the help of machine learning (QEC/ML), allows fault-tolerant code switching (Nautrup *et al.*, 2019).

Another quantum error correction method proposes a three-dimensional surface code in the form of the staged progression of one surface code being slid underneath two other surface codes in time (thus constituting a "time technology") (Brown, 2020). The method provides a new type of non-Clifford-gate error-correcting method without the need for the computational overhead of state distillation. There are two kinds of quantum gates, Clifford gates and non-Clifford gates. Clifford gates (based on elements in the Clifford algebra) are basic quantum gates (Pauli matrices, Hadamard gate, CNOT gate, and $\pi/2$-phase shift gates) that can be simulated efficiently on a classical computer (i.e. in polynomial time). Non-Clifford gates are needed for greater logical depth and more complex operations (such as the $\pi/8$ gate) and cannot be simulated efficiently on a classical computer (Rieffel & Polak, 2014, p. 318).

The non-Clifford gates rely on so-called magic state distillation which is the computationally expensive task of consolidating multiple noisy quantum states into fewer reliable states. Brown's three-dimensional surface code is an advance in circumventing the need for magic state distillation in the execution of non-Clifford gates. The non-Clifford gate uses three overlapping copies of the surface code that interact locally over a period of time. This is carried out by taking thin slices of the three-dimensional surface code and collapsing them into a two-dimensional space. The process is repeated with the help of just-in-time gauge fixing, a procedure for stacking together the two-dimensional slices on a chip, as well as dealing with any occurring errors. The three surface codes replicate the three-dimensional code that performs the non-Clifford gate functions.

#### 6.2.2.1 *AdS/QECC*

The AdS/CFT correspondence is a recognized as a quantum error correction structure, formally as an operator algebra problem (Almheiri *et al.*, 2015). An early example of AdS/QECC (quantum error correction codes) is demonstrated using tensor networks (Pastawski *et al.*, 2015). The implication of AdS/QECC is that a physical qubit in the bulk can be protected by entangling it with logical qubits on the boundary. AdS/QECC work continues to link advances in algebraic formalisms and information theory to quantum error correction. In AdS/CFT research, a key objective is bulk reconstruction, reconstructing emergent structure in the bulk.

In quantum error correction, the implementation is protecting a physical qubit in the bulk with a logical ancilla of qubits on the boundary. The structural and formal objectives inform each other in AdS/QECC applications. One finding is that conditions in which bulk and boundary relative entropies are equal do not always hold in error correction scenarios. Thus, work in quantum information theory is used to argue that for any quantum channel of information transmission, there exists an approximate recovery channel, using type 1 von Neumann algebras as the formalism (Junge *et al.*, 2018). The initial state can be corrected from the recovery channel acting as the identity on all states in the domain, to perform sufficiently approximate error correction. The AdS/QECC implication is that any low-energy bulk operator in the entanglement wedge (related area) of a boundary region can be represented as an operator acting on that boundary region, without having to assume that the bulk and boundary relative entropies are equal (Cotler *et al.*, 2019). The type 1 von Neumann algebras as the formalism are extended to arbitrary von Neumann algebras in subsequent work (Faulkner *et al.*, 2020).

#### 6.2.2.2 *QECC example: The three-qutrit code*

A good example of a QECC is the three-qutrit code. For example, there is a qubit that needs to be protected from quantum noise or for security reasons. The idea is to encode the qubit, a logical qutrit, into three physical qutrits. The logical qutrit is in the bulk and the three physical qutrits are on the boundary. A qutrit is a three-state qubit, which is a useful self-contained nine-state error-correction code system. The logical qutrit is encoded into physical qutrits A and B together, B and C together, and A and C together, as groups of boundary regions or surface states. The physical qutrit can be recovered from any pair of the surface states since they are entangled. There are three different ways to recover the qutrit since any two of three boundary states are needed to reconstruct the qutrit. The message is incoherent to an outsider if only examining one pair without knowing how the qutrits are entangled.

A typical example is sending a Greenberger–Horne–Zeilinger (GHZ) state (an entangled quantum state involving at least three entangled particles or qubits) using the three-qutrit code. Each of the three-qutrits has three states (nine total states). The three-particle GHZ state is encoded into the three-qutrit (nine-state) system and the three-qutrits are sent one at a time. The GHZ state cannot be recovered from just one qutrit, but can be reconstructed from any two of the three-qutrits (the full state can be reconstructed from six states). The receiver acts with an operator (specified ahead of time) to decode the entangled qutrits (code subspace) and access the message. The state can be recovered from any two of the qutrits by acting on them with the operator to obtain the full GHZ state (Harlow, 2017, p. 25). Applications of holographic quantum error-correcting codes are further discussed by Swan *et al.* (2020, pp. 319–36).

### 6.2.3 *Out-of-time-order correlators*

A concept frequently used in quantum information theory is evolving time backward and forward in a quantum system. As the name indicates, out-of-time-order correlation (OTOC) functions are operators used to evolve a quantum system back or forward through time, in particular to measure the scrambling time (how quickly information spreads out over the entire system so that a local measurement is not possible). The function evolves a quantum system back or forward through time so that two different states of the quantum system can be compared. The two different states are compared either by applying a function and waiting for some time for the system to evolve forward in time and then measure it, or by applying a measurement, evolving the system back in time and applying another operator at some earlier moment to measure it then. The formalism is carried out by comparing how fast two operators which are initially commuting, decay to become non-commuting (Swingle *et al.*, 2016, p. 1).

### 6.2.4 *Quantum walks and Hadamard coins*

Classical random walks are based on Markov (stochastic) processes and a coin flip, and are used to explain Brownian motion in real-life systems. Quantum random walks are the quantum version, also determined by a coin flip (a quantum coin-flip operator), and are used to find faster quantum algorithms (for search and cryptography), and involve more variables including the graph setup, the walk algorithm, the time regime (discrete or continuous), and the coin-flip operator. The quantum structure offers significant potential speedups versus classical random walks, which are confined to a classical diffusive spreading out rate. Instead, quantum walks have various regimes of ballistic, hyper-ballistic, and chaotic spreading, delivering at minimum a quadratic speedup improvement compared to classical methods (Pires *et al.*, 2019). Also, continuous-time quantum walks can be exponentially faster than classical random walks due to interference effects which enable the quantum walk to penetrate decision-tree structures more quickly (Farhi & Gutmann, 1998).

Quantum walks can be implemented on any platform, in particular optical platforms such as photonic waveguide arrays, graphene, and crystal lattices (Razzoli *et al.*, 2020). Other applications for quantum walks include coin-space entanglement and memory (in the form of elephant walks with good memory (Di Molfetta *et al.*, 2018)). Quantum walks can be performed in discrete-time or continuous-time (Childs, 2005).

A classical random walk is a mathematical object that is a stochastic (random) process describing a path of successive random steps in a space, used to facilitate the explanation of Brownian motion in systems such as stock prices, population ecologies, and superconducting materials. A random walk proceeds as a Markov process in which, at every time step, a particle moves (either left or right) to one of two neighboring sites as a result of the random outcome of a coin toss.

In quantum walks, the wavefunction describing the system evolves according to the value of an inner binary property (such as the spin or the chirality) whose state is locally updated by the action of a unitary operator (the coin operator). One of the main coin operators is the Hadamard coin or coin-flip operator, a real-valued unitary operator that performs a Hadamard transformation (flips into superposition) on the chirality of the particle. There are various coin operators (site-dependent coins, time-dependent coins, history-dependent coins, and random coins (unitary coin operators selected at random)) (Montero, 2017).

The space in which the quantum walk takes place is more complicated than that of the classical random walk as quantum walks often proceed in elaborate lattice graph structures. The lattice graphs might be embedded in a Euclidean plane to form a regular tessellation (triangular, square, and honeycomb lattice graphs). Continuous-time quantum walks in embedded lattices are of particular interest (Flamini *et al.*, 2018, p. 20). A photon propagating through a lattice shows a ballistic spread for a distance proportional to the evolution time, due to the interference of the wave packet amplitudes across the continuous-time quantum walk. In continuous walks on disordered lattices with static disorders, an Anderson localization can be produced in which the wave packet localizes on the initial sites of the lattice. An Anderson localization is the absence of the diffusion of waves in a disordered medium (a useful property of electron localization in semiconductors with implications for computation). It is also possible to manipulate Bloch oscillations (periodic oscillations between the spreading and the localization of the wave packet) on lattices with external gradient forces.

Quantum chaos formulations have important practical uses in the ballistic regimes of chaotic spreading of quantum walks that are much faster than the diffusion spreading of classical random walks. Quantum walk algorithms can be used to develop faster algorithms for search and cryptography. The advent of usable quantum chaos for computing scenarios introduces a ratcheting effect that impacts quantum information security. The risk is that lower-dimensional systems with slower-speed and chaotic dynamical behavior degradation could leave systems vulnerable to attack (El-Latif *et al.*, 2020). Quantum cryptosystem design thus makes use of the latest quantum walk protocols, similar to the way that classical algorithms incorporate the latest cryptographic standards.

## References

Almheiri, A., Dong, X. & Harlow, D. (2015). Bulk locality and quantum error correction in AdS/CFT. *J. High Energ. Phys.* 1504:163.

Bennett, C.H. & DiVincenzo, D.P. (2000). Quantum information and computation. *Nature.* 404:247–55.

Bennett, C.H. & Shor, P.W. (1998). Quantum information theory. *IEEE Trans. Inf. Theory.* 44:2724–42.

Boltzmann, L. (2011, 1896). *Lectures on Gas Theory.* Mineola NY: Dover.

Brown, B.J. (2020). A fault-tolerant non-Clifford gate for the surface code in two dimensions. *Sci. Adv.* 6(eaay4929):1–13.

Brown, B.J., Nickerson, N.H. & Browne, D.E. (2016). Fault-tolerant error correction with the gauge color code. *Nat. Commun.* 7:12302.

Brun, T.A. (2019). Quantum error correction. arXiv: 1910.03672.

Childs, A.M. (2005). Universal computation by quantum walk. *J. Quantum Inf. Comput.* 5:456–66.

Cotler, J., Hayden, P., Penington, G. *et al.* (2019). Entanglement wedge reconstruction via universal recovery channels. *Phys. Rev. X.* 9(3):031011.

Czech, B., Hayden, P., Lashkari, N. & Swingle, B. (2015). The information theoretic interpretation of the length of a curve. *J. High Energ. Phys.* 1506:157.

Davies, P.C.W. (1992). Why is the physical world so comprehensible? *CTNS Bull.* 12(2):16–21.

Di Molfetta, G., Soares-Pinto, D.O. & Queiros, S.M.D. (2018). Elephant quantum walk. *Phys. Rev. A.* 97(6):062112.

El-Latif, A.A.A., Abd-El-Atty, B., Amin, M. & Iliyasu, A.M. (2020). Quantum-inspired cascaded discrete-time quantum walks with induced chaotic dynamics and cryptographic applications. *Sci. Rep.* 10:1930.

Erhard, M., Krenn, M. & Zeilinger, A. (2020). Advances in high dimensional quantum entanglement. *Nat. Rev. Phys.* 2:365–81.

Farhi, E. & Gutmann, S. (1998). Quantum computation and decision trees. *Phys. Rev. A.* 58(2):915–28.

Faulkner, T., Hollands, S., Swingle, B. & Wang, Y. (2020). Approximate recovery and relative entropy I. general von Neumann subalgebras. arXiv:2006.08002v1.

Flamini, F., Spagnolo, N. & Sciarrino, F. (2018). Photonic quantum information processing: A review. *Rep. Prog. Phys.* 82(1):016001.

Gibbs, J.W. (1902). *Elementary Principles in Statistical Mechanics.* New York: Scribner.

Harlow, D. (2017). TASI lectures on the emergence of bulk physics in AdS/CFT. In *Proceedings of Theoretical Advanced Study Institute Summer School 2017, "Physics at the Fundamental Frontier"*, Boulder, Colorado, USA, June 4–July 1, 2017. arXiv:1802.01040, PoS(TASI2017)002.

Horodecki, M., Oppenheim, J. & Winter, A. (2007). Quantum state merging and negative information. *Commun. Math. Phys.* 269(1):107–36.

Junge, M., Renner, R., Sutter, D. *et al.* (2018). Universal recovery maps and approximate sufficiency of quantum relative entropy. *Annales Henri Poincaré*. 19:2955–78.

Kim, I.H. & Kastoryano, M.J. (2017). Entanglement renormalization, quantum error correction, and bulk causality. *J. High Energ. Phys.* 1704:040.

Kitaev, A.Y. (1997). Quantum error correction with imperfect gates. In *Quantum Communication, Computing, and Measurement*. Eds. Holevo, A.S., Hirota, O. & Caves, C.M. New York: Plenum Press, pp. 181–88.

Lee, R.S.T. (2020). *Quantum Finance: Intelligent Forecast and Trading Systems.* Singapore: Springer.

Litinski, D. (2019). A game of surface codes: Large-scale quantum computing with lattice surgery. *Quantum*. 3(128):1–37.

Montero, M. (2017). Quantum and random walks as universal generators of probability distributions. *Phys. Rev. A*. 95(6):062326.

Nautrup, H.P., Delfosse, N., Dunjko, V. *et al.* (2019). Optimizing quantum error correction codes with reinforcement learning. *Quantum*. 3(215):1–21.

Nielsen, M.A. & Chuang, I.L. (2010). *Quantum Computation and Quantum Information*. 10th-Anniversary Edition. Cambridge: Cambridge University Press.

Pastawski, F., Yoshida, B., Harlow, D. & Preskill, J. (2015). Holographic quantum error-correcting codes: Toy models for the bulk–boundary correspondence. *J. High Energ. Phys.* 6(149):1–53.

Pires, M.A., Di Molfetta, G. & Queiros, S.M.D. (2019). Multiple transitions between normal and hyperballistic diffusion in quantum walks with time-dependent jumps. *Sci. Rep.* 9(1):19292.

Razzoli, R., Paris, M.G.A. & Bordone, P. (2020). Continuous-time quantum walks on planar lattices and the role of the magnetic field. *Phys. Rev. A*. 101(3):032336.

Rényi, A. (1961). On measures of entropy and information. In *Proceedings of the 4th Berkeley Symposium on Mathematical Statistics and Probability*. University of California Press: Berkeley, CA, USA, pp. 547–61.

Rieffel, E. & Polak, W. (2014). *Quantum Computing: A Gentle Introduction*. Cambridge MA: MIT Press.

Ryu, S. & Takayanagi, T. (2006). Aspects of holographic entanglement entropy. *J. High Energ. Phys.* 0608:045.

Schumacher, B. (1995). Quantum coding. *Phys. Rev. A*. 51(4):2738–47.

Shannon, C. (1948). A mathematical theory of communication. *Bell Syst. Tech. J.* 27(3):379–423.

Swan, M., dos Santos, R.P. & Witte, F. (2020). *Quantum Computing: Physics, Blockchains, and Deep Learning Smart Networks*. London: World Scientific.

Swingle, B. (2012). Entanglement renormalization and holography. *Phys. Rev. D*. 86(065007).

Swingle, B., Bentsen, G., Schleier-Smith, M. & Hayden, P. (2016). Measuring the scrambling of quantum information. *Phys. Rev. A*. 94(4):040302.

von Neumann, J. (1932). *Mathematische Grundlagen der Quantenmechanik*. Berlin: Springer.

Weihs, G., Jennewein, T., Simon, C. *et al.* (1998). Violation of Bell's inequality under strict Einstein locality conditions. *Phys. Rev. Lett.* 81(23):5039.

Wheeler, J.A. (1990). Information, physics, quantum: The search for links. In *Proc. 3rd Int Symp Foundations of Quantum Mechanics*, Tokyo, 1989, pp. 354–68.

# Chapter 7

# Quantum Computing 101

*[Quantum computing] does not merely make computer science a branch of physics. It also makes part of experimental physics into a branch of computer science*

— Deutsch (1985, p. 115)

**Abstract**

This chapter discusses writing quantum algorithms and quantum circuits to run on quantum hardware platforms. Qubits are encoded into various physical systems such as electron spins, superconducting current, and optical lattices. Input data are modulated (written) onto qubits with basis (one-to-one) encoding or amplitude (many) encoding. Quantum programs are rerun many times to obtain probabilistic confidence of the results. Quantum computation proceeds with unitary transformations (one-off steps) to evolve quantum systems forward in time.

## 7.1 Quantum Algorithms and Quantum Circuits

Quantum computing consists of the two steps of writing a quantum algorithm and running it on a quantum circuit. A quantum algorithm is a set of instructions for performing a quantum computation. A quantum circuit is a standard computational unit used to conduct logic operations with quantum gates on a quantum information processor. Both have analogs in

Table 7.1. Quantum computing steps.

| Term | Definition |
|---|---|
| Quantum algorithm | Set of instructions to perform a quantum computation |
| Quantum circuit | Computational unit used to perform logic operations with quantum gates on a quantum information processor |

classical computing. Whereas quantum algorithm design began decades ago, activity now includes the design of quantum circuits for real-life hardware implementation or simulation (Table 7.1).

The mathematics was quickly understood for how the quantum domain operates differently from the classical domain and how to produce computational speedups. The first focus is writing programs as linear algebra vectors to offer an improvement as compared to classical algorithms (Biamonte *et al.*, 2017). Some of the first quantum algorithms were written in the 1990s, notably Shor's (1997) algorithm for factorization and Grover's (1996) algorithm for search. Initially algorithm writing was a theoretical project without much to do with practical implementation, although quantum computing has always been realizable in principle. Now, what is different is real-life instantiations, and the aim is writing and translating quantum algorithms for implementation on real-life quantum computing platforms. Since quantum algorithms are exponentially faster at performing linear algebra calculations, a low-hanging fruit task is modifying classical algorithms to incorporate quantum linear algebra subroutines to gain the quantum speedup.

## 7.2 Qubit Encoding

To perform operations on a quantum computer, input data are encoded into a quantum state using qubits. Quantum bits, or qubits, are two-level quantum systems (Schumacher, 1995). They can be physically realized in many ways such as by the states of a spin-1/2 particle, the polarization of a single-photon, two distinguished levels of a trapped atom or ion, the current states of a microscopic superconducting loop, or many other physical systems (Table 7.2).

Table 7.2. Qubit encoding in various physical systems.

| No. | System | Quantity | Qubit (One-Zero) |
|---|---|---|---|
| 1 | Electrons | Spin | Up/down |
| | | Charge | 0/1 electrons |
| 2 | Josephson junction | Charge | 0/1 Cooper pair |
| | | Current | Clock/counter-clockwise |
| | | Energy | Ground/excited state |
| 3 | Single-photon | Spin angular momentum: Polarization | H/V, L/R, diagonals |
| | | Orbital angular momentum: Spatial modes | Left/right |
| | | Waveguide propagation path | 0/1 photons |
| | | Time-bin, frequency-bin | Early/late arrival bins |
| 4 | Optical lattice | Spin | Up/down |
| 5 | Quantum dot | Spin | Up/down |
| 6 | Nuclear spin | Spin | Up/down |
| 7 | Majorana fermions | Topology | Braiding |

*Source*: Adapted from Flamini *et al.* (2018, p. 3).

Qubits can be encoded in any variety of physical systems in which a zero and a one can be clearly designated. Most qubit systems use binary state properties that can be labeled in a quantum object (atom, ion, photon) related to energy, spin, and other physical properties. The qubit states (zero and one) are literal translations of the real-life physical properties of the quantum object. One of the most straightforward ways to formulate a qubit is with an electron spin. Other systems include Josephson junctions (superconducting devices with quantum tunneling), photonic lattices, nuclear spin systems, and Majorana fermions (non-abelian anyons in topological superconductors with interspersed braid-like trajectories).

### 7.2.1 *Quantum circuit demonstrations*

Two different ways to prepare a quantum circuit (for machine learning tasks in data classification) are described in detail by Farhi and

Neven (2018) and Grant *et al.* (2018), in the respective concepts of quantum neural networks and quantum tensor networks (Table 7.3). Grant *et al.* (2018) develop a hierarchical 8-qubit quantum circuit to classify both classical data (Iris and MNIST) and entangled quantum data (self-generated) with a tensor network structure (TTN and MERA), and test the circuit with Iris data on the IBM QX4 quantum computer.

Farhi and Neven propose a "quantum neural network" that represents labeled data and is trained with supervised learning methods. Digits from the MNIST database are distinguished (the 3 and the 6). The model maps 17-element data strings to 17 qubits in the quantum circuit. The 17 qubits consist of 16 data bits of $4 \times 4$ MNIST digits (down-sampled from $28 \times 28$ pixel images) plus a data label. The bit strings representing the input data are loaded into a qubit register. The method is tested by running a simulation of a quantum device on a classical computer (but could in principle be run on NISQ devices), and in terms of size, could expand from 17 qubits to 40 qubits.

The two approaches are structurally quite similar, encoding classical data into quantum states, processing the data with quantum circuits, and measuring a target qubit with a Pauli (spin) operator at the end. Both teams employ standard machine learning techniques such as stochastic gradient descent (a loss function structure to optimize the learning process). One difference is that Grant *et al.* (2018) provide results from a real-life quantum computer while Farhi and Neven (2018) provide results from the classical simulation of a quantum computer.

The other main difference is that Farhi and Neven (2018) use a standard neural network format and Grant *et al.* (2018) employ a tensor

Table 7.3. Quantum circuit preparation.

| Approach | Data Embedding | Hardware | Data |
|---|---|---|---|
| Quantum neural network | Basis embedding (bit string) | Simulation on classical computer | MNIST (classical) |
| Quantum tensor network | Basis embedding (classical data) and amplitude embedding (quantum data) | IBM QX4 quantum computer | IRIS, MNIST (classical) and self-generated (quantum) |

network format. The tensor network format might offer greater flexibility in testing different configurations of the circuit composition. This is important since many of the steps in running a quantum circuit are fairly straightforward, namely, encoding input data into quantum states, measuring target qubits to obtain results, and repeating to generate high-confidence in the output probability distribution. However, the actual circuit design in terms of the gate set types and order, and parametrization of the unitary transformations to be employed, is much less clear, and tensor networks may offer greater visibility into circuit optimization than neural networks (traditionally a "black box" operation).

## 7.3 How Does Quantum Computing Work?

### 7.3.1 *Input, processing, output, repeat*

#### 7.3.1.1 *Quantum gate logic*

Quantum states are represented as quantum circuits to perform logic operations (Carrasquilla, 2020). This means that quantum states are translated into quantum computations that are written in terms of quantum circuits or logic operations, which are converted into probabilistic circuits (probabilistic gate logic). The quantum circuit is initialized with a simple quantum state, which is evolved into a more complicated quantum state, and measured at the end of the computation.

The theoretical basis for quantum computing is probability (Orus *et al.*, 2019). To produce a quantum circuit, the operation is first written in terms of quantum state language. The quantum state language is then translated into an initial probability distribution. In the computational operation, a sequence of matrix transformations is applied to the initial probability distribution to obtain an ending probability distribution at the conclusion of the computation. For example, the initial quantum state might be represented as a simple tensor product (such as 0 0 0 0). The state could be evolved by applying a sequence of unitary matrices that act on the initial state. The unitary matrices act locally on a few qubits at a time, iteratively repeating and extending the operation. The idea is that the probability distribution corresponding to the quantum state is evolved through time using matrix operations to compute the problem.

The specification of the unitary matrices that are to be applied in the logic gates is about the only aspect of the problem that can be chosen. At the end of the computation, the outcome is measured on a designated qubit.

#### 7.3.1.2 *Setting up a quantum computation*

In quantum computing, the primary task is to design a quantum circuit (an algorithm or sequence of steps) to represent some data, perform some operations on it, and measure the output toward a goal, such as classifying data with labels. This is the usual structure of computation, namely, the three steps of data input, processing, and output.

In quantum computing, the data input is a quantum state. The input data for the problem are packaged into a quantum state, which is the format that can be read by the quantum circuit. The input data are encoded into a quantum state, either a single-qubit state or a multi-qubit state, possibly with entanglement. Once the data have been encoded as a quantum state, the data processing phase consists of a series of unitary operations applied to the initial quantum state. The circuit performs a series of steps called unitary transformations (one by one steps with operators acting on qubits) to advance the computation. These are the logic gates of the computation, carried out with the analogs of classical computation (Boolean gates such as IF, THEN, NOT). All of the classical logic operations can be performed and encoded in the structure of the quantum computation. Finally, a measurement is performed to obtain the result of the logic operation on the data. The main difference with quantum computing is that states cannot be measured along the way, and once the state of a qubit is measured, the computation is over. Hence, there is a fourth step, repetition (repeating the running of the circuit), as many times as necessary to obtain confidence in the probability-distribution output.

In quantum computing, there are many ways to make qubits, however once produced, qubits operate per standard gate logic. The most basic standard gate logic in quantum systems entails the Hadamard gate (which acts on one qubit to put it in a superposition state), the CNOT gate (which acts on two qubits to flip one), and the Toffoli gate (which acts on three or more qubits to implement the Boolean operators). There are many other more complicated gates (Nielsen & Chuang, 2010, pp. xxx–xxxi).

Summarizing, quantum data processing is analogous to classical data processing in that the same primary steps apply, namely, acquiring input data, processing the data per programmed instructions, obtaining a result, and repeating the process as necessary. In quantum computing, the process adds some domain-specific wrinkles. The steps consist of encoding input data into quantum state, processing the operation as a series of unitary operations applied to the initial quantum state, measuring a target qubit, and repeating the process to confirm the result. The biggest unknown and hence a substantial design focus is determining the optimal circuit architecture (gate order) and parametrizations of the unitary operators (Table 7.4).

### 7.3.2 *Step 1: Data encoding (embedding)*

There are two kinds of encoding in quantum computing. There is qubit encoding and data encoding (or more accurately, data embedding). Qubit encoding is producing qubits in the physical system in which the qubits are designated (such as electron spins, photonic polarization, and ion traps). Data encoding is the method by which data are converted or modulated (written) onto qubits for computation. In data encoding, one electron spin rotation, for example, may correspond to one input value. Data encoding may be in a one-to-one relationship with a qubit, or take advantage of the multiple dimensions of the qubit (multiple rotations).

One distinction in data encoding is between basis embedding and amplitude embedding. Farhi and Neven (2018) use basis embedding (for classical data) and Grant *et al.* (2018) use both techniques (for classical and quantum data). Basis encoding is a one-to-one relation of quantum

Table 7.4. Steps in performing a quantum computation.

| No. | Step | Description |
|---|---|---|
| 1 | Acquire data | Encode input data into a quantum state |
| 2 | Process data | Process operation as a series of unitary transformations (one-by-one operations) applied to the initial quantum state |
| 3 | Obtain result | Measure a target qubit (with a Pauli (spin) operator) |
| 4 | Repeat | Repeat to obtain a high-confidence probability distribution |

states with classical bit values. One qubit is used for each data element. Each data element is associated with one qubit, and one state of the qubit, such as one electron spin rotation. The basis embedding method applies to classical data that are in the form of binary strings. The embedded quantum state is the bit-wise translation of a binary string to the corresponding states of the quantum subsystems. An input of 1001, for example, would be represented by the 4-qubit quantum state |1001>.

Amplitude embedding is the other data encoding method, and is applicable to quantum data that are already in a superposition state, or encoding data into a multidimensional state. The multiple dimensions of the data are mapped correspondingly to multiple dimensions of the qubit state, such as multiple amplitude rotations. Data are encoded into the amplitudes of the quantum state. Notably, basis embedding, one-to-one encoding (one qubit for each state), is not a scalable method. Superposition states (instead of devoting a whole qubit to each state) is ultimately a more scalable way of managing classical data, and what give quantum computing the ability to encode exponentially large number of values in a set of qubits. However, at the early stages of development of quantum computing, proof of method is most important, and one-to-one encoding on NISQ platforms is easiest to manage.

#### 7.3.2.1 *Classical data*

Grant *et al.* (2018) describe some of the differences in encoding classical and quantum data (Table 7.5). Input data may be classical or quantum. Whatever the classical data are, they are encoded into a quantum state to be run in the quantum computation. The most straightforward

Table 7.5. Classical and quantum data encoding.

| Data | Input Data [Feature Vectors; Label] | Quantum State Data Encoding |
|---|---|---|
| Classical | $n$-dimensional real-valued input vectors; label | Encode into single-state qubit rotations |
| Quantum | $2^n$-dimensional complex-valued input vectors; label | Encode into superposition states |

implementation is that classical data are written as vectors and each vector element is encoded into a qubit format. Machine learning data are typically already organized and presented in a structural form (feature vector; label) that is conducive to vector representation.

Ultimately, input data vectors are written as a wavefunction (with coefficients indicating the probability of whether a qubit is in the zero or one state) that is ready to use in a quantum algorithm. Classical data are encoded into a quantum state, the quantum format of a wavefunction. Data from classical datasets such as Iris and MNIST are already packaged in such a data vector format that is favorable to machine learning treatment. The data structure is straightforward to encode into the quantum format. In the basic formulation, the data vectors are encoded into a quantum state in a vector-to-qubit encoding method, using $N$ qubits to encode an $N$-dimensional data vector.

#### 7.3.2.2 *Quantum data*

Similar methods apply to quantum data. However, whereas classical data may have $N$-dimensional input vectors that are real numbers, quantum data may have $2^n$-dimensional input vectors that are complex numbers. Quantum data may be in the form of entangled states which are better stored in superposition states (a more efficient quantum state encoding method). For example, a quantum dataset for binary classification may be one in which the data features component is complex numbers of $2^n$-dimensional input vectors of unit length, and the classifier labels term is the usual (0,1) label. Hence, instead of real-valued single-qubit states as with classical data encoding, there are complex-valued quantum amplitudes for quantum data encoding. In contrast to classical data, quantum data (such as the output of another quantum circuit or data received from a quantum sensor) may already be in a superposition state. The quantum states can be brought into the computation directly without additional state preparation required. The point is that classical data may consist of real numbers, and quantum data may be comprised of complex numbers. The potential benefits of quantum computing can be seen in being able to manage the complex numbers of quantum data as compared to the lower-dimensional real numbers of classical data.

### 7.3.3 *Step 2: Data processing*

#### 7.3.3.1 *Circuit architecture*

Data processing refers to the circuit architecture (the design structure of gate logic type and order) and the unitary parametrization (how unitary transformations are to be applied) in the operation of the quantum gates on the quantum state data. A challenge is that guidelines have not yet been established for the type and order of unitary transformations (gate set order) to apply to the qubits in standard variety of computations.

Farhi and Neven (2018) deploy a neural network method based on either random gate selection or restricted gate selection. They obtain essentially sub-par results as compared to other machine learning classification methods, but provide an important proof of demonstration of the quantum circuit simulation method. Grant *et al.* (2018) use tensor networks instead of neural networks as the structure of the machine learning model, which involves eliciting greater structure from the underlying data and produces a hierarchical model for gate selection. Their results are on par with other classification methods. The key difference is that the tensor network structure allows quantum correlations on a particular length scale to be captured at the same layer of the network. The hierarchical model of tensor networks is thereby able to avoid the parametrization problem of random gate selection or arbitrarily restricted gate selection because tensor networks are a more robust structure that naturally incorporates more of the local information in the nearest neighbor relationships in the data.

#### 7.3.3.2 *Unitary parametrization*

The unitary parametrization is how the unitary transformations (linear advances through the computation by one regular unit) are to be set up to operate on quantum state data through the series of quantum logic gates that comprise the quantum circuit. Different unitary parametrizations of the circuit can be implemented on the basis of employing more sophisticated quantum computational formulations. Unitary parametrizations apply similarly to classical data (real-valued numbers) and quantum data (complex-valued numbers).

Grant *et al.* (2018) test an increasing order of gate complexity based on the number of qubits. There are three gate parametrizations with single-qubit rotations and a CNOT gate, standard 2-qubit gates, and 3-qubit gates (with an ancilla qubit for nonlinear operations). The first uses only single-qubit rotations and a fixed CNOT gate. This means that two arbitrary single-qubit rotations are followed by a CNOT gate (which can act to flip the qubit). The structure can be implemented with available quantum computers. The second instantiates standard 2-qubit gates. An arbitrary 2-qubit gate in the general setting requires compilation into hardware-dependent gates in available quantum computers. The third uses 3-qubit gates. The arbitrary 3-qubit gate involves adding an ancilla qubit which can be used for nonlinear operations. The circuit would also need to be compiled in currently available hardware (Table 7.6).

The aim of the table is to indicate that quantum computing is in the early phases of development. The simplest methods are being employed at first (although already elaborate compared to classical computing), with the expectation of becoming more sophisticated over time. Once techniques are proven, and hardware, and possibly error correction methods become available, it would be expected that the complexity of methods, and the types of problems that can be analyzed would grow substantially.

Table 7.6. Qubit gates and unitary parametrizations.

| Qubits | Parametrization | Description | Ease of Implementation |
|---|---|---|---|
| 1 | Single-qubit rotations and a CNOT gate | Two arbitrary single-qubit rotations followed by a CNOT gate (spin-flipping) | Available NISQ devices |
| 2 | Standard 2-qubit gates | General 2-qubit gate model | Requires hardware compilation |
| 3 | 3-qubit gates (one ancilla qubit) | One additional ancilla qubit allows a richer suite of nonlinear operations | Requires hardware compilation |

*Source*: Extended from Grant *et al.* (2018, p. 5).

### 7.3.4 *Steps 3 and 4: Results and repetition*

Measurement is different between classical and quantum computing. In classical computing, measurement samples can be taken any time, and system state and measurement are essentially synonymous. In quantum systems, however, measurement is a distinct concept. Qubits are subject to the no-cloning and no-measurement principles of the quantum domain. Viewing or measuring the qubit changes its state. In quantum computation, measurement collapses the qubit wavefunction to a specific value (one or zero). Therefore, the quantum system cannot be measured during the processing, only at the end, and the system state is obtained by measuring a designated readout qubit. For Farhi and Neven (2018), at the end of the series of gate operation progressions, a measurement is carried out on a target qubit. The measurement is performed on a specific qubit and consists of a simple Pauli (spin) measurement in a chosen direction.

In practice, multiple runs are required to approximate the expectation of the measurement outcome, and the most frequent outcome is taken as the predicted class. Having more runs increases the confidence in the result. The assumption in quantum computing is that the experiment can be repeated many times (hundreds or thousands of times) to obtain confidence in the probabilistic results. For example, if the same quantum message is sent 100 times (in the simplest setup, a zero or a one), and a certain result (say a zero) is obtained in 80% of the measurements, and the other result (a one) obtained in only 20% of the measurements, the conclusion is that it is highly likely that a zero was the value of the qubit sent in the message. The assumption is that the exact quantum state of the experiment can be recreated an arbitrary number of times to obtain confidence in the probabilistic results.

#### 7.3.4.1 *Results measurement with complexity*

Since repetition is a feature of quantum computing, many different permutations can be tested. Ascertaining the accuracy and quality of results is important. A series to tests can be performed to evaluate the accuracy of a circuit's results. Also, different circuits may be compared to see which gate logic structure is more efficient. One way to compare circuits is on the basis of complexity. Complexity is typically assessed as a function of the number of operations required to complete a task. This could be the number of queries to a data source, or the number of multiplications required to perform a task. The computational complexity (the number of unitary transforms or matrix multiplication operations) can be compared for different data encodings and gate logic circuits to see which is the best for a certain measurement outcome.

## 7.4 Advances in Quantum Computing

Some of the major events in the timeline of quantum computing are summarized in Table 7.7. The initial conceptual proposal was by

Table 7.7. Advances in quantum computing.

| No. | Event | Description | Year |
|---|---|---|---|
| *Conceptual proposal* | | | |
| 1 | Universal quantum simulator | Simulate quantum systems directly with quantum molecules | 1982 |
| 2 | Quantum computer | Fully quantum computing model for computation | 1985 |
| *Algorithm development* | | | |
| 3 | Deutsch–Jozsa algorithm | Example of a quantum algorithm being exponentially faster than classical algorithm | 1992 |
| 4 | Shor's algorithm | Efficient quantum factoring algorithm, threat to global cryptography standards | 1997 |
| 5 | Grover's algorithm | Widely applicable search algorithm | 1996 |
| *Experimental demonstrations* | | | |
| 6 | NMR implementation | 7-qubit NMR factorization of the number 15 | 2001 |
| 7 | Optical implementation | Four photonic qubit factorization of the number 15 (tomography-verified) | 2007 |
| 8 | Solid-state superconducting qubits implementation | Nine-element solid-state quantum processor-based factorization of the number 15 (tomography-verified) | 2012 |

Feynman (1982), suggesting that simulating quantum systems with quantum molecules would be more efficient than with classical system. Deutsch then developed the idea into "a general, fully quantum model for computation" (Deutsch, 1985, p. 102). With the concept of quantum computing in mind, algorithms started to be proposed that would take advantage of the unique quantum possibilities of the platform. One of the first examples of a quantum algorithm that is exponentially faster than a classical algorithm is the Deutsch–Jozsa algorithm (Deutsch and Jozsa, 1992).

One of the first events that drew substantial attention to quantum computing was Shor's articulation of a quantum algorithm for factoring large numbers. The algorithm signifies a clear speedup of quantum systems over classical systems, and a potential threat to existing cryptography if implemented (Shor, 1997). Shor's algorithm has two parts, one that casts factoring as the problem of finding the period of a function (which may be implemented classically), and one that finds the period of the function using the quantum Fourier transform (using the superposition capability of a quantum computer to be in multiple states simultaneously). Grover's search algorithm is likewise important, and although does not offer the same exponential speedup, is more widely applicable than Shor's algorithm (Grover, 1996). Grover's quantum search algorithm finds a particular register in an unordered database within a certain number of steps. Some of the first experimental demonstrations of quantum algorithms occurred in the 1990s.

Early work (Beckman *et al.*, 1996) suggested that a proof-of-principle demonstration of quantum factoring (factorization of 15) might be performed with only six trapped ions and 38 laser pulses. An initial implementation of Shor's algorithm was shown by a team at IBM using a 7-qubit nuclear magnetic resonance (NMR) system, factoring 15 into 3 × 5 (Vandersypen *et al.*, 2001). (The Deutsch–Jozsa algorithm and Grover's algorithm were likewise demonstrated elsewhere). Two optical demonstrations followed, both using four photonic qubits with linear optical equipment to factor the number 15 (Lu *et al.*, 2007) and confirming the results with tomography (Lanyon *et al.*, 2007). Both relied on the ability to generate entanglement between qubits by coherent application of a series of quantum gates.

In the experimental setup for Lu *et al.* (2007), femtosecond laser pulses pass through specialized crystals (Beta-barium borate) to produce two pairs of entangled photons. Polarizers are used to disentangle the photons and prepare them into quantum states denoting spatial modes. The photons pass through half-wave plates and are superposed on the polarizing beam splitter to implement the necessary single-qubit and 2-qubit gates. To ensure good spatial and temporal overlap, the photons are spectrally filtered and coupled by single-mode fibers. The final measurement results are read out using polarizers and single-photon detectors. Lucero *et al.* (2012) were among the first to factor the number 15 using Shor's algorithm using a nine-element quantum processor with Josephson junctions (solid-state qubits).

## 7.5 Unitary Transformation

The basic format of quantum computing is encoding data into circuits, performing unitary transformations, and measuring the result. A unitary transformation is the application of the unitary operator to evolve a quantum system forward by one linear step. Mathematically, a unitary transformation is the application of certain linear algebra matrix operations. A unitary transformation is not only the most basic step forward allowed in evolving a quantum system but also has deep philosophical roots as a concept in quantum mechanics.

- *Unitary*: Adjective: a system or state whose evolution is by the unit operator (advancing linearly by one regular unit); Noun: synonym for unit operator, unitary operator (a unitary = a unitary operator).
- *Unit operator or unitary operator*: Standard quantum mechanical system evolution operator, acting to advance a quantum system linearly by one regular unit, preserving inner products in Hilbert space.
- *Unitarity*: System property of the time evolution of a quantum state according to the Schrödinger equation as mathematically represented by a unitary operator.
- *Unitary matrix*: An $n \times n$ complex square matrix whose conjugate transpose is also its inverse, and both are equal to the identity matrix (matrix $U$ is unitary if $U^*U = UU^* = I$).

- *Identity matrix*: An $n \times n$ square matrix with ones on the main diagonal and zeros elsewhere (the main diagonal runs top left to bottom right); a primitive used in matrix operations.
- *Unitary transformation*: Application of the unitary operator to evolve a quantum system forward by one linear step.

A postulate of quantum physics is that quantum evolution is unitary. Unitary means by units, that a quantum system or state can only advance linearly by one regular unit (Susskind & Friedman, 2014, p. 98). The unit operator ("unitary operator" or simply "unitary") acts to perform the state evolution, preserving the inner products in Hilbert space. In a quantum system, movement can only occur in discrete unit-sized changes, any change is in the size of the basic unit (advancing one step at a time, not two steps or 1.3 steps). In quantum physics, unitarity is the condition that the time evolution of a quantum state proceeds according to the Schrödinger equation, as represented by a unitary operator.

With linear algebra, the unitary operator acts on the unitary matrix to perform the transform. The unitary matrix is an $n \times n$ complex square matrix whose conjugate transpose is also its inverse, and both are equal to the Identity matrix (matrix $U$ is unitary if $U^*U = UU^* = I$). The implication is that many transformations are possible given the structural equivalence of the matrix properties. The identity matrix is an even simpler matrix primitive, an $n \times n$ square matrix with ones on the main diagonal and zeros elsewhere (the main diagonal runs top left to bottom right). The unitary structure sets up well-formedness in quantum computing.

## References

Beckman, D., Chari, A.N., Devabhaktuni, S. & Preskill, J. (1996). Efficient networks for quantum factoring. *Phys. Rev. A*. 54(2):1034–63.

Biamonte, J., Wittek, P., Pancotti, N. *et al.* (2017). Quantum machine learning. *Nature*. 549(195):195–202.

Carrasquilla, J. (2020). Machine learning for quantum matter. *Adv. Phys. X*. 5(1):1797528.

Deutsch, D. (1985). Quantum theory, the Church-Turing principle and the universal quantum computer. *Proc. Roy. Soc. London A*. 400:97–117.

Deutsch, D. & Jozsa, R. (1992). Rapid solutions of problems by quantum computation. *Proc. Roy. Soc. London A*. 439(1907):553–58.

Farhi, E. & Neven, H. (2018). Classification with quantum neural networks on near term processors. arXiv:1802.06002. MIT-CTP/4985.

Feynman, R.P. (1982). Simulating physics with computers. *Int. J. Theor. Phys.* 21(6):467–88.

Flamini, F., Spagnolo, N. & Sciarrino, F. (2018). Photonic quantum information processing: A review. *Rep. Prog. Phys.* 82(1):016001.

Grant, E., Benedetti, M., Cao, S. *et al.* (2018). Hierarchical quantum classifiers. *NPJ Quantum Inf.* 4(1):1–8.

Grover, L.K. (1996). A fast quantum mechanical algorithm for database search. In *Proceedings of the Twenty-eighth Annual ACM Symposium on Theory of Computing. STOC '96*. Association for Computing Machinery: Philadelphia, Pennsylvania, USA, May 22–24, 1996, pp. 212–19.

Lanyon, B.P., Weinhold, T.J., Langford, N.K. *et al.* (2007). Experimental demonstration of a compiled version of Shor's algorithm with quantum entanglement. *Phys. Rev. Lett.* 99(25):250505.

Lu, C.-Y., Browne, D.E., Yang, T. & Pan, J.-W. (2007). Demonstration of a compiled version of Shor's quantum factoring algorithm using photonic qubits. *Phys. Rev. Lett.* 99(25):250504.

Lucero, E., Barends, R., Chen, Y. *et al.* (2012). Computing prime factors with a Josephson phase qubit quantum processor. *Nat. Phys.* 8(10):719.

Nielsen, M.A. & Chuang, I.L. (2010). *Quantum Computation and Quantum Information*. 10th-Anniversary Edition. Cambridge: Cambridge University Press.

Orus, R., Mugel, S. & Lizaso, E. (2019). Quantum computing for finance: Overview and prospects. *Rev. Phys.* 4(10):100028.

Schumacher, B. (1995). Quantum coding. *Phys. Rev. A*. 51(4):2738–47.

Shor, P.W. (1997). Polynomial-time algorithms for prime factorization and discrete logarithms on a quantum computer. *SIAM J. Comput.* 26:1484–509.

Susskind, L. & Friedman, A. (2014). *Quantum Mechanics: The Theoretical Minimum*. New York: Basic Books.

Vandersypen, L.M.K., Steffen, M., Breyta, G. *et al.* (2001). Experimental realization of Shor's quantum factoring algorithm using nuclear magnetic resonance. *Nature*. 414(6866):883–87.

# Chapter 8

# Glia Neurotransmitter Synaptome

*Given that glial cells associated with synapses integrate neuronal inputs and can release transmitters that modulate synaptic activity, it is time to rethink our understanding of the wiring diagram of the nervous system*

— Haydon (2001, p. 185)

**Abstract**

This chapter discusses neural signaling models that progress beyond those that are primarily focused on electrical action potentials, to a broader picture that also includes the action of glial cells, neurotransmitters, and synapse proteins. The connectome and the synaptome could be the "killer applications" of quantum computing for the brain. The connectome is the wiring diagram of all neural connections in the brain, and the synaptome is the similar map for synapses.

## 8.1 Glial Cells

Glia (glial cells) are nonneuronal cells in the central and peripheral nervous system that maintain homeostasis, form myelin, and provide support and protection for neurons. It is now recognized that glia are more central to brain functioning than was previously thought (Fields, 2009). First, glia have an active role in neural signaling and synapse formation and operation. Second, glia have their own calcium signaling system, with each astrocyte wrapping around more than 100,000 synapses, tiling out to cover the whole-brain in a nonoverlapping manner, and responding more slowly than electrical signaling but having greater reach. Third, glia are implicated in pathology management as astrocytes and oligodendrocytes phagocytose (engulf) unhealthy neurons. Fourth, it has been shown experimentally that neurons cannot survive without astrocytes (Jakel & Dimou, 2017). Composite models of neural signaling necessarily include both electrical action potentials and glial calcium signaling, both of which are amenable to quantum platforms as wavefunctions.

There are about as many glia as neurons, an estimated 85 billion glia and 86 billion neurons in the human brain[1] (Herculano-Houzel, 2009). There are three main kinds of glia in the central nervous system (Table 8.1). Oligodendrocytes are generally thought to be the most numerous (45–75%), followed by astrocytes (19–40%) and microglia (about 10%) (von Bartheld *et al.*, 2016, p. 11). Corroborating research finds oligodendrocytes to be the most numerous glial cells in the mouse brain with an absolute number of 17.4 million and a proportion of 40% of glia (Valerio-Gomes *et al.*, 2018). As oligodendrocytes and astrocytes both have large populations, research also often cites astrocytes as the most abundant glial cells in the mammalian brain (Allen & Eroglu, 2017).

Oligodendrocytes myelinate axons. Each oligodendrocyte may extend myelin sheaths to as many as 50 axons, and has the capacity to renew

Table 8.1. Central nervous system glial cells.

| Glial Cells | Percentage | Function |
|---|---|---|
| Oligodendrocytes | 45–75% | Provide myelination to insulate axons |
| Astrocytes | 19–40% | Calcium signaling, neurotransmitter recycling |
| Microglia | 10–20% | Destroy pathogens, phagocytose debris |
| Ependymal cells | Low | Cerebrospinal fluid and the blood-brain barrier |
| Radial glia | Low | Neuroepithelial development and neurogenesis |

[1] The implied one-to-one relationship between neurons and glia varies by brain region. In the cerebral cortex, the overall ratio is 3.72, and for gray matter 1.48. The cerebellum has only 0.23 neurons to glia, whereas the basal ganglia, diencephalon, and brainstem regions have a ratio of 11.35 to 1 (Azevedo *et al.*, 2009).

myelin sheaths three times per day (Peferoen *et al.*, 2013, p. 302). The oligodendrocyte sends out paddle-shaped extensions that wrap around the axon membrane and form sheaths that are approximately 1 mm in length. The next form of glia is the astrocytes which participate in calcium signaling, create and dismantle synapses, recycle neurotransmitters, and otherwise maintain homeostasis in the central nervous system. The third type is microglia which are the immune system of the brain.

### 8.1.1 *Astrocyte calcium signaling*

Far from being merely "glue" as the name derivation suggests, glial cells are essential to active brain operation. Astrocytes in particular, are central to neural signaling, as they are implicated in synaptogenesis, neuronal transmission, and synaptic plasticity. During disease and injury, astrocytes efficiently protect neurons by various means, including by sealing them off from neurotoxic factors and by repairing the blood–brain barrier. Initially, astrocytes were considered to be passive supporters of neurons, with metabolic support, neurotransmitter precursors, and ion buffering, however, neural signaling cannot proceed without astrocytes.

#### 8.1.1.1 *Tripartite synapse*

Given the active role of astrocytes in neural signaling, the notion of the "tripartite synapse" is proposed to describe the synapse as two neurons and an astrocyte as a functional unit (Araque *et al.*, 1999). Although synaptic activity was recorded over a century ago using electrophysiology, it was not until the 1950s with development of electron microscopy that more detailed synapse structures could be visualized in greater detail. It was then discovered that neuronal synapses are not just composed of presynaptic and postsynaptic neurons, but in many cases are also contacted by an astrocyte process (Farhy-Tselnicker & Allen, 2018).

In a tripartite synapse, the neurotransmitters released from neurons also bind to receptors on adjacent astrocytes, activating signaling pathways in the astrocytes which modulate synaptic behavior. Astrocytes regulate synapses by direct contact, and by secreting soluble factors (gliotransmitters) that target presynaptic and postsynaptic sites, thereby modulating the structure and function of both excitatory and inhibitory synapses. In addition to contacting neurons, astrocytes are interconnected with each other by gap junctions, specialized channels which allow nutrients and ions to diffuse between networks of astrocytes. Such communication further expands the range and magnitude of synaptic regulation of neurons by astrocytes.

#### 8.1.1.2 *Astrocyte tiling: Nonoverlapping territories*

A prominent organizational feature of astrocytes is that they spread out across the brain into nonoverlapping territories. Astrocytes avoid interfering with processes from neighboring cells by tiling themselves out in a process that results in a volume overlap of only 4–6% between adjacent astrocytes (Bushong *et al.* 2002). In the mature brain, the processes of astrocytes extensively infiltrate into the neural structure and wrap around synapses. In this way, astrocytes completely parcel out the gray matter in a nonoverlapping manner, forming separate anatomical domains. A single mouse cortical astrocyte is estimated to contact over 100,000 synapses, whereas a human astrocyte can contact up to 2,000,000 synapses (Oberheim *et al.*, 2009). These observations suggest that astrocytes, through their detailed processes, have the ability to sense and adhere to synapses and coordinate with neighboring astrocytes to completely cover the neural architecture (Allen & Eroglu, 2017).

In healthy functioning, astrocytes are shaped like sponge-like cells, each covering a distinct territory in the central nervous system. However, Grosche *et al.* (2013) find that there is an age-related increase in the territorial volumes of astrocytes that leads to loss of the strict organization in nonoverlapping territories. The resulting reactive gliosis has been proposed to affect to age-related pathologies such as Alzheimer's disease and amyotrophic lateral sclerosis.

#### 8.1.1.3 *Astrocyte signaling: Calcium operations*

Calcium signaling is implicated in neural signaling both in connection with action potentials and in the calcium-based signaling network with other astrocytes. The main way that calcium signaling is recognized in neural signaling is when an action potential induces the opening of calcium ion channels in the presynaptic terminal wall. This leads to the propagation of calcium ion transients through the terminal and influences a chain of operations to produce synaptic vesicle exocytosis, disgorging neurotransmitters into the synaptic cleft (Sudhof, 2004).

What is new is the understanding of the vast calcium-signaling networks of astrocytes, on an intracellular (within the astrocyte) and extracellular (among astrocytes) basis. Calcium signals are the universal response of astrocytes to various forms of stimulation. Astrocytes express numerous receptors and ion channels linked to the generation of a variety of complex cytoplasmic calcium responses. The increases in calcium levels experienced by individual glial cells can propagate across large distances in the form of calcium waves.

Calcium can propagate over greater distances than electric action potentials. The mechanism of propagation involves both intracellular and extracellular signals (via inositol and ATP, respectively). Inositol diffusion through gap junctions is important for short-range wave propagation, whereas ATP is more relevant for propagation across larger distances (Haydon, 2001). Further, calcium waves propagate directly or indirectly, directly through gap junction channels, and indirectly by releasing gliotransmitters that activate membrane receptors on neighboring cells. The major target of calcium signaling is extracellular plasma membrane proteins, but there are also many intracellular targets (Scemes & Giaume, 2006, p. 18) (Table 8.2).

Extracellular glial calcium waves produce a signaling pathway between glial cells. These spontaneous waves are propagated by ATP release. Glial calcium elevation can lead to the release of glutamate, ATP, and D-serine, altering synaptic efficacy and neuronal excitability. Glial calcium elevations also trigger the release of arachidonic acid metabolites that regulate blood vessel diameter (Kurth-Nelson *et al.*, 2009).

The calcium signals propagated by glial cells create a spreading wave of calcium ions ($Ca^{2+}$) which allows information exchange within cellular networks. The propagating calcium waves are primarily mediated by intracellular excitable media formed by calcium storage organelles within the glia. The glial calcium signals can be evoked by neuronal activity, and vice versa, they may also initiate electrical and calcium-based responses

Table 8.2. Astrocyte calcium signaling targets.

| No. | Target Location | Description | Reach |
|---|---|---|---|
| 1 | Plasma membrane proteins | Metabotropic receptors | Extracellular |
| 2 | Plasma membrane proteins | $K^+$ ($Ca^{2+}$) channels | Extracellular |
| 3 | Plasma membrane proteins | $Na^+/Ca^{2+}$ exchanger | Extracellular |
| 4 | Plasma membrane proteins | $Ca^{2+}$-ATPase | Extracellular |
| 5 | Intracellular membrane proteins | Phospholipases | Intracellular |
| 6 | Endoplasmic reticulum | Inositol-trisphosphate receptors | Intracellular |
| 7 | Cytoskeleton elements | Actin turnover proteins | Intracellular |
| 8 | Enzymes | Calcium-dependent effectors | Intracellular |
| 9 | Vesicles (gliotransmitter) | Glutamate | Intracellular |
| 10 | Gap junction channels | Same targets in neighboring cells | Extracellular |

Table 8.3. Astrocytes control the synapse life cycle.

| No. | Synapse Phase | Astrocyte-secreted Molecules and Receptors |
|---|---|---|
| 1 | Structural formation | Thrombospondins (TSPs) and hevin (both synaptogenic) |
| 2 | Functional formation | Glypican (synaptogenic) and SPARC (negative regulator) |
| 3 | Elimination | TGF-b and MERTK/MEGF10 receptor-based phagocytosis |

in adjacent neurons. Glial calcium signals thus are able to integrate glial and neuronal compartments and are therefore involved in the information processing in the brain (Deitmer *et al.*, 1998). The sequential activation of neighboring astrocytes occurs during the spreading of the calcium wave.

#### 8.1.1.4 *Astrocytes and synapse formation*

Astrocytes are also noted for their important coordination role with synapses. Astrocytes are involved in the structural formation, the functional formation, and the elimination of synapses by secreting a variety of targeted synaptogenic and then later phagocytosis-related molecules (Allen & Eroglu, 2017, p. 700) (Table 8.3).

### 8.1.2 *Glia and neuropathology*

Glia are implicated in several immune system and neuropathology functions. Although microglia are the brain's primary immune system, oligodendrocytes and astrocytes also participate in immune response, and all three cell types are in communication with each other and neurons to coordinate this response. For example, in diseases involving autoimmune attacks on myelin such as multiple sclerosis, oligodendrocytes, in conjunction with their responsibilities for myelinating axons, take on related immune system responsibilities, in communication with microglia (Falcao *et al.*, 2018).

In neurodegenerative pathologies such as Alzheimer's disease, when a neuron goes into apoptosis (cell death), microglia and astrocytes act in concert to dispatch it (Damisah *et al.*, 2020). Microglia, as the main immune system in the brain, phagocytose the soma (cell body). Astrocytes, already wrapped around synapses for signaling purposes, are thus close to the dendritic arbors, and absorb the dendrites of the phagocytosed neuron. Both types of phagocytosis (soma and dendrite) require the receptor *Mertk* to be expressed for the operation, which the microglia and the astrocyte can recognize and take action. However, because there are a number of failures of function in aging and unhealthy brains that produce inflammation (or "inflamm-aging" (Franceschi *et al.*, 2000)), microglia can be triggered to engulf living cells by mistake (Brown & Vilalta, 2015). Glia malfunction in phagocytosing declining but still living cells is not yet understood or remedied (Fakhoury, 2018; Gomes-Leal, 2019).

In the case of stroke, all three of the main glial cells are involved. In minor stroke, astrocytes repair damage and provide energy to neurons by breaking down stored glycogen to generate lactate. In the acute phase of stroke, astrocytes reduce damage through the uptake of glutamate and potassium, and by scavenging reactive oxygen species. In severe stroke, astrocytes themselves die which causes glutamate to be released due to membrane depolarization, which can lead to excitotoxicity (overstimulation, too much excitatory stimulation). This excitotoxicity can in turn lead to oligodendrocyte death as oligodendrocytes have a high metabolic rate and are particularly sensitive to excitotoxicity. In stroke recovery, astrocytes release neuroprotective agents such as erythropoietin and vascular endothelial growth factor (VEGF). Microglia are activated by damaged neurons in stroke to phagocytose debris and secrete pro-inflammatory cytokines (Scimemi, 2018).

## 8.2 Neurotransmitters and Chemical Signaling

### 8.2.1 *Glutamate (excitatory) and GABA (inhibitory)*

Neurotransmitters are chemicals used by neurons to send signals across the synaptic cleft. In the human brain, about 80% of synapses are excitatory and 20% inhibitory (Xu *et al.*, 2016). Further, glutamate (excitatory) and GABA (inhibitory) are the prominent neurotransmitters, activated in 90% of synapses in the human brain (Sapolsky, 2005, pp. 13–14). Other important neurotransmitters include acetylcholine, adrenaline, dopamine, serotonin, histamine, and melatonin, and over 200 have been discovered.

Neurotransmitters are stored in synaptic vesicles near the cell membrane in the presynaptic terminal of the sending neuron. When needed, neurotransmitters are released into the 20 nm wide synaptic cleft, where they bind to specific receptors on the membrane of the postsynaptic neuron. The synapses on the receiving neuron are either excitatory or inhibitory, and have different shapes and locations. Excitatory synapses are located prominently on the edges of dendritic spines, whereas inhibitory synapses are located on the shaft of the spines closer to the path to the cell body. The locational setup is so that the inhibitory synapses can serve as a block or brake to modulate excitatory signals if necessary on their way from the dendritic arbors to the cell's body.

The mechanism of action is that neurotransmitters bind to the dendrites on the receiving neuron, influencing the membrane in either an excitatory way by depolarizing it, or in an inhibitory way by repolarizing it. Nerve cells have a resting potential characterized by the inside of the cell being negative with respect to the outside (extracellular) solution by a little less than a tenth of a volt. Incoming excitatory signals depolarize the cell membrane, making the inside less negative, and creating a membrane potential called an excitatory postsynaptic potential (EPSP). Inhibitory signals hyperpolarize the cell membrane, making it more negative, and creating a membrane potential called an inhibitory postsynaptic potential (IPSP). Thus, incoming neurotransmitters act to increase (excitatory) or decrease (inhibitory) the transmembrane ion flow contributing to the probability that the receiving cell ultimately produces an action potential.

Neurotransmitters are central to the operation of the brain. Astrocytes (glial cells) constantly recycle glutamate and GABA. Neurons must rely on astrocytes as they are not able to synthesize glutamate directly (since they do not have the enzyme pyruvate carboxylase). About 15% of glutamate results from *de novo* synthesis and the rest from recycling (Hampe *et al.*, 2018, p. 67). Glutamatergic and GABAergic imbalances are implicated in a variety of neurological diseases related to epilepsy, autism spectrum disorders, and anxiety disorders (van Veenendaal *et al.*, 2018).

One classificatory mechanism for neurotransmitters is by size (Table 8.4). There are only a few large amino acid neurotransmitters, for example, glutamate and aspartate (excitatory), and GABA and glycine (inhibitory). Acetylcholine is the third most important neurotransmitter after glutamate and GABA as a general alert system that increases the probability of presynaptic neurotransmitter release and has either excitatory or inhibitory action. Most neurotransmitters are small molecules

Table 8.4. Neurotransmitter classes.

| Neurotransmitter Class | | Stimulus | |
|---|---|---|---|
| Type | Neurotransmitter | Excitatory | Inhibitory |
| | Glutamate | X | — |
| Large amino | Aspartate | X | — |
| acids | GABA | — | X |
| | Glycine | — | X |
| Other | Acetylcholine | X | X |
| | Dopamine | X | — |
| Small molecules | Norepinephrine | — | X |
| (monoamines) | Epinephrine | X | — |
| | Histamine | X | — |
| | Serotonin | X | X |

(single amino acids) such as dopamine, norepinephrine, histamine, and serotonin. Small molecule neurotransmitters may have both excitatory and inhibitory action (such as serotonin), or one or the other. Examples of small molecule neurotransmitters are noradrenaline (signaling a stress response) and dopamine (activating the reward system).

Another classificatory mechanism for neurotransmitters is whether they are either ionotropic (complicated) or metabotropic (less complicated). Both classes operate by binding to transmembrane-based receptors on the receiving neuron. Ionotropic neurotransmitters cause an ion channel to open in the receiving membrane, and the less powerful metabotropic neurotransmitters trigger a signaling cascade within the receiving cells (by coupling to G-proteins). The major neurotransmitters, glutamate and GABA, tend to use ionotropic receptors, and small molecules such as dopamine and noradrenaline use metabotropic receptors coupled to G-proteins (Nicholls *et al.*, 2012, p. 185). With its priority as an alert system, acetylcholine makes use of both uses both ionotropic and metabotropic binding mechanisms.

### 8.2.2 *Neurotransmitter transport*

The primary orchestration point of neurotransmitters is the presynaptic terminal. In addition to transporting inorganic ions, nerve cells have mechanisms for accumulating a variety of other substances, including those involved in synaptic transmission. Inside a neuron, neurotransmitters are transported into organelles within the cytoplasm of presynaptic nerve terminals (synaptic vesicles), where they are stored to be ready for release. After release, neurotransmitters (e.g. glutamate, GABA, norepinephrine, serotonin, and glycine) are recovered from the synaptic cleft by transporters in the plasma membranes of either the terminals themselves or adjacent glial cells. Neurotransmitter recovery processes involve transport mechanisms that use energy from the movement of sodium, potassium, or hydrogen ions down their electrochemical gradients to power transmitter accumulation. The two main types of neurotransmitter trafficking are transport from the neuron's cytoplasm into presynaptic vesicles, and neurotransmitter transmitter uptake from the synaptic cleft (intercellular medium) into the neuron cytoplasm.

### 8.2.2.1 *Transport into presynaptic vesicles: Proton gradient*

Neurotransmitters are synthesized in the presynaptic terminal cytoplasm and taken up (with endocytosis) into concentrations in presynaptic vesicles by transport mechanisms coupled to proton outflow. The transport mechanism is analogous to sodium-driven transport across the plasma membrane (used by action potentials). However, instead of a sodium gradient, a proton gradient is used (established by the transport of hydrogen ions from the cytoplasm into the vesicle by hydrogen ATPase). Three solute carrier (SLC) genetic families of proton-coupled transporters manage this process and are expressed in the lipid bilayers of secretory vesicles (*SLC17*, *SLC18*, and *SLC32*) (Table 8.5).

### 8.2.2.2 *Molecular economy*

The family of solute carrier (SLC) proteins has different forms, each of which is related to transporters that are responsible for accumulating specific neurotransmitters in vesicles. The *SLC17* protein, for example, is associated with the VGLUT1 transporter (vesicle glutamate transporter) and orchestrates glutamate. The membrane transport process is accomplished through an economy of molecular exchange. The molecular exchange ratio (stoichiometry) varies. For *SLC17*-managed transport of the excitatory neurotransmitter Glutamate, the ratio is one Hydrogen ATPase proton for one Glutamate molecule transport plus one chloride

Table 8.5. Neurotransmitter transport into vesicles.

| No. | Gene | Transporter | Neurotransmitter | Molecular Exchange Ratio |
|---|---|---|---|---|
| 1 | *SLC18* | VMAT1,2 | Norepinephrine, dopamine, serotonin | Two hydrogen ATPase protons for one monoamine or acetylcholine molecule |
| 2 | *SLC18* | VAChT | Acetylcholine | |
| 3 | *SLC32* | VGAT VIAAT | GABA, glycine | One hydrogen ATPase proton for one GABA or glycine molecule |
| 4 | *SLC17* | VGLUT1,2,3 | Glutamate | One hydrogen ATPase proton for one glutamate molecule transport plus one chloride molecule |

*Source*: Adapted from Nicholls *et al.* (2012, p. 151).

molecule. In other operations, for *SLC18*-facilitated transport, two Hydrogen ATPase protons are exchanged for one monoamine or acetylcholine molecule. For *SLC32*-related transport of inhibitory neurotransmitters GABA and glycine, the ratio is one Hydrogen ATPase proton for one GABA or glycine molecule.

#### 8.2.2.3 *Transmitter uptake from cleft: Sodium gradient*

The same kinds of processes of endocytosis are at work in neurotransmitter recycling from the synaptic cleft, involving neurotransmitter uptake from the intercellular medium to the neuron's cytoplasm. Once released from presynaptic nerve terminals into the synaptic cleft, most neurotransmitters are recovered either by the nerve terminals themselves or by adjacent glial cells. In general, such recovery serves two purposes. First, the neurotransmitter is removed from the extracellular space in the region of the synapse, which helps to terminate its synaptic action and prevents diffusion to other synaptic regions. Second, the neurotransmitter molecules recovered by the nerve terminal can be packaged again for future release. All synaptic uptake mechanisms use the electrochemical gradient for sodium to carry transmitter substances across the plasma membrane into the cytoplasm.

Two major transmitter uptake families are expressed in the cell membranes of neurons and glial cells. The *SLC1* family mediates the uptake of glutamate and neutral amino acids, and the *SLC6* family is responsible for the uptake of dopamine, serotonin, norepinephrine, glycine, and GABA. Again, each family has different forms, related transporters, and molecular exchange ratios. In the *SLC1* system, the inward transport of one glutamate ion is coupled to the influx of two sodium ions and the efflux of one potassium ion, coupled with either the extrusion of an hydroxyl ion or influx of a proton. In the *SLC6* system, the molecular exchange ratio for the uptake of each transmitter molecule is accompanied by the entry of two sodium and one chloride ion (Table 8.6).

The *SLC1* family includes several high-affinity glutamate transporters (EAAT: Excitatory amino acid transporter) for glutamate uptake. The *SLC6* family includes transporters for GABA (GAT: GABA transporter) and small molecule neurotransmitters. Both neurons and glia express transporters and participate in the neurotransmitter recovery operation.

Table 8.6. Neurotransmitter uptake from synaptic cleft.

| No. | Gene | Transporter | Neurotransmitter | Molecular Exchange Ratio |
|---|---|---|---|---|
| 1 | *SLC1* | EAAT1, EAAT2–5 | Glutamate | One $K^+$ and one $OH^-$ for one glutamate and two sodium |
| 2 | *SLC6* | GAT1,2 | GABA | One GABA, glycine, or monoamine molecule coupled to two sodium and one chloride molecule |
| 3 | | NET | Norepinephrine | |
| 4 | | DAT | Dopamine | |
| 5 | | SERT | Serotonin | |
| 6 | | GLYT1,2 | Glycine | |

*Source*: Redrawn from Nicholls *et al.* (2012, p. 151).

## 8.3 Synaptome

Although synapse proteome analysis most often focuses on postsynaptic proteins (and excitatory synapses as 80% of the brain's synapses are excitatory), presynaptic proteins are also of interest as more than 1,000 proteins function in the presynaptic nerve terminal, and hundreds are thought to participate in exocytosis (Sudhof, 2004, p. 510).

### 8.3.1 *Genome, connectome, and synaptome*

The synaptome is a map of all the brain's different synapses and the synaptosome is the synapse proteome, a list of all of the proteins that are used at the synapses in the brain (DeFelipe, 2010). The connectome is the wiring diagram of the neural connections in the brain, and the synaptome the similar map of synapses. A standard resource is the Mouse Lifespan Synaptome Atlas for the investigation of synapse function across all brain regions during the full lifespan of the mouse (Gokhale *et al.*, 2020). The synapse proteome is dynamic and changes during the lifespan, including indicating various biomarkers of the neuropathologies of aging.

The synaptome is one of latest "omics" fields (high-throughput analysis to characterize the entirety of a biological phenomenon) in the progression that includes genomics, connectomics, and synaptomics (Table 8.7). Genes encode the proteins used at synapses. The genome is all of the genetic material of an organism, and genomics aims at mapping the

Table 8.7. Brain "omics" fields.

| Field | Focus | Definition |
|---|---|---|
| Genome | Genes | All genetic material of an organism |
| Connectome | Neurons | All neural connections in the brain |
| Synaptome | Synapses | All synapses in the brain and their proteins |

chromosome location and function of each gene (Winkler, 1920). The connectome is a comprehensive map of the neural connections in the brain (a wiring diagram) (Hagmann, 2005; Sporns *et al.*, 2005). The synaptome is the description and mapping of the set of synapses in the brain, and the synaptosome their proteins (DeFelipe, 2010; Barker *et al.*, 1972).

#### 8.3.1.1 *Quantum computing-level complexity*

Synapse proteome analysis is a combinatorially complex problem as there are an estimated $2^{n-1}$ types of synapses arising from $n$ proteins (Grant, 2019a, p. 221). The possibility space is such that even 50 proteins (less than 5% of the 1,000 proteins in the synapse proteome) could potentially generate more types of synapses than there are total synapses in the human brain; 500 trillion ($5 \times 10^{14}$) possible synapses versus 242 trillion total estimated synapses (Martins *et al.*, 2019). The combinatorial complexity of synapse proteins and their structure as a $2^n$ problem immediately suggests the need for quantum computing as an analysis platform.

#### 8.3.1.2 *Synapse proteome and neuropathology*

In the human brain, about 80% of synapses are excitatory and 20% inhibitory (Xu *et al.*, 2016). Over 133 brain diseases are caused by mutations that disrupt gene encoding in the proteome of excitatory synapses in the postsynaptic density (Bayes *et al.*, 2011). Human genome sequencing applied to brain disorders indicates that synapse proteins have a larger impact on neuropathology than other brain proteins. The work isolates the postsynaptic density from the human neocortex and identifies 1,461 proteins. Human postsynaptic density mutations cause 133 diseases, 80%

affecting the central nervous system and 20% affecting the peripheral nervous system. The diseases are classified according to the clinical rubric of the International Classification of Disease (ICD-10). Four of the 22 classifications concern common neurodegenerative diseases (such as Alzheimer's, Parkinson's, and Huntington's). A synaptomic theory of brain disease has been proposed (Grant, 2019b).

### 8.3.2 *Mouse synaptome: Aging pathologies*

The first whole-brain synaptome was reported in 2018 by the Grant laboratory (Zhu *et al.*, 2018). The protein composition and morphological features of one billion individual synapses across all regions of the mouse brain were consolidated as a standardized resource. Notably, the synapse proteome is highly complex with over 1,000 conserved proteins.

Earlier work (Grant, 2007), proposed a molecular catalogue of synapses, and that synapse proteome markers could be biomarkers of aging. Further, the standard purified synaptome could be a laboratory resource, having synaptomes with identical proteomes in limitless amounts to test disease scenarios as a clonal population of uniform cells (the "clonal synapse"). Two different clonal synapse preparations, for example, could show a different signature of protein marker expression (e.g. excitatory glutamatergic synapse and inhibitory GABA synapse).

In follow-on work, the team further analyzes the molecular diversity and spatiotemporal architecture of five billion excitatory synapses at single-synapse resolution across the whole-brain mouse synaptome from birth to old age (Cizeron *et al.*, 2020). The key finding is that synapse composition in all brain regions changes during the course of a lifespan. Synaptome changes can be divided into three epochs that correspond to childhood and adolescence, early adulthood, and late adulthood. Synapse diversity expands between birth and early adulthood, differentiating brain regions, and then changes in synapse composition progressively dedifferentiate brain regions in old age. The resulting lifespan synaptome architecture indicates factors that can modify the expression of synaptic proteins (such as genetic mutation, inflammation, and pharmaceutical intervention). The work is consolidated into a Mouse Lifespan Synaptome Atlas to provide standard lifespan trajectories of various behavioral changes, psychological functions, and gene mutations that can lead to synaptic pathology in certain brain areas at certain ages.

#### 8.3.2.1 *Three phases of development, stability, and decline*

Using synaptome mapping, the work investigates excitatory synapse diversity through two leading postsynaptic scaffold proteins (PSD95 and SAP102), identifying spatiotemporal synaptome architecture in mice from birth until 18 months of age. Synapses are classified into three types, those that express PSD95, SAP102, or both, and 37 synaptome subtypes are defined on the basis of molecular and morphological features. Data are examined in 109 anatomical subregions within 12 overarching regions (isocortex, olfaction, hippocampus, cortical subplate, striatum, pallidum, thalamus, hypothalamus, midbrain, pons, medulla, and cerebellum).

Each subtype shows a unique anatomical expression pattern across the brain. The spatiotemporal lifespan trajectories of PSD95 and SAP102 puncta (point) density, intensity, and size are plotted as graphs and heatmaps to explore characteristic patterns at three scales, the whole-brain, the 12 regions, and the 109 subregions. Lifespan changes occur in three phases. During the first phase (from birth to one month old), the numbers of puncta increased rapidly. The second phase began as the rate of increase in puncta density slowed and was characterized by relative stability until six months (adulthood). The third phase, late adult life, was characterized by a decline in puncta density and an increase in synapse size.

#### 8.3.2.2 *Synapse diversity and plasticity*

The second finding regarding synapse diversity is that there are different peaks at different ages, and that old age does not preclude additional development (which is in parallel with human results). Each synapse type and subtype had a specific trajectory in each brain region and subregion, reaching peak values at different ages. Thus, the synapse composition of brain regions continues to change throughout the lifespan and is not restricted to early life development, when synapse density increases. Further, the presence of more than one peak at different ages suggests that shaping synapse composition (through processes such as transcriptional regulation, synapse pruning, and growth) is an ongoing process. The proportion of large synapses increases with age, since many small synapses are lost in the olfactory areas and thalamus in the aging brain.

#### 8.3.2.3 *EPSPs and fMRI data*

The possible outcome of EPSPs resulting from three kinds of brain waves (gamma, theta, and theta-burst) on hippocampal synapses at three ages is tested with a computational simulation approach. The finding is that the (more generic) theta waves produce a stable response at all ages, whereas the gamma and theta-burst brain waves result in different responses at different ages.

The synaptome contains three-dimensional molecular information about brain structure and function. Hence, it makes sense to relate synaptome analysis to established brain imaging methods in the clinic. The synapse proteome composition of regions of the human neocortex has been showed to correlate with functional brain imaging (Positron Emission Tomography (PET) and functional Magnetic Resonance Imaging (fMRI)) (Roy *et al.*, 2018). In the mouse synaptome work, correlation in the synaptome node degree was found with the small-world topology of brain networks in resting states (Zhu *et al.*, 2018, p. 789).

### 8.3.3 *Alzheimer's disease synaptome*

#### 8.3.3.1 *Synaptic plasticity and long-lived proteins in humans*

How the brain manages synaptic plasticity, changing the strength and structure of synapses, is not well understood. Certain forms of synaptic plasticity, such as long-term potentiation or depression, can be maintained for many months to years. The earliest events leading to these initiations involve activation of cellular signaling machinery, which can last on the order of seconds to minutes. Later phases, which can be examined experimentally over several hours, involve the synthesis, recruitment, and capture of specific proteins that produce changes in the structure and strength of the synapse.

Heo *et al.* (2018) demonstrate the existence of long-lived proteins in synapses in the human brain and support a potential role for them in synaptic plasticity. The research problem is that while cellular memories may persist for the lifetime of an organism, the majority of proteins undergo rapid degradation and synthesis to minimize the toxic effect to cells and tissues. It has been appreciated that proteins with longer half-lives exist in certain cells and tissues and this work identifies synaptic long-lived proteins by high-resolution mass spectrometry. In general, synaptic proteins exhibit slower turnover than cytosolic proteins.

Other long-lived proteins in the body have been studied. DNA, for example, employs several mechanisms to repair damage, whereas crystallin and collagen, which make up the lens of the eye and cartilage, do not, and are subject to the formation of cataracts and cartilage stiffening. Synaptic kinases may help to maintain long-lived synapse proteins. For example, the activation of $Ca^{2+}$/calmodulin-dependent protein kinase type II (CaMKII) is required for the induction of LTP and increased phosphorylation and functionality of AMPA receptors (AMPARs), and autophosphorylation of CaMKII has been proposed to maintain LTP and long-term memory.

The work finds 164 synaptosomal long-lived proteins in mice. Long-lived proteins retain at least 50% of a label after a seven-week chase period, corresponding to a relative isotope abundance turnover ratio of 2.0 or less, thus indicating a half-life of several weeks or months. This is in comparison to other proteins with a relatively high turnover ratio (such as PSD95 at 2.69 and amyloid beta A4 protein at 5.61). The research identifies several synaptome proteins that have not been previously been identified with longevity, including type-II regulatory subunits of PKA (protein kinase A), several components of the extracellular matrix, and all five members of the collapsin response mediator proteins (CRMP) family of microtubule binding proteins. CRMP5 in particular showed almost no turnover during the seven-week chase period (Heo *et al.*, 2018, p. E3829).

### 8.3.3.2 *Alzheimer's disease synaptome and intervention*

Synaptome analysis is a new and promising method of attack for possibly combating Alzheimer's disease (AD). Genomic analysis has been an indicator of the potential risk of developing the disease, but there have only been vague phenotypic indicators used to diagnose the pathology, often after the fact (WHO, 2021, 146). It is now known that synapse loss is the best indication of AD (Spires-Jones & Hyman, 2014; Terry *et al.*, 1991). The two proteins involved in AD are amyloid-beta plaques and tau proteins (Serrano-Pozo *et al.*, 2011). Tau-related pathology manifests in intracellular neurofibrillary tangles composed of hyperphosphorylated tau proteins. Amyloid-beta plaques comprised of the apolipoprotein (apoE) protein are extracellular and accumulate in synapses, leading to synapse loss (Koffie *et al.*, 2012). The single biggest risk factor for AD is the inherited genetic profile for the apoE epsilon 4 allele (APOE4); one copy of the APOE4 variant is associated with a three-fold increase in disease risk, and two copies with a ten-fold increased risk (Corder *et al.*, 1994).

Hesse *et al.* (2019) conduct a proteomic analysis of the human "synaptoneurosome" from the temporal and occipital cortices of human Alzheimer's disease patient and control subjects with known APOE gene status (for $n = 33$ total subjects). The analysis identifies over 5,500 proteins in the human synaptoneurosome and highlights disease, brain region, and APOE-associated changes in multiple molecular pathways. In Alzheimer's disease patients, synaptic and mitochondrial function proteins are decreased, and neuroimmune interactions and intracellular signaling proteins are increased. The apolipoprotein E4 risk gene is associated with exacerbated changes in synaptic proteins in Alzheimer's disease. Notably, the work incorporates glial processes closely associated with the synapse, which is key for understanding the role of nonneuronal cells in synapse degeneration, an important emerging research topic (Henstridge & Spires-Jones, 2019). The method uses high-resolution imaging with wave-modeling based array tomography (Jackson *et al.*, 2019).

Analysis investigating pathway alterations in the 1,532 proteins that were changed more than 20% in Alzheimer's disease indicate a clear upregulation of pathways involved in immune response and cellular signaling, and downregulation of pathways involved in synaptic function including long term potentiation, glutamate signaling, and calcium signaling. As pathological severity increases, pathways involved in synaptic function are also decreased (including glutamate, GABA, and CREB signaling), and synaptic long-term potentiation and long-term depression, and proteins are decreased in pathways implicated in mitochondrial function.

Synapse degeneration is an important precursor to synapse loss in Alzheimer's disease. It is likely that there is some degree of synaptic remodeling or compensation taking place as some synaptic proteins are increased and others are decreased. The increase in immune system-related synaptic proteins may indicate the development of pathology. For example, the synaptic receptor TMEM97 is increased in synapses, whose disruption is protective and being tested for efficacy in human Alzheimer's disease as a therapeutic (Izzo *et al.*, 2014). Also notably increased (21%) in Alzheimer's disease as compared to controls is clusterin, which has been shown within individual synapses containing amyloid-beta in Alzheimer's disease (Jackson *et al.*, 2019). The work further supports the hypothesis that proteins may be removed from synapses in Alzheimer's disease and cleared from the brain via the cerebrospinal fluid. Overall, the research demonstrates that specific synaptic proteins and their signaling pathways are identified that become differentially upregulated or downregulated versus controls in Alzheimer's disease and that these early warning indicators might possibly be targeted by therapeutics.

Another project addresses the multiscalar nature of neural signaling (Jolivet *et al.*, 2015). Activity-dependent metabolic coupling in the neuron-glia-vasculature ensemble is modeled, integrating the respective timescales at which energy metabolism and neuronal excitability occur. The healthy brain coordinates the temporal regimes but the disruption of normal metabolic processes is suggested to underlie the progression of neurodegenerative diseases such as Alzheimer's disease.

## References

Allen, N.J. & Eroglu, C. (2017). Cell biology of astrocyte-synapse interactions. *Neuron*. 96:697–708.

Araque, A., Parpura, V., Sanzgiri, R.P. & Haydon, P.G. (1999). Tripartite synapses: Glia, the unacknowledged partner. *Trends Neurosci.* 22(5): 208–15.

Azevedo, F.A., Carvalho, L.R., Grinberg, L.T. *et al.* (2009). Equal numbers of neuronal and non-neuronal cells make the human brain an isometrically scaled-up primate brain. *J. Comp. Neurol.* 513(5):532–41.

Barker, L.A., Dowdall, M.J. & Whittaker, V.P. (1972). Choline metabolism in the cerebral cortex of guinea pigs. *Biochem. J.* 130:1063–80.

Bayes, A., van de Lagemaat, L.N., Collins, M.O. *et al.* (2011). Characterization of the proteome, diseases and evolution of the human postsynaptic density. *Nat. Neurosci.* 14:19–21.

Brown, G.C. & Vilalta, A. (2015). How microglia kill neurons. *Brain Res.* 1628(Pt B):288–97.

Bushong, E.A., Martone, M.E., Jones, Y.Z. & Ellisman, M.H. (2002). Protoplasmic astrocytes in CA1 stratum radiatum occupy separate anatomical domains. *J. Neurosci.* 22:183–92.

Cizeron, M., Qiu, Z., Koniaris, B. *et al.* (2020). A brainwide atlas of synapses across the mouse life span. *Science*. 369:270–75.

Corder, E.H., Saunders, A.M., Risch, N.J. *et al.* (1994). Protective effect of apolipoprotein E type 2 allele for late onset Alzheimer disease. *Nat. Genet.* 7:180–4.

Damisah, E.C., Hill, R.A., Rai, A. *et al.* (2020). Astrocytes and microglia play orchestrated roles and respect phagocytic territories during neuronal corpse removal in vivo. *Sci. Adv.* 6(26):eaba3239.

DeFelipe, J. (2010). From the connectome to the synaptome: An epic love story. *Science*. 330:1198–201.

Deitmer, J.W., Verkhratsky, A.J. & Lohr, C. (1998). Calcium signaling in glial cells. *Cell Calcium*. 24(5–6):405–16.

Fakhoury, M. (2018). Microglia and astrocytes in Alzheimer's disease: Implications for therapy. *Curr. Neuropharm.* 16:508–18.

Falcao, A.M., van Bruggen, D., Marques, S. *et al.* (2018). Disease-specific oligodendrocyte lineage cells arise in multiple sclerosis. *Nat. Med.* 24: 1837–44.

Farhy-Tselnicker, I. & Allen, N.J. (2018). Astrocytes, neurons, synapses: A tripartite view on cortical circuit development. *Neural Dev.* 13(1):7.

Fields, R.D. (2009). *The Other Brain: From Dementia to Schizophrenia, How New Discoveries about the Brain Are Revolutionizing Medicine and Science*. New York: Simon and Schuster.

Franceschi, C., Bonafe, M., Valensin, S. *et al.* (2000). Inflamm-aging. An evolutionary perspective on immunosenescence. *Ann. NY Acad. Sci.* 908:244–54.

Gokhale, R., Qiu, Z., Koniaris, B. & S.G.N. Grant. (2020). *The Mouse Lifespan Synaptome Atlas*. Available at: www.brain-synaptome.org. Accessed March 15, 2021.

Gomes-Leal, W. (2019). Why microglia kill neurons after neural disorders? The friendly fire hypothesis. *Neural Regen. Res.* 14(9):1499–502.

Grant, S.G.N. (2007). Toward a molecular catalogue of synapses. *Brain Res. Rev.* 55:445–9.

Grant, S.G.N. (2019a). Synapse diversity and synaptome architecture in human genetic disorders. *Human Molec. Genet.* 28(R2):219–25.

Grant, S.G.N. (2019b). The synaptomic theory of behavior and brain disease. *Cold Spring Harb. Symp. Quant. Biol.* 83(037887):1–12.

Grosche A., Grosche, J., Tackenberg, M. *et al.* (2013). Versatile and simple approach to determine astrocyte territories in mouse neocortex and hippocampus. *PLoS ONE.* 8(7):e69143.

Hagmann, P. (2005). From diffusion MRI to brain connectomics. *Thesis.* Lausanne: EPFL.

Hampe, C.S., Mitoma, H. & Manto, M. (2018). GABA and Glutamate: Their transmitter role in the CNS and pancreatic islets. *New Developments in Neurotransmission Research.* London: IntechOpen Limited, pp. 65–89.

Haydon, P.G. (2001). Glia: Listening and talking to the synapse. *Nat. Rev. Neurosci.* 2:185–93.

Henstridge, C.M. & Spires-Jones, T. (2019). Beyond the neuron — cellular interactions early in Alzheimer's disease pathogenesis. *Nat. Rev. Neurosci.* 20(2):94–108.

Heo, S., Diering, G.H., Na, C.H. *et al.* (2018). Identification of long-lived synaptic proteins by proteomic analysis of synaptosome protein turnover. *Proc. Natl. Acad. Sci.* 115(16):E3827–36.

Herculano-Houzel, S. (2009). The human brain in numbers: A linearly scaled-up primate brain. *Front Hum. Neurosci.* 3:31.

Hesse, R. Hurtado, M.L., Jackson, R.J. *et al.* (2019). Comparative profiling of the synaptic proteome from Alzheimer's disease patients with focus on the APOE genotype. *Acta. Neuropath Comm.* 7:214.

Izzo, N.J., Xu, J., Zeng, C. *et al.* (2014). Alzheimer's therapeutics targeting amyloid beta 1-42 oligomers II: Sigma-2/PGRMC1 receptors mediate Abeta 42 oligomer binding and synaptotoxicity. *PLoS One.* 9(11):e111899.

Jackson, R.J., Rose, J., Tulloch, J. *et al.* (2019). Clusterin accumulates in synapses in Alzheimer's disease and is increased in apolipoprotein E4 carriers. *Brain Commun.* 1(1):fcz003.

Jakel, S. & Dimou, L. (2017). Glial cells and their function in the adult brain: A journey through the history of their ablation. *Front Cell Neurosci.* 11:24.

Jolivet, R., Coggan, J.S., Allaman, I. & Magistretti, P.J. (2015). Multi-timescale modeling of activity-dependent metabolic coupling in the neuron-glia-vasculature ensemble. *PLoS Comput. Biol.* 11(2):e1004036.

Koffie, R.M., Hashimoto, T., Tai, H.C. *et al.* (2012). Apolipoprotein E4 effects in Alzheimer's disease are mediated by synaptotoxic oligomeric amyloid-beta. *Brain.* 135:2155–68.

Kurth-Nelson, Z.L., Mishra, A. & Newman, E.A. (2009). Spontaneous glial calcium waves in the retina develop over early adulthood. *J. Neurosci.* 29(36):11339–46.

Nicholls, J.G., Martin, A.R., Fuchs, P.A. *et al.* (2012). *From Neuron to Brain.* 5th Edition. Sunderland, MA: Sinauer Associates, Inc.

Oberheim, N.A., Takano, T., Han, X. *et al.* (2009). Uniquely hominid features of adult human astrocytes. *J. Neurosci.* 29:3276–87.

Peferoen, L., Kipp, M., van der Valk, P. *et al.* (2013). Oligodendrocyte-microglia cross-talk in the central nervous system. *Immunology.* 141:302–13.

Roy, M., Sorokina, O., Skene, N. *et al.* (2018). Proteomic analysis of postsynaptic proteins in regions of the human neocortex. *Nat. Neurosci.* 21:130–38.

Sapolsky, R. (2005). *Biology and Human Behavior: The Neurological Origins of Individuality.* 2nd Edition. New York: The Teaching Company.

Scemes, E. & Giaume, C. (2006). Astrocyte calcium waves: What they are and what they do. *Glia.* 54(7):716–25.

Scimemi, A. (2018). Astrocytes and the warning signs of intracerebral hemorrhagic stroke. *Neural Plasticity.* 2018(7301623):1–11.

Serrano-Pozo, A., Frosch, M.P., Masliah, E. & Hyman, B.T. (2011). Neuropathological alterations in Alzheimer disease. *Cold Spring Harb. Perspect. Med.* 1(1):a006189.

Spires-Jones, T.L. & Hyman, B.T. (2014). The intersection of amyloid beta and tau at synapses in Alzheimer's disease. *Neuron.* 82:756–71.

Sporns, O., Tononi, G. & Kotter, R. (2005). The human connectome: A structural description of the human brain. *PLOS Computational Biology.* 1(4):e42.

Sudhof, T.C. (2004). The synaptic vesicle cycle. *Annu. Rev. Neurosci.* 27: 509–47.

Terry, R.D., Masliah, E., Salmon, D.P. *et al.* (1991). Physical basis of cognitive alterations in Alzheimer's disease: Synapse loss is the major correlate of cognitive impairment. *Ann. Neurol.* 30:572–80.

Valerio-Gomes, B., Guimaraes, D.M., Szczupak, D. & Lent, R. (2018). The absolute number of oligodendrocytes in the adult mouse brain. *Front Neuroanat.* 12:90.

van Veenendaal, T.M., Backes, W.H., Tse, D.H.Y. *et al.* (2018). High field imaging of large-scale neurotransmitter networks: Proof of concept and initial application to epilepsy. *NeuroImage: Clinical.* 19:47–55.

von Bartheld, C.S., Bahney, J. & Herculano-Houzel, S. (2016). The search for true numbers of neurons and glial cells in the human brain: A review of 150 years of cell counting. *J. Comp. Neurol.* 524(18):3865–95.

WHO. (2021). Global status report on the public health response to dementia. Geneva: World Health Organization. 1–251. https://www.who.int/health-topics/dementia.

Winkler, H.L. (1920). *Verbreitung und Ursache der Parthenogenesis im Pflanzen und Tierreiche* (*Distribution and Cause of Parthenogenesis in the Plant and Animal Kingdoms*). Jena Germany: Verlag Fischer.

Xu, J.-C., Fan, J., Wang, X. *et al.* (2016). Cultured networks of excitatory projection neurons and inhibitory interneurons for studying human cortical neurotoxicity. *Sci. Transl. Med.* 8(333):333ra48.

Zhu, F., Cizeron, M., Qiu, Z. *et al.* (2018). Architecture of the mouse brain synaptome. *Neuron.* 99(e710):781–99.

# Chapter 9

# Black Hole Information Theory

*Philosophy [i.e. physics] is written in this grand book — I mean the universe — which stands continually open to our gaze, but it cannot be understood unless one first learns to comprehend the language and interpret the characters in which it is written. It is written in the language of mathematics ... without which ... one is wandering around in a dark labyrinth*

— Galileo Galilei (1623, pp. 237–38)

**Abstract**

This chapter discusses black holes as a model system and information-theoretic format for foundational physics. The AdS/CFT correspondence was proposed to study black holes and might likewise be applied to the brain. The information-theoretic correspondence formulation uses entropy to study the UV–IR (short-range and long-range) correlations in a system. A geodesic (shortest-length curve) through the bulk provides a measure of boundary region entanglement.

## 9.1 Black Holes

A black hole is a region of spacetime in which gravity is so strong that nothing can escape from it, not even electromagnetic radiation such as light. The most basic example is a Schwarzschild black hole which does not rotate and has no charge. The next definitions are for a charged (Reissner–Nordstrom) and a rotating (Kerr) black hole, and there are many others. The no-hair theorem is the claim that black holes can be characterized by three physical properties: Mass, charge, and angular momentum (and no others, i.e. no additional "hair"). The black hole information paradox arises in that material (information) is absorbed by black holes, and black holes evaporate over time (via Hawking radiation), but it is not known what happens to the information. The information might stay inside the black hole perhaps in a transformed manner, evaporate in the Hawking radiation, or create a firewall or ring of information (soft hair) around the edge of the black hole horizon.

To solve the black hole information paradox and many other problems, black holes ensue as an active research frontier. Anti-de Sitter (AdS) black holes (i.e. model black holes) are a realization of holographic superconductivity (Gubser, 2008; Hartnoll *et al.*, 2008). AdS black holes become superconductors in the presence of "scalar hair". This is a scalar field close to the black hole horizon, held in place by the gravitational pull toward the interior of the AdS space combined with electrostatic repulsion from the horizon (Hartnoll *et al.*, 2020). The holographic correspondence as a model system is used to understand more about superconducting materials and black hole interiors. Other work posits that real-life black holes might have stretched horizons containing quantum information, as a form of quantum hair (soft hair), around the black hole horizon. So far, most observational data support the "no hair" hypothesis. However, a quantum information layer of condensate (hair) might occur in the excited states of high-energy cataclysmic events such as black hole mergers, and might possibly be measured in the altered profile of outgoing radiation (spacetime ripples). Such hypotheses might be tested with a more sensitive version of LIGO (Crowell & Corda, 2020).

### 9.1.1 *Black holes as a model system*

Black holes are a good model system, serving as the "*C. elegans* of theoretical physics". This is in the sense that they require understanding general relativity and quantum mechanics together, provide a venue for interrogating many not-yet-understood problems in physics, and admit a quantum-information theoretic interpretation with many tools and formalisms for applied study such as entropy, entanglement, quantum states, information scrambling, chaos, thermal system analysis, and the holographic correspondence. Research results in black hole physics (from both empirical and model systems) contribute wide-ranging foundational physics knowledge that may have an impact on quantum computing (including superconducting materials) and neuroscience investigation (most directly imaging technologies such as EEG and fMRI).

#### 9.1.1.1 *Quantum gravity and black hole evaporation*

A theory of quantum gravity is needed to explain black holes. Black holes are precisely the site of conflict between general relativity and quantum mechanics as the two main theories of physical reality. On the one hand, general relativity predicts black holes and suggests the "no-hair" theorem that black holes can be fully described by the three macroscopic properties of mass, charge, and angular momentum (Einstein, 1916). On the other hand, black holes have also been found to have an entropy associated with them. The entropy is proportional to the area of the black hole (the event horizon of the black hole) (Bekenstein, 1973; Hawking, 1975). General relativity does not allow for a microscopic description since black holes are characterized exclusively by their macroscopic parameters. This suggests that there are some underlying microscopic degrees of freedom that are not being described in general relativity and that perhaps the theory is incomplete. The incompleteness of general relativity is one of the first indications that it is necessary to develop a quantum theory of gravity. Such a quantum theory of gravity would explain the underlying microscopic quantum mechanical degrees of freedom that give rise to observed macroscopic parameters that include gravity, and space and time.

A further conflict concerns the status of information in the black hole. General relativity indicates that information inside a black hole cannot escape. However, a core tenet of quantum mechanics is that information cannot be destroyed. In describing the dynamics of black holes, Hawking found that they emit radiation (photons). The so-called Hawking radiation carries energy which means that the mass of the black hole has to decrease as a function of time, and eventually evaporates until nothing is left.

The point is that it is not possible to explain black hole entropy or evaporation in the classical picture with general relativity alone, and that quantum mechanics is also needed.

General relativity and quantum mechanics share a similar property, though, in that their equations are intractable. Both Einstein's field equations in the formulation of general relativity and the Schrödinger wave-function equation in quantum mechanics involve partial differential equations which are difficult to compute. Hence, into this conflict comes the AdS/CFT correspondence which provides a calculable model between the gravity theory in the bulk (general relativity) and the gauge theory on the boundary (quantum mechanics) (Maldacena, 1999). The correspondence is a solvable model of quantum gravity from either direction. Some of the standard interpretations of the bulk-boundary relationship are listed in Table 9.1.

#### 9.1.1.2 *Black hole in a box*

The AdS/CFT correspondence is a model to study quantum gravity without having to address the complications of quantum gravity directly. A strategy used in physics to cope with complicated systems is to put the problem in a box. Some well-known examples are the "gas in a box" and the "particle in a box" methods as bounded models for examining a finite number of the numerous particles that comprise a gas or a subset of the movement of a particle. The box can grow and become distorted, but putting the problem in a box limits the system and makes it easier to evaluate. System attributes that are infinite can be made finite, and other limitations placed on the model such that the problem can be addressed. The AdS/CFT correspondence effectively packages AdS space as a

Table 9.1. AdS/CFT bulk-boundary configurations.

| No. | Bulk | Boundary | Reference |
|---|---|---|---|
| 1 | Gravity theory | Gauge theory | Maldacena (1999) |
| 2 | Black hole | Thermal state | Shenker and Stanford (2014) |
| 3 | Quantum gravity | Quantum state of an exotic superconducting material | Hayden *et al.* (2016) |

representative box (shaped as a hyperbolic sphere with negative curvature) for quantum gravity (Harlow, 2017, p. 5).

The problem is that quantum gravity does not easily fit into a rectangular box as in the "particle in a box" or the "gas in a box" strategies. The correspondence therefore uses a special box for quantum gravity which is different from the regular universe. The familiar everyday universe is described by de Sitter space, with three spatial dimensions and one time dimension. AdS space is a simpler toy version of de Sitter space. Instead of extending forever, AdS space is bounded and has negative curvature. The Escher *Circle Limit* drawings depict this kind of space as a circle or globe tiled with identical fish, large and sparse in the center, and becoming smaller and more profuse when reaching the boundary. AdS space is in this configuration, having a curved boundary with increasing numbers of fish as the boundary is reached.

The AdS/CFT correspondence provides a simpler version of the real-life universe with which to examine problems such what happens to information in a black hole. The hyperbolic (negatively curved) geometry of AdS space is likened to the Escher figures and also a can of soup. The "soup" or bulk volume inside the can is the quantum gravity region, which is complicated and messy, and the boundary is the can itself, a more cleanly solvable theory in one less dimension than the bulk. The quantum gravity bulk is filled with the matter and force particles that have gone into creating the black hole. The boundary is the event horizon or quantum field theory which can be interpreted as the quantum state of some material on the boundary in one less dimension.

### 9.1.2 *Hologram decoding dictionaries*

The AdS/CFT correspondence encodes a higher-dimensional space (the bulk) in a one less dimensional space (the boundary), and therefore has a holographic format. An important precursor to the AdS/CFT correspondence is the holographic principle (Susskind, 1995), which applies the concept of holography to physics. The holographic principle states that the information stored in a spatial volume $V_d$ is encoded in its boundary area $A_{d-1}$, measured in units of the Planck area (Erdmenger, 2018, p. 14). The boundary is a hologram. The hologram format allows a three-dimensional image to be encoded into a two-dimensional film. In the bulk-boundary correspondence, there is a three-dimensional space encoded into two dimensions of space, or in a simpler example, two dimensions of space encoded into one. There can be many varieties.

The correspondence is used to investigate how structure arises in the bulk to form gravity, space, and time. Calculating from the boundary, an extra radial dimension emerges from the bulk, often interpreted as space. The bulk has one more dimension than the boundary, an extra dimension of space, the radial dimension which emerges when computing the AdS/CFT correspondence from the boundary theory. Since the correspondence is a tool for identifying the emergence of bulk microscopic structure and relating it to macroscopic manifestations on the boundary, a question naturally arises as to how the bulk of degrees of freedom are encoded on the boundary. In information-theoretic terms, the question is one of finding dictionary mappings to decode the hologram of how the bulk degrees of freedom are encoded in the boundary degrees of freedom.

One of the first holographic dictionaries is the Ryu and Takayanagi (2006) formula for entanglement entropy. The formula states that the entanglement entropy of a boundary region is equal to the area of a minimal surface in the bulk (effectively hanging down from the boundary region). Another holographic dictionary is quantum error correction codes (Pastawski *et al.*, 2015). This idea describes how a bulk physical qubit can be protected by an ancilla of boundary logical qubits via the bulk-boundary entanglement relationship.

A third holographic dictionary mapping is called (informally) the "fish-counting metric" or (formally) the bulk minimal curve (Hayden & Penington, 2019, p. 24; Czech *et al.*, 2015). The work draws from the Escher's *Circle Limit* pictures in which AdS space has a curved geometry and there are many more fish are at the edge of the boundary. The shortest path between any two points on the boundary passes through the bulk. Instead of tracing along the boundary through many fish, the shortest path between the points is a curve through the bulk that touches as few fish as possible. Hence, the "fish-counting metric" is the shortest distance between any two points in AdS space, which is a bulk curve that is the curved space equivalent of a straight line (a geodesic).

The bulk can contain anything complex that is not straightforward to analyze directly such as black holes, gravity, or the particles in a room. The AdS/CFT correspondence provides a model for studying how this complexity behaves. The premise of the correspondence is that the bulk degrees of freedom are encoded in the boundary. The "fish-counting metric" can be applied to concertize the bulk and boundary degrees-of-freedom (parameters) relationship. The shortest distance between two points on the boundary is a minimal curve in the bulk. Changing the system, such as by putting a heavy black hole in the bulk can bend the curve, so instead of being a regular curve, it becomes distorted. The bulk geometry is not fixed and can be manipulated to characterize the system. For example, increasing the entanglement of a field in the bulk changes its minimal surface behavior topologically, which via the duality, relates to scaling dimensions in the boundary calculation (Hayden *et al.*, 2016).

## 9.2 Practical Quantum Communications Protocols

A practical application of the AdS/CFT correspondence is employing the model to calculate the entropy of a boundary state to develop a quantum communications protocol for information transfer. The correspondence can be applied in either direction, as a known boundary theory to calculate an unknown bulk, or as a known bulk theory to calculate an unknown boundary. One of the quintessential applications of the correspondence is interrogating unknown bulk structure such as trying to define a theory of quantum gravity with a known quantum field theory from the boundary. Another standard application of the correspondence is in condensed matter physics, using classical gravity as a known bulk theory to investigate the properties of unknown materials such as novel superconductors on the boundary. The quantum field theories that characterize strongly interacting novel superconductors in the boundary area unknown, but they can be studied through their entanglement relationship with classical gravity in the bulk. The idea is to use the AdS/CFT correspondence to understand more about such novel superconducting materials so that they may be used in quantum computing and quantum communications. The information-theoretic frame for investigation is setting up the problem to calculate entropy. The problem is phrased as transmitting the quantum state of the material in the most efficient way possible, based on its entropy. Entropy is the fewest number of qubits needed to send a quantum information state from one location to another.

The AdS/CFT correspondence can be used to calculate entropy. One holographic dictionary mapping is the Ryu and Takayanagi (2006) formula for computing the entanglement entropy of a boundary region as being equal to the area of a corresponding minimal bulk surface. Another holographic dictionary mapping is the fish-counting metric which establishes the shortest distance between two boundary points as the shortest-length geometric curve (geodesic) through the bulk (Czech *et al.*, 2015). The shortest bulk curve method can be interpreted as a measure of entropy. The correspondence translates boundary problems such as calculating entropy into geometric questions in the bulk. The bulk domain is one of a classical theory of gravity or geometry (geometry is Einsteinian relativity). The correspondence indicates that entropy can be evaluated by a geometrical quantity. This could be with the Ryu–Takayanagi formula of the minimal area of a corresponding bulk surface or as the shortest-length curve through the bulk.

In the quantum communications example, there is an exotic superconducting material on the boundary. It is complex, quantum mechanical, and has many degrees of freedom. In the black hole analogy, it is a ring of exotic material around the outside of the black hole whose physics is supposed to encode quantum gravity. The idea is to calculate properties about the exotic material such as its entropy which relates to the information diversity of the microscopic degrees of freedom. The prescribed method for obtaining the quantum mechanical (von Neumann) entropy is to sum over all the minimal measurement bases of the material. However, this is difficult to compute for the exotic superconducting material. Instead, the shortest bulk curve method can be applied as a more expedient formula for calculating entropy. In this bulk-to-boundary application of the AdS/CFT correspondence, the complexity is in the boundary in the difficult entropy calculation. The strategy is thus to solve the boundary theory from the bulk theory.

### 9.2.1 *UV–IR information compression*

The correspondence-based entropy calculation can be used to develop an information compression protocol for use in quantum communications.

In general, entropy is the measure of the interrelatedness of subsystems within a system, how related one area is to another within the system. The interrelations are measured as short-range (UV) and long-range (IR) correlations. If the task is to send the information of the system from one location to another, the entropy, or interrelatedness of the subsystems, can be interpreted as an efficient compression of the UV–IR correlations. This captures the detail and complexity of the system. The AdS/CFT correspondence provides a structure with which to interpret the UV–IR correlations of a system. In the bulk-boundary setup, the boundary material has short-range (UV) correlations with the portions of the bulk closest to the boundary, and long-range (IR) correlations with the deep bulk interior. UV (ultraviolet) and IR (infrared) are frequently used terms in physics, not always meant literally to designate short and long wavelengths, but as a heuristic for the nearest and farthest ranges or extremes of a system.

In the nonquantum picture, information compression protocols are used in applications such as audio and video media streaming. If a video service is transmitting a movie to an end-user, the most efficient protocol is to compress and send the whole movie. This incorporates all of the possible correlations in the movie content and provides the best compression. Both the short-range (UV) correlations and the long-range (IR) correlations are exploited. However, for live streaming, a different information compression protocol is needed. In a typical movie, the scene does not change much between individual image frames, suggesting that the short-range correlations are the most relevant. Short-range correlations are those that are local in time in the movie. For example, these could be small changes in character movements, moment to moment in the scene. An information protocol might send only the changes between the image frames on a short-time basis (UV). The long-range (IR) correlations are those that are over long-time intervals in the course of the movie. For example, the faces of the main characters do not change, but their expressions do. This information could be compressed as long-range correlations in an information compression protocol (Table 9.2).

Video delivery services tend to start streaming the content immediately instead of waiting to compress and send all of the UV and IR correlations at once. As a result, information compression protocols typically only make use of the short-term UV correlations and do not include the

Table 9.2. UV–IR correlations (short- and long-range).

| Correlation Range | Movie Information Compression Example |
|---|---|
| UV (ultraviolet): Short-range correlations | Changes in character movements moment to moment in a scene |
| IR (infrared): Long-range correlations | Change in facial expressions of the main characters over the course of the movie |

long-term IR correlations. The longer the window to compress the file, the more UV and IR correlations can be included. For real-time streaming, only short-range correlations are exploited, and over a narrow time window. The fixed-size time window advances as the movie is streamed.

A similar information compression protocol can be defined for sending the quantum state of an exotic superconducting material. The cost of sending the information is the number of qubits that need to be sent, which can be calculated as the length of the bulk curve. The correspondence-based entropy calculation is used to find the shortest curve, which equates to the cost of sending the information. With the correspondence, an information compression protocol can be developed to identify the optimal configurations of the short-range and long-range correlations in the quantum system of the superconducting material to send. Unlike in the movie example, the right mix of UV–IR correlations to transport the quantum state of the exotic material is unknown. The video streaming setup is similarly employed to have a fixed-size window ratcheting over the quantum system to perform entropy (correlation) calculations. As with the movie, the most efficient protocol incrementally constrains the quantum information contents. The full long-distance (IR) correlations the material has with the depths of the bulk interior are not accessed as much as the short-distance (UV) correlations the material has with the portions of the bulk closest to the boundary, in a finite window at every step. The sequence of windows is given by intervals calculated from the entropy curves.

A specific information compression protocol setup for the quantum system is as follows. At each point on the bulk curve, a tangent circle is created. In flat space, every point on a curve has a tangent line. In curved space, there is a tangent geodesic (shortest path on a curved surface). The tangent geodesics are circular shapes that intersect the boundary at two points. For each point on the curve, there is a tangent circle and that intersects the boundary at two points, and which defines an interval. These intervals are analogous to the ratcheting intervals in the video streaming information compression protocol. The sequence of intervals can be used to define or to constrain a streaming compression protocol for an efficient means of sending quantum information (Balasubramanian *et al.*, 2014).

The collections of intervals from the tangent geodesics of the curve are used to define a streaming compression protocol. This is the minimal qubit cost to transmit qubits containing the quantum information state of the exotic superconducting material in an information compression procedure. The qubits could be compressed and sent generally or via quantum teleportation. In quantum teleportation, the cost of sending qubits is even more prominent as entangled Bell pairs need to be created. The minimal number of entangled Bell pairs required to teleport would be the number of qubits in the compression as they have a one-to-one relationship (one Bell pair for each qubit sent by quantum teleportation). The minimum compression rate is the entropy. The practical result is that the entropy counts the minimum number of qubits required to compress and send the information in the material, computed as the minimal length of the bulk curve and its related correlations.

#### 9.2.1.1 *UV–IR correlations for interrogating bulk structure*

The information compression protocol based on entropy and UV–IR correlations is not only a practical method for sending quantum information states but also has theoretical benefits for interrogating emergent bulk structure. The geometry of the bulk is translated into entropy as an information-theoretic formulation on the boundary, to constitute the information compression protocol. The UV and IR constraints on the information compression protocol reflect the structure of the bulk. The key point is that the boundary entropy has information about the bulk geometry, and can be constructed from the bulk geometry using shortest-length curves. The broader impact of this advance is that it provides a framework that reveals how the points inside the bulk are related to points on the boundary. How the long-range correlations are related between the boundary and the deeper points inside the bulk is a tool for investigating different kinds of structural emergence in the bulk such as quantum gravity, and space and time.

## References

Balasubramanian, V., Chowdhury, B.D., Czech, B. *et al.* (2014). A hole-ographic spacetime. *Phys. Rev. D.* 89(8):086004.

Bekenstein, J.D. (1973). Black holes and entropy. *Phys. Rev. D.* 7(8):2333–46.

Crowell, L. & Corda, C. (2020). Quantum hair on colliding black holes. arXiv:2007.01106v1.

Czech, B., Hayden, P., Lashkari, N. & Swingle, B. (2015). The information theoretic interpretation of the length of a curve. *J. High Energ. Phys.* 1506:157.

Einstein, A. (1916). The foundation of the general theory of relativity. *Annalen der Physik.* 354(7):769.

Erdmenger, J. (2018). Introduction to gauge/gravity duality. In *Proceedings of Theoretical Advanced Study Institute Summer School 2017, "Physics at the Fundamental Frontier"*, Boulder, Colorado, USA, June 4–July 1, 2017. arXiv:1807.09872v1, PoS(TASI2017)001.

Galilei, G. (1957, 1623). Il Saggiatore (The Assayer). Trans. S. Drake. *Discoveries and Opinions of Galileo.* New York: Anchor.

Gubser, S.S. (2008). Breaking an Abelian gauge symmetry near a black hole horizon. *Phys. Rev. D.* 78(6):065034.

Harlow, D. (2017). TASI lectures on the emergence of bulk physics in AdS/CFT. In *Proceedings of Theoretical Advanced Study Institute Summer School 2017, "Physics at the Fundamental Frontier"*, Boulder, Colorado, USA, June 4–July 1, 2017. arXiv:1802.01040, PoS(TASI2017)002.

Hartnoll, S.A., Herzog, C.P. & Horowitz, G.T. (2008). Holographic superconductors. *J. High Energ. Phys.* 0812:015.

Hartnoll, S.A., Horowitz, G.T., Kruthoff, J. & Santos, J.E. (2020). Diving into a holographic superconductor. arXiv:2008.12786v2.

Hawking, S.W. (1975). Particle creation by black holes. *Commun. Math. Phys.* 43(3):199–220.

Hayden, P., Nezami, S., Qi, X.L. *et al.* (2016). Holographic duality from random tensor networks. *J. High Energ. Phys.* 11(9):1–57.

Hayden, P. & Penington, G. (2019). Learning the Alpha-bits of black holes. *J. High Energ. Phys.* 12(007):24.

Maldacena, J.M. (1999). The large N limit of superconformal field theories and supergravity. *Intl. J. Theor. Phys.* 38(4):1113–33.

Pastawski, F., Yoshida, B., Harlow, D. & Preskill, J. (2015). Holographic quantum error-correcting codes: Toy models for the bulk/boundary correspondence. *J. High Energ. Phys.* 6(149):1–53.

Ryu, S. & Takayanagi, T. (2006). Aspects of holographic entanglement entropy. *J. High Energ. Phys.* 0608:045.

Shenker, S.H. & Stanford, D. (2014). Multiple shocks. *J. High Energ. Phys.* 1412:046.

Susskind, L. (1995). The world as a hologram. *J. Math. Phys.* 36(11):6377–96.

# Part 3

# Connectivity

# Chapter 10

# Quantum Photonics and High-Dimensional Entanglement

*The photon ... is the only elementary particle of energy, whereas there are hundreds of elementary particles of matter*

— Nair (2006, p. 321)


**Abstract**

This chapter discusses quantum computing in global networks as opposed to standalone machines. Global networks are built on photonic transfer, an expertise honed over decades. Optical qubits can be encoded and entangled in many ways, leading to the high-dimensional entanglement of qudits (quantum information digits) and the sending of GHZ (Greenberger–Horne–Zeilinger) states (entangled quantum states involving at least three qubits or particle states). Gaussian boson sampling is an optical NISQ device, and can be interpreted with graph theory.


## 10.1 Quantum Photonics

### 10.1.1 *Technical benefits and qudits*

Photonics is likely to be a significant contributor to quantum computing, a U.S. National Science Foundation roadmap suggests (Awschalom *et al.*, 2019). Global quantum networks for computing, communications, and sensing (Table 10.1) may be implemented with all-optical components from the outset or optical-electrical interconnects, and linked to cloud-based quantum repeaters, routers, and switches.

Quantum optical platforms suggest better-than-classical performance in computation, communication, and sensing (Nunn *et al.*, 2013), and also outperform other quantum methods. Optical systems do not need to be supercooled (like superconducting chips) as quantum effects in optical systems can be easily observed at room temperature. Optical circuits also do not require error correction. Light has numerous degrees of freedom that can be used to encode, entangle, and transmit quantum information, and optical signals can be generated and detected efficiently. Photonic processing is well understood from global fiberoptic telecommunications networks. The capacity of optical transmission is leveraged with dense multiplexing techniques, encoding strategies that might be applied likewise to quantum processing. The terms optical and photonic are used interchangeably, and mean the manipulation of information with light.

Even without quantum computing, optical networking is expecting substantial growth due to traffic from cloud-based services and 5G roll-outs. Gartner estimates that worldwide cloud services spending will increase 18% in 2021 (Costello & Rimol, 2020) and IDC indicates that more than 59 zettabytes of data were created worldwide in 2020 (Reinsel, 2020). Cisco forecasts that by 2023, global mobile devices will grow from 8.8 billion in 2018 to 13.1 billion, with 1.4 billion being 5G capable (and that a 5G connection will generate nearly 3× more traffic than a 4G connection) (Cisco, 2020, p. 1, 33).

Harnessing the quantum aspects of light (particularly entanglement) has been necessary to the realization of global fiberoptic telecommunication networks. Such networks have been employing quantum principles since the 1960s (Glauber, 1963). Photons are the ideal carriers of quantum information over long distances. The contemporary focus is adding even more quantum aspects and upgrading the communications network

Table 10.1. Quantum networks.

| Computing | Communication | Sensing |
|---|---|---|
| Processing | Transmission | Capture |

infrastructure to be more oriented to quantum computation (including with quantum key distribution, quantum routers, quantum teleportation, and distilled entanglement). It is possible that one or more equipment manufacturing companies might emerge as the "Cisco of quantum networks" in providing quantum internet components.

Quantum photonics has been a well-established industry for decades and is poised to be central to facilitating a potential transition to quantum networks for computing and communication. Quantum optical systems are prominent candidates for the quantum future because they link quantum computation and quantum communication in the same framework. The U.S. National Science Foundation workshop roadmap emphasizes the development of quantum optical interconnects for next-generation information technologies (Awschalom *et al.*, 2019). Although there are many ways to make qudits (quantum information digits) for quantum computing on standalone machines, for a larger architecture of networked machines, electrical signals must be converted to optical signals. Hence, there are two methods in development for quantum computing networks. One is creating an all-optical platform from the beginning with continuous qubit optical interfaces. The other is building a microwave superconducting platform (in the model of semiconductors) that is later interfaced to optical networks with electrical-optical interconnects. Both approaches could develop simultaneously.

Quantum optics is a proven method in the communications field. In many ways it is easier and less costly to manipulate light than other physical systems. Some of the first demonstrations of Shor's algorithm were in optical systems, using four photonic qubits to factor the number fifteen (Lu *et al.*, 2007; Lanyon *et al.*, 2007). Another argument in favor of photonics is that the platform is a natural fit for the realization of qudits (quantum information digits beyond the two-valued qubit). The qudit structure often provides the best packaging of information and draws from established methods in greater than two-channel multiplexing (Imany *et al.*, 2019). Also, it is easy to realize quantum photonics with existing off-the-shelf linear optics equipment. Such quantum computing with linear optics (combined with adaptive measurement) might be a blueprint for universal for quantum computation (Knill *et al.*, 2001).

#### 10.1.1.1 *Bosons and fermions*

There are many practical reasons for optics (widely used in global telecommunications, well-understood, off-the-shelf equipment), and there are also quantum mechanical reasons. The two basic types of quantum mechanical particles are bosons (force particles such as photons) and fermions (matter particles such as electrons and quarks). In some cases, bosons can be easier to treat because they clump together (unlike matter particles which repel per the Fermi exclusion principle). Bosons are also attractive because they have symmetric wavefunctions (meaning it is possible to easily swap in another particle), whereas fermions have antisymmetric wavefunctions. Boson wavefunction amplitudes are nonnegative and do not have the "sign problem" of fermions in which positive and negative terms need to be canceled out in computations. This means that Monte Carlo analysis can be applied more easily to approximate bosonic ground states than fermionic ground states.

However, bosonic wavefunction amplitudes are more difficult to calculate than fermionic amplitudes and are in a more difficult computational complexity class, #P-complete versus P (Aaronson & Arkhipov, 2013, pp. 13–14). Fermionic amplitudes are given by determinants of $n \times n$ matrices (determinants are in the P class of computational complexity). Bosonic amplitudes are given by permanents (permanents are #P-complete). Overall, in some ways, bosons are better for quantum computation, and in other ways, fermions are. Boson sampling, for example, is an implementation of the "harder job" of calculating bosonic wavefunction amplitudes. Quantum computing is proceeding forward with both fermionic (matter-based) and bosonic (photon-based) systems, two respective examples are Gaussian boson sampling to demonstrate quantum advantage (Zhong *et al.*, 2020), and Majorana fermions to simulate the minimal realization of the AdS/CFT correspondence with the SYK model (Garcia-Alvarez *et al.*, 2017).

## 10.2 Boson Sampling

Boson sampling is the statistical method of sampling from the output distribution of photon scattering. The probability distribution of many bosons whose quantum waves interfere with one another is calculated in a way that essentially randomizes the position of the particles. The typical experimental setup is an interferometer implementing a Haar-random (narrow-range) transformation on $n$ indistinguishable bosons (photons). The problem is computationally complex as it is difficult to evaluate the permanent (the statistical value of positive terms in a matrix expansion) in the scattering amplitudes. The boson sampling problem is in the complexity class #P-hard due to the complexity of the permanent. Boson sampling is theoretically interesting because it is believed to be intractable for a classical computer, and can thus serve as a means of establishing quantum advantage (better-than-classical performance). Such as a real-life claim of quantum advantage has been made using Gaussian boson sampling (Zhong *et al.*, 2020) in an ongoing implementation of the theoretical proposal (Aaronson & Arkhipov, 2013).

Boson sampling is a promising route for demonstrating quantum advantage as it uses existing off-the-shelf equipment (single-photon sources, passive beam splitter networks and single-photon detectors). In the original boson sampler design, $N$ single-photon Fock states are launched into an $N^2$-mode interferometer. This is a good test for quantum computing because the mathematics required to calculate bosonic statistics is classically intractable (an equation with many unknown variables must be calculated). Technically, computing the probability of measuring a specific photon pattern at the output depends upon the permanent of a submatrix of the interferometer unitary. The permanent is in the #P complexity class (Valiant, 1979, p. 189). This class, #P, is based on counting the number of functions that are solutions to an NP-hard problem (a problem whose number of solutions increases exponentially with the number of variables, and that cannot be calculated efficiently with classical computing, but whose possible answers can be easily verified). Since the permanent is #P-hard (in the #P complexity class), sampling from the distribution of bosonic statistics is an intractable problem for classical computers. There is no classical shortcut for the computation as boson sampling is a #P-hard problem (Ball, 2020).

### 10.2.1 *Gaussian boson sampling*

Reliable photon generation and detection equipment are crucial to calculating boson statistics. In early boson sampling experimental efforts, reliable (perfectly deterministic) sources of single photons were not available. Efforts thus made use of post-selected photon-pair states to confirm results, but the method does not scale to high numbers of photons. A key innovation is Gaussian boson sampling (Hamilton *et al.*, 2017). The advance came from noticing that while earlier methods such as scattershot boson sampling make use of Gaussian input states, they discard their Gaussian nature, retaining only a specific number of post-selected single photons from the complete distribution, which constrains the input squeezers to a low gain regime.

Instead, the new idea is a boson sampling method that takes advantage of the full Gaussian nature of the input states. This is achieved by using squeezed input states with a higher gain. High-gain squeezed states are incorporated as a nonclassical input resource and nonclassical methods are also used to compute the bosonic statistics. The probability of measuring specific photon patterns from a general Gaussian state (a state whose distribution is Gaussian) in the Fock basis is related to a matrix function called the hafnian, a classically intractable #P-class problem that is solved with quantum computation. The speedup results from instead of having to post-select Gaussian states from output results, reliably generating Gaussian states in the first place. The high-gain squeezed states as a nonclassical resource for producing photons increases the probability of obtaining Gaussian states. The method relates the probability of measuring specific photon patterns from a general Gaussian state in the Fock basis to the hafnian matrix function (which computes the number of perfect matchings in the graph of an adjacency matrix).

Gaussian boson sampling is established as a special-purpose model of photonic quantum computation in which a multi-mode Gaussian state is prepared and then measured in the Fock basis (multiparticle Hilbert space). A Gaussian state is a state whose distribution function in phase space or density operator in Fock space is in the Gaussian form. A Gaussian state can be prepared from the vacuum by a sequence of single-mode squeezing, multi-mode linear interferometry, and single-mode displacements. Fock-basis measurements can be implemented by using photon-number resolving detectors. A basic Gaussian state with zero mean can be prepared using only state squeezing followed by linear interferometry, and there is a high probability that the required kinds of outputs can be observed. The result is a more efficient boson sampling method as compared to other approaches.

#### 10.2.1.1 *Gaussian boson sampling demonstration*

One of the first experimental demonstrations of Gaussian boson sampling was reported by Zhong *et al.* (2019), and then sharpened to a claim of quantum advantage a year later (2020). The boson sampling problem is that it is difficult to evaluate boson scattering amplitudes (due to the matrix expansion term (permanent)). There is no shortcut for performing the calculation on a classical computer. However, a quantum computer can sidestep the brute-force calculation by simulating the quantum process directly, allowing bosons to interfere and then sampling from the resulting distribution (Ball, 2020). Here, the quantum advantage experimental setup is as follows. Gaussian boson sampling was achieved by sending 50 indistinguishable single-mode squeezed states into a 100-mode ultralow-loss interferometer with full connectivity and sampling the output using 100 high-efficiency single-photon detectors.

Photons are used as qubits, encoding states (modes) that make use of two degrees of freedom encoding (horizontal and vertical polarization and spatial position). The states are then pumped into an optical network effectively consisting of 300 beam splitters and 75 mirrors to create the interference. Within 200 seconds, over 3 million events of 43-photon coincidence were obtained as the photon distribution output. Photodetectors capable of registering single photons measure the distribution, which in effect encodes calculations that are classically intractable. The team estimates that a $10^{14}$ quantum advantage is obtained as the problem would take 2.5 billion years to calculate on China's TaihuLight supercomputer (the world's fourth most powerful supercomputer as of November 2020 with 125 Pflop/s (Top500, 2020)). The Gaussian boson sampling protocol not only significantly enhances the photon generation probability, compared to standard boson sampling with single-photon Fock states, but also supports potential applications in dense subgraph problems and quantum chemistry.

#### 10.2.1.2 *Gaussian boson sampling as a NISQ device*

Gaussian boson sampling is not only a theoretical platform for the demonstration of quantum advantage, but also a NISQ device (available quantum computer that does not require error correction) with practical applications. A number of problems can be encoded with Gaussian boson sampling methods. Relevant Gaussian boson sampling algorithms have been developed for applications such as how proteins dock to one another and to probe spectral analysis in quantum chemistry. Sparrow *et al.* (2018), for example, exploit a natural mapping between vibrations in molecules and photons in waveguides to demonstrate a reprogrammable photonic chip as a simulation platform for a range of dynamic quantum behavior in various chemical molecules. The time evolution of vibrational excitations in the harmonic approximations for four-atom molecules (including $H_2CS$, $SO_3$, HNCO, HFHF, $N_4$, and $P_4$) is simulated, and also energy transport and thermal relaxation. The results highlight the power of simulation tools for molecular quantum dynamics and the field of femtochemistry.

### 10.2.2 *Gaussian boson sampling/graph theory*

An emerging field of application is Gaussian boson sampling/graph theory (GBS/GT), using Gaussian boson sampling to study problems in graph theory. The output of sampling is graphs, and thus it is a natural connection to apply Gaussian boson sampling to graph theory problems. Sampling output is in the form of various different kinds of graphs including random graphs, matched graphs, and Erdos–Renyi graphs. A body of work is developed by Schuld *et al.* (2019) and other team members, formalizing the relationship between Gaussian boson sampling and graph theory. The work relies on Gaussian boson sampling being a NISQ device for studying quantum computational phenomena (Table 10.2).

First, graph matching polynomials are used to study the relationship between distributions defined over classes of samples from a GBS device (Bradler *et al.*, 2019). A new graph polynomial is introduced called the displaced GBS polynomial (whose coefficients are the coarse-grained photon-number probabilities of an arbitrary undirected graph encoded in

Table 10.2. Gaussian boson sampling/graph theory.

| No. | Gaussian Boson Sampling (GBS) | Graph Theory |
|---|---|---|
| 1 | Distributions classes over GBS samples | Graph matching polynomials |
| 2 | Gaussian boson sampling | Hardware-induced graph kernel |
| 3 | GBS hafnian for probability sampling | Graph density (dense subgraphs) |
| 4 | Quantum light state graph encoding | Graph isomorphism invariants |
| 5 | Adjacency matrix hafnian output | Undirected graph perfect matching |
| 6 | Proportional sampling of GBS | Densest *k*-subgraph approximation |

a GBS device). Notably, there is a duality between the displaced (arbitrary) GBS polynomial and a certain matching polynomial that is a prism over the graph (the Cartesian graph product of the graph with a single-weighted edge). The graph polynomial relationship provides greater insight into the functioning of Gaussian boson sampling, and suggests how Gaussian boson sampling might be simulated classically. The method is also used in the second example of constructing feature maps in a quantum kernel learning application (Schuld *et al.*, 2019). The work proposes how a new type of coarse-grained quantum statistics might be used to construct feature maps and makes use of a quantum hardware-induced graph kernel.

Third, Gaussian boson sampling is used to identify dense subgraphs (Arrazola & Bromley, 2018). Focusing on the NP-hard densest *k*-subgraph problem, stochastic algorithms are found to be enhanced through GBS, which selects dense subgraphs with high probability. The findings incorporate a link between graph density and the number of perfect matchings (enumerated by the hafnian) which is the relevant quantity determining sampling probabilities in GBS.

Fourth, a connection is made between a Gaussian boson sampler and the graph isomorphism problem (Bradler *et al.*, 2018b). The setup encodes graphs into quantum states of light, whose properties are then probed with photon-number-resolving detectors. A proof is given that the probabilities of different photon detection events in this scheme can be combined to provide a complete set of graph invariants. Two graphs are isomorphic if and only if their detection probabilities are equivalent.

Fifth, a famous hard graph problem of computing the number of perfect matchings (the number of unique and complete pairings of the vertices of a graph) is tackled (Bradler *et al.*, 2018a). A method is proposed for estimating the number of perfect matchings of undirected graphs based on the relationship between GBS and graph theory. The probability of measuring zero or one photons in each output mode is directly related to the hafnian of the adjacency matrix, and thus to the number of perfect matchings of a graph. The result is a set of encodings for translating the adjacency matrix of a graph into a Gaussian state, along with strategies for boosting the sampling success probability.

Sixth, quantum approximate optimization with Gaussian boson sampling is proposed (Arrazola *et al.*, 2018). Difficult optimization problems are often approached by finding approximate solutions. Here, proportional sampling is proposed for improving the performance of stochastic algorithms used for optimization. An NP-Hard problem, Max-Haf, is introduced to demonstrate that GBS can be used to enhance any stochastic algorithm for this problem.

#### 10.2.2.1 *Application tools for boson sampling/graph theory*

Realizing the need for standardized software development tools to facilitate the use of Gaussian boson sampling as a NISQ device, Bromley *et al.* (2020) introduce the GBS application layer of Strawberry Fields. The project is an open-source Python library for photonic quantum computing, available at github.com/XanaduAI/strawberryfields. The application layer is built with the goal of providing users with the capability to implement and test GBS algorithms using only a few lines of code. Specifically, the toolkit contains modules dedicated to dense subgraph identification, maximum clique, graph similarity, point processes, and vibrating spectra. The project addresses one the most substantial roadblocks to quantum computing by providing easy-to-use tools for writing quantum algorithms.

## 10.3 Space-Division Multiplexing Innovation

Quantum photonics is the science of generating, manipulating, and detecting light in regimes in which it is possible to coherently control photons (as individual quanta of the light field) (Pearsall, 2017). The high demand for global communications networks makes quantum photonics an active research frontier. Activity began in the 1950s–1960s when it was realized that light requires a quantum formulation, and that the classical picture (only electromagnetic fields) would be insufficient to describe it. A key advance is the coherent state, an oscillatory quantum state. This is a state with dynamics closely resembling the oscillatory behavior of a classical harmonic oscillator, in particular for the manipulation of quantum light (bosons) (Glauber, 1963). It was further demonstrated that light could be emitted one photon at a time, which has given rise to global fiberoptic telecommunications networks and single-photon manipulation.

There are various ways to write (modulate) information onto light. Traffic is often received as analog electrical signals which are converted to optical signals for transport and then reconverted back to analog electrical signals for delivery at the other end. A key piece of technical equipment is optical-to-electronic interconnects for traffic ingress and egress. All signals are typically multiplexed to fit as much information as possible onto a communications fiber. The different techniques to optimize multiplexing are based on time, wavelength, polarization, phase, and space. Demand continues to grow for transmitting increasing amounts of information over longer distances and a key focus is on expanding the capacity and information transmission rates in fibers (Xavier & Lima, 2020). The same kinds of light manipulation techniques are used for different applications; data multiplexing activities are generally kept separate from those involving entanglement generation and management.

### 10.3.1 *Information multiplexing*

The optical fiber is the central unit in the communications infrastructure. A variety of multiplexing techniques are used for encoding information onto the fiber are based on time, wavelength, and space (Table 10.3).

Time-division multiplexing (TDM) has been used for decades as a method for increasing channel capacity by transmitting and receiving independent signals over a common signal path by means of synchronized switches at each end of the transmission line. Wavelength division multiplexing (WDM) is another technique for increasing transmission capacity

Table 10.3. Multiplexing in global fiberoptic networks.

| No. | Multiplexing Method | Year |
|---|---|---|
| 1 | Time-division multiplexing (TDM): Time synchronization between sender-receiver | 1880 |
| 2 | Wave-division multiplexing (WDM): Multiplex onto forward direction of wave movement | 1990 |
| 3 | Space-division multiplexing (SDM): Multiplex onto sideways direction of wave movement | 2013 |

that involves multiple data channels being multiplexed using different wavelengths over a single fiber (Brackett, 1990).

Space-division multiplexing (SDM) is the most recent advance (Richardson *et al.*, 2013). The technique was known, and has become technologically feasible. Space-division multiplexing is the spatial analog of wave-division multiplexing. Whereas waves propagate forward and can be multiplexed (divided into channels) on this basis, there is also the transverse (sideways) dimension of waves. The insight is to multiplex data onto both the forward-propagating and transverse direction of the optical modes of a light beam to increase the spatial density of the communications fiber. The transverse optical modes are electromagnetic field patterns of the radiation encoded in the plane perpendicular (transverse) to the radiation's propagation direction. New optical fiber designs and components help to realize space-division multiplexing as multiple co-existing data channels based on light propagation over distinct transverse optical modes.

In particular, space-division multiplexing draws from recent progress in fiber research. There are improvements to conventional fibers and high-precision fabrication methods have been developed to produce fibers with hollow cores and other complex microstructures. State-of-the art space-division multiplexing technology as of 2019 was on the order of 266.1 terabits per second transmission over a six-mode fiber (Wakayama, *et al.*, 2019). This compares to TeleGeography's estimated total global internet bandwidth capacity of 295 terabits per second ($10^{12}$ bps) in 2017 (Rebatta, 2017). The implication is that just one fiber can provide the entire backbone capacity of recent moments of internet traffic.

Simultaneously, there have been developments in quantum information processing, with novel protocols and devices for computing, communication, and sensing. Quantum networks could lead to the full-fledged implementation of the quantum internet and other novel kinds of quantum networks. Technological advance, demand, and a more intense potential era of quantum networks are motivating the deployment of space-division multiplexing. However, one barrier to increasing information transmission rates with space-division multiplexing is that many installed fibers are a basic technology that is only designed to support the fundamental Gaussian propagation mode (single-mode transmission). Fortunately, in some cases, space-division multiplexing might be run as an overlay to existing technologies. The installed plant of fiber cables is a mix of legacy and upgrade technologies, with some being more conducive to space-division multiplexing than others.

Any fiber that can support more than one transverse (perpendicular) optical mode of propagation is possibly suitable for space-division multiplexing. The most direct approach is to embed several single-mode cores into a single fiber cladding to produce a multi-core fiber. If the transverse core separation is large enough, the fibers can be approximated as independent fibers in most applications. Another alternative is to use a fiber with only a single core, but which is capable of supporting more than one transverse mode for light propagation. Existing multi-mode optical fibers are less conducive to space-division multiplexing as they already run their own complicated expansion technology supporting hundreds of modes which require complex auxiliary optoelectronic systems to reconstruct the original wavefront.

Space-division multiplexing can also be implemented with quantum techniques, particularly to reach terabit per second data rates (Wang *et al.*, 2012). One quantum strategy is the multiplexing of data channels using transverse optical modes carrying orbital angular momentum (OAM) (Gibson *et al.*, 2004). A certain kind of light beam (Laguerre-Gaussian) is used to carry discrete OAM modes. Each associated photon carries a fixed amount of OAM ($l\hbar$, where $\hbar$ is Planck's constant divided by $2\pi$).

#### 10.3.1.1 *Spacetime states*

Foundational physics advance continues to encourage progress in quantum computation and communications networks. New ideas might be applied to substantially extend the capacity and information rates of global communications networks. Zhang *et al.* (2020) use theoretical physics to expand the possibilities of multiplexing. The research presents a unified approach to space and time integration in quantum theory, by building quantum states across spacetime instead of only on spatial slices. Instead of distinguishing measurements on the same system at different times, measurements are taken on different systems at one time and spacetime states are constructed on the basis of these measurement statistics. The work proposes six possible definitions for spacetime states in continuous variables, based on four different measurement processes: Quadratures, displaced parity operators, position measurements and weak measurements. The central idea is to treat different instances of time as different quantum modes. The formalisms used are the pseudo-density matrix formulation and the path integral formulation. These definitions lead to practically useful network properties, and theoretically help to illuminate the differences between spatial and temporal correlations. The operational meaning of the spacetime states can be confirmed with tomography or other similar methods.

### 10.3.2 *Personal brain networks*

Advances in communications (high-capacity secure network transfer with quantum optical networks and personal area network protocols) and neuroscience (individual connectomes with the Virtual Brain project and wavelet interpretation algorithms) could come together in the idea of personal brain networks. Such personal brain networks could noninvasively acquire and monitor personal neurological data continuously, and transfer these data for secure processing, storing, and permissioned sharing. Personal connectomics could develop from the Virtual Brain (VirtualBrain.org) connectome-based brain simulation platform which has over fifty individual human connectomes (Triebkorn *et al.*, 2020). Personal connectomes might be analyzed with ultrafast wavelet-based data management techniques that increase the capacity of optical networks (Cincotti *et al.*, 2005). Such methods propose an optical wavelet packet division multiplexing (WPDM) scheme in which data signals are waveform-coded onto wavelet atom functions for transmission.

This consists of compact integrable architectures to perform the discrete wavelet transforms and the wavelet packet decomposition of an optical digital signal. The implication is the possibility of using wavelet technology for personal local networks, including personal brain networks (with appropriate security). Neuroscience imaging signals are already wavelet-processed (Puckett *et al.*, 2020), and having a secure personalized data collection method via optical networking technology could speed the development of personalized connectomes and other applications.

Khalid *et al.* (2019) discuss Visible Light Communication as a model for next-generation wireless communication in local area networks. The method is designed to relieve radio-frequency (RF) congestion by using a visible light band for transmission. The RF spectrum has become crowded with the demand for high-speed multi-media mobile services. Particularly with an eye to 5G roll-out, innovations in broadband technology are needed. One research program examines new ideas for data transmission on a highly localized basis. Visible Light Communication is such a local data communication technology based modulating the intensity of light to transmit information, mostly by means of Light Emitting Diodes. The IEEE has confirmed Visible Light Communication as the standard for data transmission in Wireless Personal Area Networks (WPANs) (IEEE protocol 802.15.17) (Sarbazi & Uysal, 2013). Hence, the major pieces are in place for an early prototype of personal brain networks with neuroscience-based brain wavelet interpretations, optical-frequency personal area network data collection, and high-speed optical network-based data multiplexing for external transfer.

## 10.4 Photonic Qubit Encoding

Encoding photons in quantum computing and quantum communications networks can be achieved with two classes of methods, those based on the physics of angular momentum and those based on technology. The physics-based methods build qubit technology around the quantum mechanical behavior of particles, namely, by using polarization to encode spin angular momentum (SAM) and spatial modes to encode OAM. The technology-based encoding methods use waveguide paths and time and frequency bins to generate and structure qubits, and are often used in boson sampling

(Zhong *et al.*, 2020). Polarization is the established workhorse method but can only send one qubit, so there is attention to developing the other methods, all of which can transmit multiple qubits including qudits (quantum digits with more than two values). The technology-based methods in particular may be able to expand arbitrarily in the number of qudits in waveguide transmission and time and frequency-binning (Table 10.4).

### 10.4.1 *Physics: Angular momentum*

Physics-based photonic qubit encoding involves the natural angular momentum attributes of particle movement. Angular momentum is a quantized measure of a particle's rotational activity in rolling, spinning, and orbiting. Qubit encoding makes use of two forms of angular momentum, SAM and OAM. SAM is associated with the circular polarization of a particle's momentum. OAM is related to the spatial structure of the particle's wave movement in a helical orbit.

#### 10.4.1.1 *Polarization: SAM*

Polarization is the most frequently used method for photon encoding. In SAM encoding, three pairs of polarization (opposite) states are used to encode information in the particle's rotational movement: Horizontal and vertical, left and right, and opposite diagonals. The techniques for producing polarization qubits are straightforward to implement and have become

Table 10.4. Photon encoding methods.

| No. | Encoding Method | Qubit Encoding | Qubit Capacity |
|---|---|---|---|
| *Physics-based encoding: Angular momentum* | | | |
| 1 | Polarization: Spin angular momentum | H/V, L/R, Diagonals | Single |
| 2 | Spatial modes: Orbital angular momentum | Left/right | Multiple |
| *Technology-based encoding: Time and frequency bins* | | | |
| 3 | Propagation path in waveguide | 0/1 (qubit) 0/1/2 (qutrit) | Multiple |
| 4 | Time-bin, frequency-bin | Early/late arrival bins | Multiple |

*Source*: Adapted from Flamini *et al.* (2018, p. 3).

the standard method used in most applications for the encoding and manipulation of quantum information. Polarization qubits can be coupled easily to other degrees of freedom to produce hybrid entangled states. In advanced transmission, polarization qubits are coupled to other degrees of freedom possessed by single photons such as OAM, propagation path, and time-frequency (energy) to create high-dimensional entangled states. Polarized qubits are an efficient resource for quantum computation and quantum communications networks. However, the shortcoming is that polarization qubits can only carry one qubit of information, and as quantum information networks expand, other methods such as OAM are needed to transmit multiple qubits.

#### 10.4.1.2 *Spatial Modes: OAM*

OAM (with allowable states: Left and Right) is a growing method of photon encoding as the technique can be used to send multiple qubits. In OAM encoding, attention is given to the particle's helical spiraling orbit along a line of propagated movement through space (visualized as if the particle were tracing a DNA strand's helical shape). The spatial distribution of the front of the propagating wave (wavefront) is measured by two terms, an internal origin-independent term associated with the helical (twisted) wavefront, and an external origin-dependent term. Quantum information processing based on OAM makes most use of the internal twisted wavefront term. Qubit values are encoded as Left and Right in relation to the helical movement of the wavefront.

The mathematics of OAM is nontrivial. OAM is carried by optical vortices (singularities) that are described by a phase term (angular coordinate) and an unbounded integer. An integral is evaluated around the vortex (singularity) for a field with the phase term. A key measure is another term which is used to measure topological charge ($q$) that counts the number of helices in the phase profile (and which can be manipulated with so-called $q$-plates). An important attribute for qubit management is that single photons are assessed as carrying quantized values of OAM given by the topological charge (the number of helices in the phase profile).

Various techniques are used to produce OAM states. Most frequently employed are spatial light modulators (which can modify the intensity or phase of the light beam at each point), cylindrical lenses, and diffraction gratings in the form of holograms. Spatial light modulators are widely used in optical communication and optical tweezers. A newer innovation is spiral wave plates, whose thickness increases in a transparent spiral structure so that light experiences a phase gradient during the propagation. However, spiral wave plates are limited by cost, wavelength selectivity, and reliable qubit generation as compared to other methods. Another tool is $q$-plates ($q$ referring to topological charge), which apply a plate structure to manipulate photons. $Q$-plates are proving useful for generating multiple degree of freedom entanglement in qubits with polarization and OAM.

#### 10.4.1.3 *Polarization versus OAM encoding*

One trade-off between polarization and OAM is that polarization is a straightforward established method whereas orbital angular moment is a more complicated emerging model. However, only one qubit at a time can be sent with polarization, and multiple qubits transmitted with OAM encoding, so there is interest in developing the technology. Another trade-off between the two techniques is the ease and reliability of qubit recognition. Polarization encoding only requires resolving two components (easily managed with the existing equipment of waveplates and polarizing beam splitters), but the number of OAM modes is potentially unbounded and difficult to characterize. The same methods are used to produce and recognize OAM qubits, and continue to be developed, as mentioned, for example, spatial light modulators, spiral phase plates, and $q$-plates. Once generated and identified, OAM states can be manipulated with a high degree of control such that quantum information can be encoded in an essentially infinite Hilbert space. Hence, it is possible that, if unlocking technology to control OAM qubits, it could be a scalable technology of the future.

### **10.4.2 *Technology: Path and time-frequency bins***

#### 10.4.2.1 *Propagation path waveguide encoding*

Path encoding is the representation of qubits in terms of their occupying modes in the waveguide and propagating along these paths.

Waveguide arrays inherently use a spatial separation and coupling method between modes, so are a natural structure for designating qubits and qudits. Qubits (optical modes) are generated and encoded directly into an available location in the waveguide path or fiber. Encoding is generic, a 0 or 1 (or more for qudits) based the assigned location in the waveguide path. Due to the structured setup, path-encoded qubits and qudits map directly onto existing photonic integrated circuits. Photonic integrated circuits have high stability and complexity, and this allows the configuration of most of the relevant features of applications in quantum computing and communication technologies. Accurate control over path-encoded qubits for universal manipulation is possible with relatively low cost and technological requirements as compared to the other encoding methods.

#### 10.4.2.2 *Time-based encoding: Time, frequency, energy*

The Heisenberg uncertainty principle implicates the special relationship of conjugate pairs such as location-momentum and time-energy. The canonical interpretation is being able to know a particle's location but not its speed, and vice versa. The relationship is structured as a gradient of being able to know more about a particle's location by knowing less about its speed. Aside from location-momentum, the other main conjugate pair is time-energy. In this context, the time and energy relationship is translated as time-frequency or the wave energy as measured by frequency, and is likewise structured as a gradient (more time precision is less energy (frequency) precision).

Time-based encoding is deployed by different mechanisms. One is that the particle wave's time is encoded into bins (two or arbitrarily more), one arriving before the other. Analogously, the second mechanism is that the particle wave's frequency (energy) is encoded into bins (two or arbitrarily more), also arriving at different intervals. Imany *et al.* (2019), for example, make use of 16-bins each of time and frequency divisions for 32 total bins. This manner of qubit or qudit encoding is labeled as Early/late arrival in time or frequency (with as many designations as needed), per being directed by the photonic device into the different time and frequency. A further mechanism is that through their conjugate pair relationship, the particle wave's time and frequency attributes can be entangled together or converted into one another.

Describing time-bin encoding in more detail, time is a natural and effective resource for writing information onto single-photon quantum states. Time-bin encoding involves coding time into different bins. The standard method uses an encoder (interferometer) with one arm that is longer than the other. The allowed qubit states are Early Time and Late Time, to distinguish between the photons taking the short path and those taking the longer path. The temporal delay must be smaller than one wavelength, and longer than the coherence length of each photon, to allow a reliable discrimination of the arrival times. Proper dynamic control of the temporal delay is needed to compensate for mechanic and thermal instabilities, but in general, the precision of using time as a degree of freedom offers various advantages over other encoding schemes. Time-bin encoding is suitable for integrated photonic devices, in which photons can be generated, manipulated and measured without the need for external encoding devices. Time-encoded qubits are resilient to the noise that can damage polarization qubits (such as depolarizing media or decoherence and mode dispersion). Time-frequency encoding offers advantages over polarization and spatial-mode encodings because multiple spectral modes are supported in the waveguides and optical fibers with minimal dispersion, and zero cross-talk. Further, time-bin encoding has been proposed as a suitable scheme for quantum walks and boson sampling.

Frequency-bin encoding proceeds in the same manner of using early-late arrival bins. Such methods have been demonstrated in quantum computing (to operate cluster states) and quantum communications networks. Particularly for quantum communications applications, frequency-encoded qubits are in parallel with existing methods and thus might be useful in applications such as quantum key distribution and quantum state teleportation. For example, time-frequency quantum key distribution protocols suggest taking advantage of the low decoherence risk available in frequency-based qubits (Nunn *et al.*, 2013).

# 10.5 High-dimensional Quantum Entanglement

## 10.5.1 *Theoretical development*

### 10.5.1.1 *Qudits and optimal information content*

In high-dimensional entanglement, particles or qubits are entangled in more than one dimension (such as polarization, spatial modes, propagation path, and time-frequency bins). High-dimensional quantum entanglement is necessary to produce qudits. The basic unit of quantum information is the qubit (quantum information bit). A *qubit* is a two-state quantum mechanical system used for computing, as the quantum version of the classical bit. However, qubits are just one example of the broader class of *qudits* (quantum information digits). As a quantum mechanical entity, a unit of quantum information can exist in any number of states. A qubit is a binary quantum information bit taking the values of 0 and 1, and exists in a superposition of 0 and 1 before measurement. A *qutrit* is a trinary quantum information bit taking the values of 0, 1, and 2, and exists in the 0, 1, and 2 states until measured. Qudits can scale to arbitrarily large quantum systems. At least as many as seven-qudit systems have been tested (Fonseca *et al.*, 2018).

For simplicity and ease of implementation, the binary qubit has been the focus of quantum information implementation. However, optical systems are now taking greater advantage of higher-dimensional qudits. In computation theory, there may be an optimal qudit number for a given system. DNA appears to be one example of an optimal encoding system (Szathmary, 2003). The four-digit information code (ATCG; adenine, thymine, cytosine, and guanine) contains the genetic instructions used in the development and functioning of all known living organisms. Technically, there are five bases as RNA adds an intelligence and security layer by transcribing T (thymine) as U (uracil) so that DNA and RNA strands are readily identifiable.

Systems of greater complexity may have a more than binary information encoding structure. In certain computational tasks, it is known that greater-than-binary structures are optimal. For example, the three-qutrit code is an efficient self-contained nine-state holographic quantum error correction code (Harlow, 2017). Likewise in information theory, quantum communication protocols based on larger alphabets may offer certain advantages (Hayden & Penington, 2019). Quantum error correction and information theory point to the benefit of higher information capacity also possibly conferring increased resistance to noise (an ancilla of extra bits may be effectively built into high capacity information encoding structures). Such functionality could be helpful in quantum key distribution in cryptography, for example.

Several physical systems already allow for the encoding of higher-dimensional quantum information in the form of qudits. Quantum photonics is one of the first and most developed. All three of the primary approaches to quantum computing (photonics, trapped ions, and superconducting circuits) allow for qudit-based information encoding which could substantially speed the development of the industry. Other qudit-enabled physical systems include a variety of benchtop quantum experimental setups such as Rydberg atoms, polar-molecules, cold atomic ensembles, and solid-state defects (Erhard *et al.*, 2020).

#### 10.5.1.2 *Greenberger–Horne–Zeilinger (GHZ) state*

Quantum computing is not constrained to the qubit, or to the notion of entanglement being applicable to just two particles and one dimension. This broader landscape has been acknowledged from the beginning. However, concretization has led to a focus on the simplest and most practical formulations as the first step. Works by Einstein *et al.* (1935) and Schrödinger (1935) examine in particular how quantum systems are related to the position and momentum of two strongly correlated (entangled) particles. Toward the practical agenda of realization, Bohm (1951) proposed the idea of investigating two entangled spin-1/2 particles (i.e. two-state systems called qubits). Bell (1964) formulated an experimentally testable theorem, which has become central to Bell pair entanglement in quantum communications.

Now in photonics, there is starting to be more of an emphasis on higher-dimension multi-particle systems, which increase the Hilbert space exponentially. A well-known multi-particle system formulation is the GHZ (Greenberger–Horne–Zeilinger) state (Greenberger *et al.*, 1989).

The GHZ state is an entangled quantum state involving at least three subsystems (particle states or qubits). The multi-particle state is used to encode quantum information and test quantum systems, as a standard target state or "Hello world" application in multi-particle systems. The GHZ state is useful as more than a demonstration case, its multi-particle entanglement might be used for quantum error correction schemes. Shor (1995, p. 2) notes that entanglements of three or more qubits can always be accomplished by a sequence of two-bit entanglements.

A key difference between the two-dimensional qubit and the GHZ state is that the *N*-partite observables do not form a commuting set of observables and are non-Hermitian. However, all observables have the multi-partite and high-dimensional GHZ state as a common eigenstate, thus still predict an outcome with certainty. All attempts to generalize the GHZ argument use local unitary observables and thus have complex eigenvalues. This is in contrast to the prevailing view in physics that physical observables must have real eigenvalues (Dirac, 1981). GHZ states point to the need to clarify the general definitions of the properties a physical observable should obey.

From an experimental standpoint, GHZ states consist of three or more entities that are entangled with one another. The GHZ argument for three and more particles in two dimensions has been generalized to an arbitrary number of local dimensions or degrees of freedom (Ryu *et al.*, 2013). The GHZ state has been demonstrated in more than two dimensions, in that a three-dimensional three-party GHZ state was realized using the OAM of optical states (Erhard *et al.*, 2018b). A four-party GHZ state with 32 dimensions in each of two degrees of freedom (time and frequency) has also been realized (Imany *et al.*, 2019). The method encodes high-dimensional units of information (qudits) in time and frequency degrees of freedom using on-chip sources. Specifically, two frequency-bin entangled photons (each carrying two 32-dimensional qudits) are used to realize a four-party high-dimensional GHZ occupying a Hilbert space equivalent to that of 20 qubits.

These experiments highlight the need to investigate high-dimensional entanglement and related research questions (such as whether physical observables must have real eigenvalues as Dirac suggested or might have complex eigenvalues as suggested by generalizations of the GHZ multi-particle entanglement theory). One practical use is to understand superconducting materials and how they may be used to build quantum computing systems. It is known that exotic phenomena arise if the quantum system size (in terms of number and dimensionality) grows to extensive numbers. Some examples of exotic phenomena are superconductivity, superfluids, and Bose–Einstein condensates. These systems are not well-understood and pose significant theoretical as well as experimental challenges. Novel physics might be revealed a deeper understanding of these large and highly correlated quantum systems.

### 10.5.2 *Experimental implementation*

High-dimensional entanglement refers to particles or qubits that are entangled in more than one dimension. The number of particles could be one or more, and the key point is that they are entangled on the basis of more than one dimension. The same techniques used to encode photonic qubits in general are also used to entangle them on the basis of one or more dimensions. The first question is whether a single-photon or a multi-photon system is being entangled. The second question is which dimensions (degrees of freedom) of entanglement are being used in the system, which could be polarization, spatial modes, propagation path, and time-frequency bins, or a combination of them (Table 10.5). The first step in producing high dimensional entanglement states is creating photons and photon pairs. The standard method for creating photon pairs is with a laser pulse to a nonlinear crystal. The second step is entangling them within one or more degrees of freedom.

Table 10.5. High-dimensional quantum entanglement.

| No. | Degrees of Freedom | Description | Qubit Encoding |
|---|---|---|---|
| 1 | Polarization | Spin angular momentum | H/V, L/R, Diagonals |
| 2 | Spatial modes | Orbital angular momentum | Left/right |
| 3 | Propagation path | Path of waveguide travel | 0/1 (qubit), 0/1/2 (qutrit) |
| 4 | Time-frequency bins | Successive bins | Early/late arrival bins |
| 5 | Hybrid entanglement | Multimode entanglement | Various |

#### 10.5.2.1 *Polarization: Spin angular momentum*

It is relatively straightforward to entangle photonic qubits on the dimension of polarization. Also, polarization qubits couple readily to all other degrees of freedom used in hybrid entangled states, namely, OAM, propagation path, and time-frequency (energy) together in high-dimensional entangled states. As such, polarization is often the first designated degree of freedom used in hybrid entanglement.

#### 10.5.2.2 *Spatial modes: OAM*

OAM entanglement is an active experimental research frontier (Erhard *et al.*, 2018a). The OAM describes the wavefront of photons (spatial modes) as they spiral in a helical motion. The main feature of these modes is singularities within the phase, which can be manipulated. The amount of OAM corresponds to the direction and number of windings of the phase around the singularities. At the singularity, the phase is not defined, which results in a doughnut-shaped intensity distribution.

A quantum state of two photons generated within a nonlinear crystal can be described according to their amount of OAM. The exact distribution of the complex coefficients describing the OAM of the photon pair is called the *spiral-spectrum*, and depends on the length of the crystal and other factors. Entangled spatial states are created by manipulating the crystal pumping process that generates the photon pair. This is accomplished by counteracting the spiral-spectrum (that describes the photon wavefront) with a corresponding superposition of different OAM quanta in the pump beam. The process can be incorporated into automated filtering techniques. More technically, a helical (twisted) phase structure leads to a quantized amount of OAM characterized in terms of $\hbar$ (the reduced Planck's constant). Photons with $+1\hbar$ of OAM have a phase structure that varies azimuthally from 0 to $2\pi$, and leads to a vortex along the beam axis. OAM modes exist in a superposition between $+1\hbar$ and $-1\hbar$ (encoded as Left and Right) (Allen *et al.*, 1992).

The nonlinear crystal is pumped to produce a photon pair which is aligned based on OAM, such that the resulting quantum state is a coherent superposition of the photon pair. The result of creating OAM-entangled photon pairs in a single nonlinear crystal is that the two-dimensional spatial field of the photons can be relayed into the entangled two-photon quantum states. OAM is straightforward to create and interpret. First, OAM entanglement can be generated with a single nonlinear crystal. Since OAM is conserved within the production process, it can be used to yield high-dimensionally entangled photon pairs directly. Second, there are several known techniques for manipulating and measuring OAM photon states.

#### 10.5.2.3 *Propagation path waveguide encoding*

Another way to create high-dimensionally entangled photon pairs is in the transmission waveguide after pair production has occurred. The waveguide propagation path encoding method also relies on momentum in the sense of the intrinsic momentum conservation of photons. The momentum conservation property allows the coherent emission of a single-photon pair on a cone. The photon pair takes up opposite positions on the emission cone due to momentum conservation. Evenly spaced on the emission cone, the photon pair can be collected with single-mode fiber pairs to create a $d$-dimensionally entangled quantum state of two photons in their respective fibers or waveguide paths. Quantum information encoded in the waveguide path degree of freedom uses off-the-shelf bulk optical elements (standard beam splitters and phase-shifters) and existing integrated optics (silicon chips with interferometric stability).

#### 10.5.2.4 *Time-based encoding: Time, frequency, energy*

Quantum information stored in time-bins or frequency-bins related to single photons is well-suited to entanglement generation for transmission over large distances using free-space links or optical fibers. One way to create entanglement between two photons in the time-bin domain is to use two indistinguishable laser pulses separated by a fixed time difference. Each laser pulse can create a photon pair within the nonlinear crystal. If there is in principle no information available in which of the two pulses the photon pair A-B has been created, the resulting state can be written as a superposition of the two creation times (denoted as Early and Late). Likewise, frequency-bins are created by early-late arrival designations.

Given the conjugate pair trade-off status of time and frequency (energy), the two degrees of freedom are a natural place to begin the hybrid entanglement of multiple degrees of freedom. Starting from time-bin encoding (with allowed states of Early Time and Late Time arrival), the scheme can be extended to multiple states by correlating the arrival time with the frequency (energy) of the photon. Ansari *et al.* (2020), for example, demonstrate two-photon quantum correlations in the time-frequency domain. Similarly, Kaiser *et al.* (2016) present an experimental method for measuring time-energy entanglement in wavelength division multiplexed (WDM) quantum networks. A related application is Nunn *et al.* (2013) who make use of time-to-frequency conversion in their time-frequency quantum key distribution scheme with entangled photon pairs. Finally, Imany *et al.* (2019) realize a four-party GHZ state with 32 dimensions, 16 each in two degrees of freedom (time and frequency).

#### 10.5.2.5 *Hybrid entanglement: Multiple degrees of freedom*

Multiple degrees-of-freedom entanglement extends beyond the time-frequency conjugate pair relationship to include any variety of degrees of freedom, often starting with polarization as the cornerstone. The general concept is achieving high-dimensional quantum states that entangle single photons on the basis several degrees of freedom simultaneously. One demonstration employs the polarization, OAM, and time-frequency degrees of freedom to create a 12-dimensionally entangled quantum state in three degrees of freedom (Barreiro *et al.*, 2005). In a similar demonstration, Wang *et al.* (2018) created an 18-qubit entangled state, a GHZ state encoded in six photons with three degrees of freedom (polarization, path, and spatial modes). One advantage of hybrid degrees of freedom is that they can use deterministic CNOT gates, which are important super-dense coding and super-dense quantum teleportation applications. Various configurations of the polarization, spatial, and time-frequency degrees of freedom can be employed to generate strong and verifiable two-photon entanglement. These correlations could enable applications such as quantum state teleportation, quantum key distribution, and remote state preparation.

### 10.5.2.6 *Degrees of freedom conversion*

A further flexibility in degrees of freedom entanglement involves the possibility of converting one degree of freedom to another. In such an approach, entanglement created in waveguide path of travel degree of freedom, for example, can be converted directly into OAM entanglement (Fickler *et al.*, 2014). This is achieved by using the mode sorter between OAM and the waveguide path in reverse. To generate a three-path entangled two-photon state, a nonlinear crystal can be used to produce pairs of photons that illuminate a three-slit mask. The consecutive mode sorter is then used to transform the path information to OAM states while maintaining the entanglement encoded in the path of travel degree of freedom. Such interfaces allow the creation and manipulation of quantum states locally on-chip using the path degree of freedom, and then the further downstream connection to distant chips via a quantum link encoded in the OAM degree of freedom.

### 10.5.2.7 *Planck's constant*

The expressions $h$ and $\hbar$ (h-bar) are widely used in quantum mechanics to refer to Planck's constant. Planck's constant is the amount of change in energy per change in frequency (in particle wave movement). Planck's constant is measured in Joules/second per cycle units, and its value is $6.626 \times 10^{-34}$ Joules/second (a very small number). The other formulation of Planck's constant is $\hbar$, which is the reduced Planck's constant, measured in units of Joules/second Radians, $1.055 \times 10^{-34}$ Joules/second/radian. Planck's constant divided by $2\pi$ results in the name h-bar, representing $h$ divided by $2\pi$. The term $\hbar$, (instead of $h$), is often used as a more natural simplified expression of angular frequency in physics.

Planck's constant is based on the idea that energy is quantized (into discrete packets or tiers). Energy is discrete and also based on frequency or oscillation waves. A formula can be written as $E = hf$ to denote the relationship that Energy (E) is equal to a constant ($h$) multiplied by frequency (f). Per observed spectra, the value of Planck's constant can be computed as $6.626 \times 10^{-34}$ joule-seconds. The constant $h$ is a proportionality constant (energy divided by frequency) that describes the relationship between energy and frequency, the amount of change in energy per change in frequency. In the same format, Einstein later associated energy directly to the electromagnetic wave in Special Relativity (1905) with the formula $E = mc^2$, that energy is equal to mass multiplied by the speed of light squared. The formula directly associates energy with a quantum or minimal element of the energy of the electromagnetic wave.

## References

Aaronson, S. & Arkhipov, A. (2013). The computational complexity of linear optics. *Theor. Comput.* 9(4):143–252.

Allen, L., Beijersbergen, M.W., Spreeuw, R.J.C. & Woerdman, J.P. (1992). Orbital angular momentum of light and the transformation of Laguerre-Gaussian laser modes. *Phys. Rev. A*. 45:8185.

Ansari, V., Donohue, J.M., Brecht, B. & Silberhorn, C. (2020). Remotely projecting states of photonic temporal modes. *Opt. Express*. 28(19):28295–305.

Arrazola, J.M. & Bromley, T.R. (2018). Using Gaussian boson sampling to find dense subgraphs. *Phys. Rev. Lett.* 121(3):030503.

Arrazola, J.M., Bromley, T.R. & Rebentrost, P. (2018). Quantum approximate optimization with Gaussian boson sampling. *Phys. Rev. A*. 98(1):012322.

Awschalom, D., Berggren, K.K., Bernien, H. *et al.* (2019). Development of Quantum InterConnects for next-generation information technologies. U.S. National Science Foundation workshop (2019) Alexandria, VA. arXiv: 1912.06642.

Ball, P. (2020). Physicists in China challenge Google's 'quantum advantage'. *Nature*. 588:380.

Barreiro, J.T., Langford, N.K., Peters, N.A. & Kwiat, P.G. (2005). Generation of hyperentangled photon pairs. *Phys. Rev. Lett.* 95(26):260501.

Bell, J.S. (1964). On the Einstein Podolsky Rosen paradox. *Physics Physique Fizika*. 1(3):195–200.

Bohm, D. (1951). *Quantum Theory*. London: Prentice-Hall.

Brackett, C.A. (1990). Dense wavelength division multiplexing networks: Principles and applications. *IEEE J. Sel. Areas Commun.* 8:948–64.

Bradler, K., Dallaire-Demers, P.-L., Rebentrost, P. *et al.* (2018a). Gaussian boson sampling for perfect matchings of arbitrary graphs. *Phys. Rev. A*. 98(3): 032310.

Bradler, K., Friedland, S., Izaac, J. *et al.* (2018b). Graph isomorphism and Gaussian boson sampling. arXiv:1810.10644.

Bradler, K., Israel, R., Schuld, M. & Su, D. (2019). A duality at the heart of Gaussian boson sampling. arXiv:1910.04022v1.

Bromley, T.R., Arrazola, J.M., Jahangiri, S. *et al.* (2020). Applications of near-term photonic quantum computers: Software and algorithms. *Quantum Sci. Technol.* 5(3):034010.

Cincotti, G., Moreolo, M.S. & Neri, A. (2005). Optical wavelet signals processing and multiplexing. *EURASIP J. Appl. Signal Process.* 10:1574–83.

Cisco. (2020). Cisco Annual Internet Report, 2018–2023. *Cisco White Paper.* https://www.cisco.com/c/en/us/solutions/collateral/executive-perspectives/annual-internet-report/white-paper-c11-741490.html.

Costello, K. & Rimol, M. (2020). *Gartner Forecasts Worldwide Public Cloud End-User Spending to Grow 18% in 2021.* Gartner, Inc. https://www.gartner.com/en/newsroom/press-releases/2020-11-17-gartner-forecasts-worldwide-public-cloud-end-user-spending-to-grow-18-percent-in-2021.

Dirac, P.A.M. (1981). *The Principles of Quantum Mechanics.* Oxford: Oxford University Press.

Einstein, A., Podolsky, B. & Rosen, N. (1935). Can quantum-mechanical description of physical reality be considered complete? *Phys. Rev.* 47:777–80.

Erhard, M., Fickler, R., Krenn, M. & Zeilinger, A. (2018a). Twisted photons: New quantum perspectives in high dimensions. *Light. Sci. Appl.* 7:17146.

Erhard, M., Malik, M., Krenn, M. & Zeilinger, A. (2018b). Experimental Greenberger–Horne–Zeilinger entanglement beyond qubits. *Nat. Photon.* 12:759–64.

Erhard, M., Krenn, M. & Zeilinger, A. (2020). Advances in high dimensional quantum entanglement. *Nat. Rev. Phys.* 2:365–81.

Fickler, R., Lapkiewicz, R., Huber, M. *et al.* (2014). Interface between path and orbital angular momentum entanglement for high-dimensional photonic quantum information. *Nat. Commun.* 5:4502.

Flamini, F., Spagnolo, N. & Sciarrino, F. (2018). Photonic quantum information processing: A review. *Rep. Prog. Phys.* 82(1):016001.

Fonseca, A., Rosier, A., Vertesi, T. *et al.* (2018). Survey on the Bell nonlocality of a pair of entangled qudits. *Phys. Rev. A.* 98(4):042105.

Garcia-Alvarez, L., Egusquiza, I.L., Lamata, L. *et al.* (2017). Digital quantum simulation of minimal AdS/CFT. *Phys. Rev. Lett.* 119(4):040501.

Gibson, G., Courtial, J., Padgett, M.J. *et al.* (2004). Free-space information transfer using light beams carrying orbital angular momentum. *Opt. Express.* 12:5448–56.

Glauber, R.J. (1963). The quantum theory of optical coherence. *Phys. Rev.* 130(6):2529–39.

Greenberger, D.M., Horne, M.A. & Zeilinger, A. (1989). Going beyond Bell's theorem. *Bell's Theorem, Quantum Theory and Conceptions of the Universe*. Berlin: Springer, pp. 69–72.

Hamilton, C.S., Kruse, R., Sansoni, L. *et al.* (2017). Gaussian boson sampling. *Phys. Rev. Lett.* 19(17):170501.

Harlow, D. (2017). TASI lectures on the emergence of bulk physics in AdS/CFT. In *Proceedings of Theoretical Advanced Study Institute Summer School 2017, "Physics at the Fundamental Frontier"*, Boulder, Colorado, USA, June 4–July 1, 2017. arXiv:1802.01040, PoS(TASI2017)002.

Hayden, P. & Penington, G. (2019). Learning the Alpha-bits of black holes. *J. High Energ. Phys.* 1912:007.

Imany, P., Jaramillo-Villegas, J.A. & Alshaykh, M.S. (2019). High-dimensional optical quantum logic in large operational spaces. *NPJ Quantum Information.* 5(59):1–10.

Kaiser, F., Aktas, D., Fedrici, B. *et al.* (2016). Optimal analysis of ultra-broad-band energy-time entanglement for high bit-rate dense wavelength division multiplexed quantum networks. *Appl. Phys. Lett.* 108:231108.

Khalid, A., Asif, H.M., Kostromitin, K.I. *et al.* (2019). Doubly orthogonal wavelet packets for multi-users indoor visible light communication systems. *Photonics*. 6(85):1–23.

Knill, E., Laflamme, R. & Milburn, G.J. (2001). A scheme for efficient quantum computation with linear optics. *Nature*. 409:46–52.

Lanyon, B.P., Weinhold, T.J., Langford, N.K. *et al.* (2007). Experimental demonstration of a compiled version of Shor's algorithm with quantum entanglement. *Phys. Rev. Lett.* 99(25):250505.

Lu, C.-Y., Browne, D.E., Yang, T. & Pan, J.-W. (2007). Demonstration of a compiled version of Shor's quantum factoring algorithm using photonic qubits. *Phys. Rev. Lett.* 99(25):250504.

Nair, C.R. (2006). Photon as a black hole. In *Modern Mathematical Physics. Proceedings, 4th Summer School, Dedicated to Irina Ya*, Arefeva's Jubilee, Belgrade, Serbia, September 3–14, 2006, SFIN A1, pp. 321–6.

Nunn, J., Wright, L.J., Soller, C. *et al.* (2013). Large-alphabet time-frequency entangled quantum key distribution by means of time-to-frequency conversion. *Opt. Express.* 21:15959–73.

Pearsall, T. (2017). *Quantum Photonics*. Berlin: Springer.

Puckett, A.M., Schira, M.M., Isherwood, Z.J. *et al.* (2020). Manipulating the structure of natural scenes using wavelets to study the functional architecture of perceptual hierarchies in the brain. *NeuroImage*. 221:117173.

Rebatta, A. (2017). 295 Tbps: Internet traffic and capacity in 2017. *TeleGeography*. https://blog.telegeography.com/295-tbps-internet-traffic-and-capacity-in-2017.

Reinsel, D. (2020). IDC's Global DataSphere Forecast shows continued steady growth in the creation and consumption of Data. *IDC Report: Worldwide Global DataSphere Forecast, 2020–2024: The COVID-19 Data Bump and the Future of Data Growth* (Doc #US44797920).

Richardson, D.J., Fini, J.M. & Nelson, L.E. (2013). Space-division multiplexing in optical fibers. *Nat. Photon.* 7:354–62.

Ryu, J., Lee, C., Zukowski, M. & Lee, J. (2013). Greenberger-Horne-Zeilinger theorem for n qudits. *Phys. Rev. A.* 88(4):042101.

Sarbazi, E. & Uysal, M. (2013). PHY layer performance evaluation of the IEEE 802.15.7 visible light communication standard. In *Proceedings of the 2013 2nd International Workshop on Optical Wireless Communications (IWOW)*, Newcastle upon Tyne, UK, October 21, 2013, pp. 35–9.

Schrödinger, E. (1935). Die gegenwärtige situation in der quantenmechanik. *Naturwissenschaften.* 23:823–8.

Schuld, M., Bradler, K., Israel, R. *et al.* (2019). A quantum hardware-induced graph kernel based on Gaussian boson sampling. arXiv:1905.12646.

Shor, P.W. (1995). Scheme for reducing decoherence in quantum computer memory. *Phys. Rev. A.* 52(4):R2493.

Sparrow, C., Martin-Lopez, E., Maraviglia, N. *et al.* (2018). Simulating the vibrational quantum dynamics of molecules using photonics. *Nature.* 557:660.

Szathmary, E. (2003). Why are there four letters in the genetic alphabet? *Nat. Rev. Genet.* 4:995.

Top500. (2020). The list: November 2020. *Top500.* https://www.top500.org/lists/top500/2020/11/1/. Accessed March 15, 2021.

Triebkorn, P., Zimmermann, J., Stefanovski, L. *et al.* (2020). Identifying optimal working points of individual Virtual Brains: A large-scale brain network modelling study. BioRxiv: 009795.

Valiant, L. (1979). *Theor. Comput. Sci.* 8(2):189–201.

Wakayama, Y., Soma, D., Beppu, S. *et al.* (2019). 266.1-Tbit/s transmission over 90.4-km 6-mode fiber with inline dual C + L-band 6-mode EDFA. *IEEE J. Lightwave Technol.* 37:404–10.

Wang, X.-L., Luo, Y.-H., Huang, H.-L. *et al.* (2018). 18-qubit entanglement with six photons' three degrees of freedom. *Phys. Rev. Lett.* 120(26):260502.

Wang, J., Yang, J.-Y., Fazal, I.M. *et al.* (2012). Terabit free-space data transmission employing orbital angular momentum multiplexing. *Nat. Photon.* 6:488–96.

Xavier, G.B. & Lima, G. (2020). Quantum information processing with space-division multiplexing optical fibers. *Commun. Phys.* 3(9):1–11.

Zhang, T., Dahlsten, O. & Vedral, V. (2020). Different instances of time as different quantum modes: Quantum states across space-time for continuous variables. *New J. Phys.* 22(023029):1–19.

Zhong, H.-S., Peng, L.-C., Li, Y. *et al.* (2019). Experimental Gaussian boson sampling. *Sci. Bull.* 64:511–5.

Zhong, H.-S., Wang, H., Deng, Y.-H. *et al.* (2020). Quantum computational advantage using photons. *Science*. 370(6523):1460–3.

# Chapter 11

# Optical Machine Learning and Quantum Networks

*Today, the second quantum revolution is in full swing and promises to revolutionize areas such as computation, communication, metrology, and imaging*

— Erhard *et al.* (2020, p. 1)


**Abstract**

This chapter discusses quantum optical machine learning as the corresponding version of quantum machine learning for optical platforms to test and develop quantum algorithms. Quantum networks as the centerpiece of global quantum computing are presented in the context of a full-stack protocols proposal including heralded (confirmed) entanglement generation, quantum teleportation, and end-to-end qubit delivery. A global quantum clock network of entangled network-wide GHZ (Greenberger–Horne–Zeilinger) states is proposed.


## 11.1 Quantum Optical Machine Learning

Optical quantum computing is an approach to quantum computing that uses all-optical components, in the three input-processing-output steps of single-photon sources, photonic integrated circuits, and single-photon

Table 11.1. Quantum optical machine learning.

| No. | Advance | Description |
|---|---|---|
| 1 | Optical quantum computing | All-optical component quantum computer |
| 2 | Optical neural networks | Machine learning on optical networks |
| 3 | Quantum optical neural networks | Machine learning on quantum optical networks |

detectors (O'Brien, 2007). Optical neural networks are a neural network implementation using optical components (Shen *et al.*, 2017). Quantum optical neural networks are machine learning applications run on quantum optical networks (Steinbrecher *et al.*, 2019) (Table 11.1).

### 11.1.1 *Optical quantum computing*

It was understood that scalable all-optical quantum computing would be a possibility at least as early as 2001, but advances in equipment were necessary to make it feasible (O'Brien, 2007, p. 1567). Such experimental developments in integrated photonics and nanofabrication have indeed enabled integrated circuits with many thousands of optoelectronic components (Harris *et al.*, 2018). Photonics has experienced a componentry revolution similar to that of electronics in a strong effort toward the miniaturization of optical components and dielectric materials in the 2010s (Flamini *et al.*, 2018, p. 6). Integrated optical circuits have special design needs and architectures built with directional couplers that have additional geometries to account for deformation-induced wave phase shifts. Rendering these and other aspects reconfigurable by using fused silicon materials has been a substantial advance. The result is low propagation losses, low birefringence, full operations from visible to infrared, good coupling efficiency with single mode fibers, and low temperature dependence. There have also been advances in the precision of photon generation and detection equipment.

The upshot is that a number of components are readily implementable using state-of-the-art integrated quantum photonics. The most important capability is that matrix multiplication can be realized across optical modes via arrays of beam splitters and programmable phase shifts. Another important feature is the incorporation of optical nonlinearities.

Both optical linearities and nonlinearities play a role in optical quantum computing. The nuance is that on the one hand, the first step in realizing optical circuits is optical linearity, the ability to perform linear transformations. An example is encoding qubits in the polarization of photons and then implementing arbitrary linear operations on the two polarization modes by using a series of wave plates. On the other hand, nonlinear transforms are also useful in optical circuits and not typically possible in nonoptical quantum circuits. Optical quantum computing offers a substantial advantage over other quantum computing methods as nonlinear processing is automatically included.

### 11.1.2 *Optical neural networks*

Optical neural networks can be realized in integrated photonic circuits or in free space. Integrated photonic circuits are preferable as they are smaller and programmable. In general, neural network architectures are structured as a series of linear and nonlinear activations. In each layer, information propagates through the neural network via linear combination (matrix multiplication), followed by a nonlinear activation function applied to the result from the linear combination. Particularly in contemporary deep neural networks, the nonlinear activation function is important for being able to access the hidden layers of the network (otherwise they are engaged as a single linear layer) to deliver the promise of machine learning in finding higher-order relationships in input data. In optical neural networks, optical linear activation is realized with waveguide interconnects (or free space interconnects in the free space model). Optical nonlinear activation is achieved with a saturable absorber, a Kerr medium, or a nonlinear optical thermal effect (Pierangeli *et al.*, 2018).

Shen *et al.* (2017) demonstrate a quantum neural network with a programmable nanophotonic processor in a cascaded array of 56 programmable Mach–Zehnder interferometers. The implementation is based on the idea that a matrix can be decomposed into components which can be instantiated in an optical architecture using a beam splitter, phase shifter, and attenuator. By tuning the phase shifter (which can perform summation operations) in the interferometers, it is possible to compute matrix multiplications for any size of input. Nonlinear activation is achieved with a saturable absorber.

The intuition is that with photonics (operating at the speed of light), optical neural networks might offer an intrinsic speed advantage over conventional neural networks which are limited by electronic clock rates. In principle, optical neural networks could be three orders of magnitude faster than electronic neural networks (*Ibid.*, p. 441). A speed advantage might be provided in three ways. First, neural networks rely heavily on matrix multiplication. Matrix multiplication inputs such as linear transformations (and certain nonlinear transformations) can be performed at the speed of light. Experimentally, optical processing has been detected at extremely fast rates exceeding 100 GHz in photonic networks, using germanium waveguide photodetectors on silicon (Vivien *et al.*, 2012).

Second, inherent optical nonlinearities in materials and components can be used to directly implement the nonlinear operations used in neural networks. Nonlinear operations are more readily implemented in optical networks than in electronic networks. Third, once a neural network is trained, the architecture can be passive in the sense that the computation on the optical signals can be performed without any additional energy input. The idea is that in optical neural networks, matrix multiplication is (almost) free. The architecture of optical neural networks demonstration is comprised of three optical processing units (Table 11.2).

First, there is an optical inference unit which is used to perform arbitrary unitary matrix multiplications on the input optical signals. The unitary matrix is obtained through the network of the 56

Table 11.2. Optical machine learning components.

| No. | Processing Unit | Operation |
|---|---|---|
| 1 | Optical interference unit | Perform unitary matrix multiplication on optical signal inputs |
| 2 | Optical amplification unit | Generalize the unitary matrix to arbitrary matrix operations |
| 3 | Optical nonlinearity unit | Apply the nonlinear activation function (via saturable absorber) |

interferometers. Second, there is an optical amplification unit which is used to generalize the unitary matrix to arbitrary matrix operations. In general, any arbitrary matrix can be generated using optical interference and linear amplification. Third, there is an optical nonlinearity unit which is used to apply the nonlinear activation function with the saturation absorption method. Saturable absorption is based on the fact that many materials respond to external light signals in a nonlinear way with respect to light intensity. Such saturable absorption, as one of the most commonly used optical nonlinearities, is deployed as a saturable absorber nonlinear function. The optical neural network is tested on the MNIST handwriting dataset ($N = 786$) and achieves a less than 10% error rate. With these three units, the optical neural network is able to perform computations in a way that is mathematically equivalent to that of a traditional artificial neural network.

#### 11.1.2.1 *All-optical waveguide platforms*

Shen *et al.*'s (2017) nanophotonic integrated circuits are a good demonstration; however, they require directional couplers and phase modulators that occupy too much space to expand optical neural networks to more than 1,000 neurons. Thus, large-scale and fast programmable photonic neural networks had not been achieved as of 2020 (Sui *et al.*, 2020). An active research trajectory supporting this work is the investigation of nano-optical components and nonlinear materials that can be integrated in optical waveguides such as black phosphorus (a two-dimensional material with high electron mobility) (Cheng *et al.*, 2020) and plasmonic nanolasers (Vyshnevyy & Fedyanin, 2018). In other research, Feldmann *et al.* (2019) demonstrate an all-optical neurosynaptic system that is capable of supervised and unsupervised learning. The work uses wavelength division multiplexing (WDM) to implement a scalable circuit architecture for photonic neural networks. Through WDM, a photonic neural network circuit is realized that performs optical pattern recognition. Photonic spiking neural networks (SNNs) have also been demonstrated in the form of neuromorphic silicon photonic networks that perform machine learning (Tait *et al.*, 2017).

#### 11.1.2.2 *All-optical reservoir computing*

The work discussed so far from Shen *et al.* (2017), Tait *et al.* (2017), and Feldmann *et al.* (2019) all relies upon integrated optical waveguide platforms. An alternative method, all-optical reservoir computing, uses fiber components based on a semiconductor optical amplifier array on a chip, with a neural network format based on directional couplers, fibers, and amplifiers (Sui *et al.*, 2020, p. 70778). One innovative proposal with reservoir computing is for a living optical neural network to combat brain tumors (Pierangeli *et al.*, 2018). The idea is to harness brain tumor pathologies as a novel architecture to study. The work uses an approach to learning machines that does not require training the network but instead employs large-scale random mixing with trained input and output. The architecture is an optical reservoir computing structure, with lasers accessing living three-dimensional brain tumor models, and organizing their componentry to detect similar cancer morphodynamics (with laser-induced hyperthermia that is inaccessible by other optical imaging techniques). Shining coherent light into biological tissue produces a wavefront-shaping method that can be used to characterize the sample. Uses of the technique include probing the effects of chemotherapy inhibiting tumor growth and developing a cytotoxicity assay.

### **11.1.3** ***Quantum optical machine learning***

Optical neural networks process classical and quantum information at the speed of light, and are compatible with silicon technology, but lack scalability and require expensive componentry (Krenn *et al.*, 2016). Thus, given the implicated capabilities of quantum computing and existing quantum optics methods, a natural step is quantum optical neural networks. Steinbrecher *et al.* (2019) propose and test such a model for quantum optical neural networks. The blueprint provides an architecture for machine learning running optical quantum computers. The work maps the features of classical neural networks onto the quantum domain to realize quantum optical machine learning. The quantum optical neural network setup is used to perform a range of quantum information processing tasks with the aid of machine learning. The method relies on the ability to train the learning system using only a subset of all possible inputs (input–output pairs from some family of quantum states). To validate and benchmark the system, a Greenberger–Horne–Zeilinger (GHZ) state is prepared and machine learning is applied to both Ising and Bose–Hubbard Hamiltonians. The quantum optical machine learning network is then tested on newly developed protocols for quantum optical state compression, quantum reinforcement learning, and one-way quantum repeaters.

An important application of quantum optical machine learning could be quantum circuit design. In quantum computing, a considerable challenge is finding the best circuit to compute a problem given the quantum state inputs. The circuit is the circuit architecture (gate order) and the parameterizations of the unitary operators. Machine learning could be applied to learn representations of quantum systems in which circuit decompositions are unknown, and to find optimal compiled implementations of known circuits.

Machine learning is a foundational infrastructural technology that is leading to sophisticated algorithm design and dedicated hardware development, particularly for quantum computing platforms. It may be possible to enhance the capabilities of machine learning by leveraging features unique to quantum computing as a physical platform. This work argues that many of the features that are natural to quantum optics (such as mode mixing and optical nonlinearity) can be mapped directly to neural networks, and the system trained to implement both coherent quantum operations and classical machine learning tasks.

The benefit of this work is that it establishes the generic infrastructural technology of machine learning on the optical quantum computing platform. This means the possibility of applying machine learning to the other quantum optical topics discussed here such as boson sampling, global photonic networks, and tabletop ion traps, ultracold atoms, and superconducting materials to extend these platforms, for example in the idea of bosonic quantum simulators. Future work is implied as the machine learning architecture only accommodates discrete variables and there is some industry development to also include continuous variable quantum neural networks (Killoran *et al.*, 2019).

#### 11.1.3.1 *GHZ state preparation and Hamiltonian simulation*

The quantum optical neural network is validated by making sure that it can learn elementary quantum tasks, such as quantum state preparation, measurement, and quantum gates. Specifically, Bell-state projection, GHZ state generation, and the implementation of the controlled NOT (CNOT) gate are demonstrated as being representative of optical quantum information processing tasks.

Next, the learning model is demonstrated for both Ising and Bose–Hubbard Hamiltonians. The task involves quantum simulation to mimic the evolution of known quantum systems of interest described a Hamiltonian. First an Ising model is tested. In the $n = 2$ spin case, the quantum optical neural network is trained on a set of 20 random two-photon states and tested on 50 different states to reliably converge to an optimum. In the $n = 3$ spin case, there is a relatively high average test error (10.1%). The higher error in the larger system motivates the need to implement more sophisticated training methods such as backpropagation and layer-wise training to train a deeper quantum optical neural network.

A Hamiltonian more natural to photons in optical modes is also examined, in the Bose–Hubbard model. The learning task involves identifying the optimal number of layers required to express a strongly interacting Bose–Hubbard model on a square lattice. Increasing the number of layers reduces the error on the test set, suggesting that deeper networks can express a richer class of quantum functions such as Hamiltonians. Five layers are found to provide a reasonable trade-off between error (1%) and computational tractability.

#### 11.1.3.2 *New protocols*

The work develops new protocols for quantum optical state compression, reinforcement learning, and one-way quantum repeaters. A quantum optical autoencoder protocol is proposed for the application of quantum information compression. A reinforcement learning protocol is designed for the classical machine learning controls task of balancing an inverted pendulum. A one-way quantum repeater protocol is developed as a quantum error correction code based on loss tolerance as the analog to forward error correction in classical communications (Table 11.3).

#### 11.1.3.3 *Quantum optical autoencoder*

Photons play a central role in quantum communications networks, either as information carriers or by mediating other interactions. However, photon transmission is sensitive to loss and hence there is a research focus on increasing the communication rate by reducing the photon number while maintaining the information content. Quantum autoencoders are proposed as an information compression technique (by encoding a family of quantum states onto a lower-dimensional manifold called the latent space) (Romero *et al.*, 2017). Similar to classical autoencoders, a quantum autoencoder likewise learns to generalize from a small training set and is able to compress other states from the same family of data that it has not previously seen. Quantum autoencoders have been proposed for applications in quantum communications networks, and as a subroutine to augment variational algorithms in finding more efficient device-specific ansatzes (guesses as to optimal wavefunction operation).

The work defines a protocol for a quantum autoencoder to learn a compressed representation of quantum states. The quantum optical autoencoder encodes input states in the Fock basis (Hilbert space of multiple qubits). A choice of a family of states that is relevant to quantum chemistry on NISQ processors is selected, the set of ground states of molecular hydrogen. The training states are the set of four ground states of Hydrogen ($H_2$). The method demonstrates a convergence to a fidelity of over 90%. Such a quantum optical autoencoder protocol might be used for quantum information compression in quantum networks to more efficiently and reliably exchange information between nodes.

Table 11.3. Quantum optical machine learning protocols.

| No. | Protocol | Application |
|---|---|---|
| 1 | Quantum optical autoencoder | Quantum information compression |
| 2 | Reinforcement learning | Control task: Balancing an inverted pendulum |
| 3 | One-way quantum repeater | Quantum loss tolerance codes QECC |

#### 11.1.3.4 *Quantum reinforcement learning*

A standard reinforcement learning problem is the challenge of balancing an inverted pendulum. Classical deep reinforcement learning uses a policy network to solve the problem. A policy network is an iterative sampling process (somewhat similar to Monte Carlo analysis) in which a network takes an observation vector as input and outputs a probability distribution over the space of allowed actions. Then the probability vector is sampled to choose an action, a new observation is taken, and the process is repeated to find the best balancing scheme (Barto *et al.*, 1983).

Machine learning outputs are in the form of probability distributions, so policy networks are a natural application. This work involves the setup of a cart moving along a frictionless track, with a pole on a hinge attached to the top. The network received four input values at each time step (the position of the cart, its velocity, the angle of the pole with respect to the track, and the time derivative of that angle) and decides whether to apply a unit of force in the plus or minus direction. The simulation runs until a boundary condition is reached (the cart goes off the track or the pole falls over). The fitness goal is the maximum number of time steps before failure.

Five training cycles (with different starting conditions) are applied using a six-layer quantum optical neural network. For each cycle, a batch size of 100 is used to determine the approximate gradient, and the fitness is averaged over 80 distinct runs of the network. Hyperparameters (layer depth, batch size, and averaging group) are tuned using linear sweeps to direct the network. The result is that overall network fitness increases with each training generation, suggesting that the network consistently learns to balance the pole for longer times, generalizing examples it has previously seen to new instances of the problem.

#### 11.1.3.5 *One-way quantum repeaters*

In classical communications networks, a number of error correction techniques are used to recover lost or damaged information. However, these generally do not apply to quantum communications because quantum information cannot be copied or measured per the no-cloning and no-measurement principles. Loss still occurs in quantum networks, though, and therefore loss correction techniques are important for quantum communications over long distances and to protect qubits in photonic quantum computing (Pant *et al.*, 2017). A one-way quantum repeater is designed to protect against such loss, and performs a role similar to that of forward error correction in classical communications. A one-way quantum repeater is essentially a quantum error correcting code for restoring quantum information given a certain loss tolerance. In quantum networks, the idea is to distribute the information over several qubits in such a way that even if loss or errors occur, the original information can be reconstructed. A single physical qubit is encoded in an ancilla (extra qubits) of logical qubits in a code structure such that the original message can be recompiled from a subset of safely received qubits.

In this work, the physical qubits with the original message and the logically encoded ancilla qubits are sent through a lossy channel. The quantum optical machine learning network uses a cost function to learn the best error correcting code structure for an example problem. The result is a (4,2) code, a two-mode code such that there can be single-photon recovery (within a maximum loss tolerance of four qubits) to repair a quantum state without having to issue a new round trip communication between the sender and the receiver. Due to the complexity of the problem, a backpropagation method was developed and gradient-based optimization methods were used to achieve accuracy in the training. The network reached numerical precision at 50 layers. An explicit optical construction of a one-way quantum repeater was previously unknown. Quantum repeaters are also used to create high-fidelity entanglement.

## 11.2 Global Quantum Networks

This section discusses an experimentally tested quantum network stack implementation. The work highlights a real-life demonstration of theoretical concepts and suggests that quantum networks are more of a near-term than may have been thought. Entanglement, for example, is not merely a quantum mechanical property, but a concretized protocol used in the long-distance network transfer of qubits.

Dahlberg *et al.* (2019) present a proposal for global quantum networks, the two central aspects of which are a full protocol stack of quantum network layers and the ability to certifiably transmit long-distance entanglement. The plan draws from novel networking architectures such as software-defined networks, data center protocols, content delivery networks, and cloud computing, and extends the team's roadmap for the quantum internet (Wehner *et al.*, 2018).

### 11.2.1 *End-to-end qubits*

A global communications network is necessarily optical. Dahlberg *et al.* (2019) therefore select nitrogen vacancy in diamond as a currently available state-of-the-art quantum optical processing platform that can produce end-to-end entangled qubits. In the nitrogen vacancy platform, qubits are created by exploiting atomic structures in the nitrogen vacancy centers in diamond lattices (Childress & Hanson, 2013). In a diamond lattice, a so-called nitrogen vacancy center is formed by replacing a carbon atom with a nitrogen atom, and by removing a neighboring carbon atom (thereby creating a vacancy). The vacancy structure allows electrons to be trapped to form a spin-one system. Two of the levels of the spin-one state are used as a qubit. Around the vacancy center, there is also an abundance of carbon-13 atoms which interact with the qubit (via electron spin) and can be manipulated to perform gate logic and serve as memory qubits.

Quantum gates are realized by applying microwave pulses to the electron spin of the carbon atom. The carbon atom spin rotates around the $X$-axis of a Bloch sphere (the Hilbert space of the qubit) in the positive (or negative) direction, with an angle that depends on the total number of pulses. With this manipulation, it is possible to perform quantum gates (unitary operations) on the carbon atom that are controlled by the state of the electron spin. Controlled rotations around other axes of the carbon atom are also performed in a similar manner. In addition, the carbon atom naturally rotates continuously around the $Z$-axis of the Bloch sphere, so other quantum gates can be applied on this basis by waiting for the appropriate rotation of the carbon atom.

#### 11.2.1.1 *Quantum network stack with entanglement*

The proposed quantum network architecture specifies a full-stack protocol for quantum hardware and software, particularly link layer protocols to produce entanglement and to deliver end-to-end qubit transmission. The quantum network stack is analogous to the Open Systems Interconnection (OSI) network stack, which is the standard model of interoperable layers in communications and computing systems (Sunshine, 1989). The OSI model is comprised of seven layers ranging from the most basic physical infrastructure to end-user application data (in layers of physical, data link, network, transport, session, presentation, and application). In the quantum network stack, the lower four tiers address the hardware-based physical treatment and transport specific to quantum entanglement, and there is no change to the top three layers (Table 11.4).

### 11.2.2 *Long-distance entanglement*

Reliable entanglement production and deliver is the central objective of the quantum network stack. The sheer physicality of quantum elements provides an advantage over classical networks in which abstraction is only available at higher layers. In quantum networks, entanglement is an inherently connected property at the lowest physical levels. The link layer is primarily responsible for producing entanglement between two nodes that

Table 11.4. Quantum network stack with entanglement.

| No. | OSI Stack | Unit | Description | Entanglement |
|---|---|---|---|---|
| 1 | Application | Data | End-user | End-user data presentation layers |
| 2 | Presentation | Data | Syntax | — |
| 3 | Session | Data | Synchronization | — |
| 4 | Transport | Segments | End-to-end connection | Qubit transmission |
| 5 | Network | Packets | Packets | Long-distance entanglement |
| 6 | Link | Frames | Frames | Robust entanglement generation |
| 7 | Physical | Bits | Physical infrastructure | Attempt entanglement generation |

*Source*: Adapted from Dahlberg *et al.* (2019, p. 2).

share a direct physical connection via an optical fiber. This is in opposition to classical networks in which the notion of a connection between a sender and a receiver must be abstracted and can only be managed at higher levels in the stack. Classical bits are distinct (not entangled) and shared states are established with higher-tier protocols. The disadvantage of quantum networks, however, is that new equipment and network reconfiguration may be needed in order to produce and distribute entanglement on a network-wide basis. A "TCP/QIP" protocol can be envisioned to establish the transfer of "quantum internet protocol" traffic.

Quantum information is more secure than classical information since it cannot be copied or measured, and entanglement confers additional security. It is not necessarily possible to factorize joint qubit states into single qubit states, and this attribute is used to produce and identify entangled states. One way to generate entangled qubits in the quantum network is by computing the joint state of qubits as given by the tensor product of their individual states. The receiving end would have information about decoding the tensor product method used.

#### 11.2.2.1 *Heralded (confirmed) entanglement*

Entangled pairs are produced and connected over short-distance intervals to form longer-range entanglement in an operation known as entanglement swapping (Zukowski *et al.*, 1993). A related procedure is entanglement distillation which increases the quality of entanglement. For example, if node A is entangled with B (a repeater node), and B with C, then B can perform entanglement swapping to create long-distance entanglement between the qubits at A and C. The procedure can be used iteratively to create entanglement through long chains of quantum repeaters (Munro *et al.*, 2015). Other proposals for long-distance quantum networks avoid entanglement swapping by using quantum error correction, but require more densely placed repeater stations. Dahlberg *et al.* (2019) streamline the efficiency of entanglement swapping with the new wrinkle of heralded entanglement. Heralded entanglement incorporates a heralding (announcement) signal confirming that entanglement has been established before proceeding with the transmission. The heralded entanglement method can be used with all forms of optical qubits.

#### 11.2.2.2 *Use cases for quantum network entanglement*

Two of the main use cases for quantum network entanglement are "measure directly" and "create and keep". In the "measure directly" use case, applications are characterized by the fact that they consume the delivered pairs (by measuring them) as soon as they are available and do not store them. This is relevant for cryptography applications that use the entangled pairs to produce stronger than classical correlations such as in quantum key distribution and secure identification. In the "create and keep" use case, applications are those that need to store entangled pairs as a coordination credential. This is relevant for applications that need to send qubits via quantum teleportation (Bennett *et al.*, 1993) or perform operations that depend on back and forth communication with another node such as sensing and metrology (for example, in the quantum network of clocks (Komar *et al.*, 2014).

#### 11.2.2.3 *Smart routing and SLA certification*

Network-produced entanglement is a feature of the quantum network. The network layer is responsible for producing and routing entanglement between nodes on an automated or on-demand basis. Stored network intelligence can indicate the preferences and service level for smart routing decisions for the formation of long-distance links from pairwise links. The quantum smart network functionality allows time-controlled heralded entanglement nodes, for example, to perform certain preprogrammed actions in each time step. Service Level Agreements (SLAs) are a key feature in the quantum protocol stack to provide the certification of quantum functionality and performance metrics (Lipinska *et al.*, 2020).

#### 11.2.2.4 *Status of long-distance quantum entanglement*

Experimental demonstrations of quantum entanglement transmission are constantly being exceeded. Short-lived entanglement has been produced over terrestrial distances of at least 100 km by sending photons on standard telecom fiber, and from space, at a distance of over 1,203 km with a satellite transmission (Yin *et al.*, 2017). Basic applications can be realized using these kinds of point-to-point links, but the nodes would need to be concatenated for the transmission of qubits over longer distances using entanglement swapping. In order to enable long-distance quantum communication and the execution of complex quantum applications, long-lived entanglement between two quantum nodes that are capable of storing and manipulating qubits is needed. To do so efficiently, a confirmation of entanglement generation through heralded entanglement is necessary. The record for producing heralded entanglement is 1.3 km, achieved by the same team in other work, also with the nitrogen vacancy solid-state platform (Hensen *et al.*, 2015). Heralded long-lived entanglement generation has also been demonstrated using remote ion traps (Moehring *et al.*, 2007) and neutral atoms (Hofmann *et al.*, 2012). The nitrogen vacancy platform, though, appears promising as several other capabilities have been demonstrated, qubit lifetimes of 1.46 seconds (Abobeih *et al.*, 2018), entanglement production faster than it is lost, and entanglement-based qubit teleporting between separated nitrogen vacancy centers.

## 11.3 Global Quantum Clock Network

### 11.3.1 *GHZ state and optical oscillators*

The prospect of global quantum networks raises the issue of a world clock. The need for real-time global clocks in the worldwide smart network infrastructure has been noted (dos Santos, 2019, p. 156). Such a quantum metrology application could serve as a real-time global timekeeper. Komar *et al.* (2014) propose a protocol for a global quantum network of clocks that brings together advances in quantum science and precision metrology. The enabling advances are the ability to transmit long-distance entanglement via satellite, and similarly, to deliver stable optical oscillators over long distances with coherent optical links. The basic idea is a "blockchain for atomic clocks" in the sense of having a global decentralized network for ultra-precise time-keeping.

The work develops a cooperative quantum protocol on the basis of entangled GHZ states for the operation of a network consisting of geographically remote optical atomic clocks. The Global Positioning System (GPS) is a familiar contemporary application enabled by time accuracy, and a global quantum clock network is another. Atomic clocks exist but are not connected in a global network, which is needed for quantum network applications such as end-to-end qubit delivery and entanglement.

Placing tighter constraints on physical constants and their variation has resulted in precise measurements of gravitational potential and gravitational wave detection, and the accuracy. The stability of optical clocks used in these measurements continues to improve, such that they now outperform microwave-based counterparts by orders of magnitude. The frequency stability of an optical clock, described as the fraction of the clock's frequency fluctuations relative to its nominal operating frequency, reaches below an instability of $10^{-18}$ (has a precision of better than one part in $10^{18}$ being inaccurate) (McGrew *et al.*, 2018). Optical atomic clocks (based on optical transitions in atoms and ions such as ytterbium, strontium, and aluminum) exploit an operating frequency that can exceed 1,000 THz, evaluated on the basis of femtoseconds, which allows for an extremely precise measurement of time.

As impressive as this is, existing optical atomic clocks are starting to reach the quantum limit of the available numbers of atoms within such lattice-based clocks, and instability limits of $10^{-18}$ might be further extended with quantum entanglement. Local clock atoms could access a wider range of partner atoms, and time-keeping resolution, through quantum correlated states.

#### 11.3.1.1 *Cooperative quantum clock network*

The idea of the global quantum clock network is a cooperative clock protocol in which individual parties (satellite-based atomic clocks from different countries) allocate resources jointly in a global network involving entangled quantum states. In addition to operating their own clocks locally, the different nodes use network-wide entangled states to interrogate their respective local oscillators. The acquired information is sent to an alternating central node where it is used to stabilize a center-of-mass mode of the different local oscillators. Such a mechanism yields an ultra-precise clock signal immediately accessible to all network members.

The global quantum clock network has a number of dispersed atomic clocks constituting the network nodes, each based on a large number of atoms (clock qubits) serving as the frequency reference at different geographical locations. Each clock has its own independently operated local oscillator. The clock keeps the time by periodically interrogating its qubits, and using the measurement data to stabilize the local oscillator frequency at the reference frequency of the atomic transition. In the conventional approach, each local oscillator interrogates its own qubits. Instead, in the cooperative approach, each network node allocates some of its qubits toward the formation of entangled states with other network nodes. When interrogated within the quantum measurement scheme, entangled network states provide ultra-precise information about the deviation of the center-of-mass frequency of all the local oscillators from the atomic resonance, and the network rebalances accordingly.

Each clock cycle consists of three phases: Preparation of the clock atom state (initialization), interrogation by the local oscillator (measurement), and correction of the frequency according to the measurement outcome (feedback) (Table 11.5). In the interrogation cycle, one of the nodes at random plays the role of the coordinating center which initiates the cycle, forms entangled GHZ states, collects teleportation measurement data from the other nodes via classical channels, and local oscillator signals via optical links, to coordinate and feedback the center-of-mass signal. Stability feedback is based on the center-of-mass clock signal generated by the network, and securely distributed to the individual nodes. After a few cycles, the local oscillators (nodes) achieve an accuracy resulting from interrogating the atoms in the entire network.

Table 11.5. Quantum world clock protocol.

| No. | Phase | Description | Enabling Advance |
|---|---|---|---|
| 1 | Initialization | Entangle all network nodes in GHZ states | Quantum entanglement |
| 2 | Measurement | Interrogate local oscillator and send status | Quantum teleportation |
| 3 | Feedback | Update local oscillator center-of-mass frequency | Optical oscillators |

#### 11.3.1.2 *Step 1 initialization: Prepare network-wide GHZ states*

In the initialization phase, network-wide entangled states are prepared. The most logical choice is to prepare a single network-wide GHZ state. Each node contains an identical number of clock atoms (qubits). The central node has access to ancilla qubits besides the clock qubits. The central node creates a fully entangled state of one half of the ancilla qubits and its first clock qubit. Technically, this can be realized with a single qubit rotation (on the first clock qubit) and a series of CNOT gates (between the first clock qubit and each ancilla qubit). The result is a GHZ state. In parallel, the central node uses the other half of its ancilla qubits to create single Bell pairs with each other node in the network (such as by using quantum repeater techniques to prepare high-fidelity entanglement). The result is that one part of the pair is stored at the center node, and the other part is stored at a remote node, forming entangled quantum states across the network. Each network node is entangled with the center.

The next step is for the central node to perform separate Bell measurements on its ancilla qubit pairs. The act of measuring teleports the state of the ancilla qubit to the first clock qubit in the remote nodes (up to a local single-qubit rotation), which is performed after the measurement outcomes are sent to the node via classical channels. The result of the individual teleportations is a collective GHZ state stretching across the first qubits of all of the network nodes.

In the final entanglement step, all of the nodes (including the central node) extend the entanglement (from their Bell pair) to all of their remaining clock qubits. To do this, each node performs a series of CNOT gates controlled on its first clock qubit and targets the other qubits. At the end of the protocol, all of the different nodes share a common GHZ state. The entanglement distribution can be achieved either via polarization-entangled photons or frequency-entangled photons.

#### 11.3.1.3 *Step 2: Interrogation of local nodes*

The second phase is that each node conducts a multi-period self-interrogation. During each time interval, clock qubits may pick up a relative phase. Due to the nonlocal character of the state, the phases accumulate in the total state of the atoms. The collective phase is computed at the end of each interrogation period. Specifically, to extract the phase information acquired by the different GHZ states, after each interrogation period, the individual nodes measure their respective qubits, and evaluate the parity of the measurement outcomes. The nodes then send the parity information to the central node via a classical channel. The central node evaluates network parity by extracting individual phase information according to a secure protocol with its own measurement outcome figuring into the decoding the phase information sent from the nodes. The central node is randomly assigned for each clock updating cycle.

#### 11.3.1.4 *Step 3: Feedback and local node clock updating*

With the local time measurement parameters of each node known by the central node, the final step is updating the network nodes to the shared world time. At each node, the measured value of the oscillator phase field indicates the center-of-mass detuning amount (error), which the central node uses to stabilize the overall network. Each node sends its local oscillator field to the center via phase-stable optical links, and the central node synthesizes the center-of-mass frequency by averaging the frequencies with equal weights. This can be implemented via the heterodyne beat of the local oscillator in the central node against each incoming laser signal. Synthesizing the beat frequencies allows the local oscillator of the central node to phase track the center-of-mass of each contribution. The central node distributes the stabilized clock signal to the network by sending individual respective error signals to the nodes, and also corrects its own local oscillator.

#### 11.3.1.5 *Time trust in the cooperative clock system*

The advantage of the proposed quantum clock network is the ability to maintain and synchronize the time standards across multiple parties in real-time. There is no delay and all participants have constant access to the ultra-stable clock signal. There is an incentive structure inherent to the distributed architecture such that each node profits from clock stability enhanced by a factor proportional to the total number of parties in the network. Further, the distributed scheme confers trust as each party has full access to their local clocks, and need not depend on one external clock.

### 11.3.2 *Paper clocks*

Surprisingly, at present, world time is calculated after the fact. International Atomic Time is a global time scale computed by taking the weighted average of 300 atomic clocks at 60 time laboratories around the world. The most stable clocks have the highest weight. Coordinated Universal Time (UTC) is based on International Atomic Time. No clock keeps the official version of UTC, because it is a "paper" time scale that can only be calculated after the data from the various international contributors are received. What is used as "time" in practice is a prediction (real-time version) of UTC that is often within a few nanoseconds of the official UTC calculations (Lombardi, 2002, 5). The international contributors and their offsets are published on a monthly basis.

## References

Abobeih, M.H., Cramer, J., Bakker, M.A. (2018). One-second coherence for a single electron spin coupled to a multi-qubit nuclear-spin environment. *Nat. Commun.* 9(1):2552.

Barto, A.G., Sutton, R.S. & Anderson, C.W. (1983). Neuron like adaptive elements that can solve difficult learning control problems. *IEEE Trans. Syst. Man. Cybernet.* 13:834–46.

Bennett, C.H., Brassard, G., Crepeau, C. *et al.* (1993). Teleporting an unknown quantum state via dual classical and Einstein-Podolsky-Rosen channels. *Phys. Rev. Lett.* 70(13):1895.

Cheng, Z. Cao, R. Guo, J. *et al.* (2020). Phosphorene-assisted silicon photonic modulator with fast response time. *Nanophotonics*. 9(7):1973–9.

Childress, L. & Hanson, R. (2013). Diamond NV centers for quantum computing and quantum networks. *MRS Bulletin*. 38(2):134–8.

Dahlberg, A., Skrzypczyk, M., Coopmans, T. *et al.* (2019). A link layer protocol for quantum networks. In *SIGCOMM '19. Proceedings of the 2019 Conference of the ACM Special Interest Group on Data Communication*, Beijing, China, August 19–23, 2019, pp. 1159–73.

dos Santos, R.P. (2019). Consensus algorithms: A matter of complexity? In *Blockchain Economics*. Eds. Swan, M., Potts, J., Takagi, S., Witte, F. & Tasca, P. London: World Scientific.

Erhard, M., Krenn, M. & Zeilinger, A. (2020). Advances in high dimensional quantum entanglement. *Nat. Rev. Phys*. 2:365–81.

Feldmann, J., Youngblood, N., Wright, C.D. *et al.* (2019). All-optical spiking neurosynaptic networks with self-learning capabilities. *Nature*. 569(7755): 208–14.

Flamini, F., Spagnolo, N. & Sciarrino, F. (2018). Photonic quantum information processing: A review. *Rep. Prog. Phys*. 82(1):016001.

Harris, N.C., Carolan, J., Bunandar, D. *et al.* (2018). Linear programmable nanophotonic processors. *Optica*. 5:1623–31.

Hensen, B., Bernien, H., Dreau, A.E. *et al.* (2015). Loopholefree Bell inequality violation using electron spins separated by 1.3 kilometres. *Nature*. 526 (7575):682–86.

Hofmann, J., Krug, M., Ortegel, N. *et al.* (2012). Heralded entanglement between widely separated atoms. *Science*. 337(6090):2–75.

Killoran, N., Bromley, T.R., Arrazola, J.M. *et al.* (2019). Continuous-variable quantum neural networks. *Phys. Rev. Res.* 1(3):033063.

Komar, P., Kessler, E.M., Bishof, M. *et al.* (2014). A quantum network of clocks. *Nat. Phys.* 10(8):582.

Krenn, M., Malik, M., Fickler, R. *et al.* (2016). Automated search for new quantum experiments. *Phys. Rev. Lett.* 116(9):090405.

Lipinska, V., Thinh, L.P., Ribeiro, J. & Wehner, S. (2020). Certification of a quantum network functionality. *Quantum Sci. Technol.* 5:035008.

Lombardi, M.A. (2002). *NIST Time and Frequency Services*. NIST Special Publication 432:1–71. (U.S. National Institute of Standards and Technology).

McGrew, W.F., Zhang, X., Fasano, R.J. *et al.* (2018). Atomic clock performance enabling geodesy below the centimeter level. *Nature*. 564:87–90.

Moehring, D.L., Maunz, P., Olmschenk, S. *et al.* (2007). Entanglement of single-atom quantum bits at a distance. *Nature*. 449(7158):68.

Munro, W.J., Azuma, K., Tamaki, K. & Nemoto, K. (2015). Inside quantum repeaters. IEEE *J. Sel. Topics Quantum Electron*. 21(3):78–90.

O'Brien, J.L. (2007). Optical quantum computing. *Science*. 318:1567–70.

Pant, M., Krovi, H., Englund, D. & Guha, S. (2017). Rate-distance tradeoff and resource costs for all-optical quantum repeaters. *Phys. Rev. A*. 95(1):012304.

Pierangeli, D., Marcucci, G., Moriconi, C. *et al.* (2018). Deep optical neural network by living tumor brain cells. arXiv:1812.09311.

Romero, J., Olson, J. P. & Aspuru-Guzik, A. (2017). Quantum autoencoders for efficient compression of quantum data. *Quantum Sci. Technol.* 18(2):023023.

Shen, Y., Harris, N.C., Skirlo, S. *et al.* (2017). Deep learning with coherent nanophotonic circuits. *Nat. Photon.* 11:441–6.

Steinbrecher, G.R., Olson, J.P., Englund, D. & Carolan, J. (2019). Quantum optical neural networks. *NPJ Quantum Inf.* 5(60):1–9.

Sui., X., Wu, Q., Liu, J. *et al.* (2020). A review of optical neural networks. *IEEE Access.* 8:70773–83.

Sunshine, C.A. (1989). *Computer Network Architectures and Protocols*. London: Springer Science & Business Media, p. 35.

Tait, A.N., de Lima, T.F., Zhou, E. *et al.* (2017). Neuromorphic silicon photonic networks. *Sci. Rep.* 7(1):7430.

Vivien, L., Polzer, A., Marris-Morini, D. *et al.* (2012). Zero-bias 40gbit/s germanium waveguide photodetector on silicon. *Opt. Express.* 20:1096–1101.

Vyshnevyy A.A. & Fedyanin, D.Y. (2018). Lasing threshold of thresholdless and non-thresholdless metal-semiconductor nanolasers. *Opt. Express.* 26(25): 33473–83.

Wehner, S., Elkouss, D. & Hanson, R. (2018). Quantum internet: A vision for the road ahead. *Science.* 362(6412):eaam9288.

Yin, J., Cao, Y., Li, Y.-H. (2017). Satellite-based entanglement distribution over 1200 kilometers. *Science.* 356(6343):1140–4.

Zukowski, M., Zeilinger, A., Horne, M.A. & Ekert, A.K. (1993). Event-ready-detectors: Bell experiment via entanglement swapping. *Phys. Rev. Lett.* 71: 4287–90.

# Chapter 12

# Connectome and Brain Imaging

*New recording technologies are producing an amazing explosion of data on neural activity. These data reveal the simultaneous activity of hundreds or even thousands of neurons*

— Recanatesi *et al.* (2019, p. 1)

**Abstract**

This chapter discusses neuroscience as a "big data" field. Since the fruit fly connectome was only finished in 2018, next-generation methods such as quantum computing are likely necessary for the human connectome and a potential future era of personalized connectomics and disease management. Imaging relies on electron microscopy as the workhorse technique, light sheet microscopy (nonliving samples), and light field microscopy and calcium signaling (living samples), including whole-brain activity recording in behaving organisms. A significant advance is molecular-scale resolution in expansion light field microscopy.

## 12.1 Connectomics

Connectomics is the production and study of connectomes, the comprehensive map or "wiring diagram" of all of the neural connections in the brain. One aim of connectomics is to connect brain structure with function. The first connectome was completed for the roundworm (*Caenorhabditis elegans*), initially with electron micrographs (White *et al.*, 1986), and later extended to a full neural circuitry database (Yamamoto & Achacoso, 1992). The fruit fly (*Drosophila*) connectome was completed in 2018 using an electron microscopy and volume reconstruction approach (Zheng *et al.*, 2018). Notably, about one half of the reconstructed cells were previously unknown, despite a substantial amount of prior work characterizing fruit fly cell types using a variety of methods (molecular genetics, light microscopy, and sparse neuroanatomical labeling techniques) (Scheffer *et al.*, 2020). For the mouse (*Mus musculus*), partial connectomes have been completed, including for the retina (Briggman *et al.*, 2011) and the primary visual cortex (Bock *et al.*, 2011). The status of connectome projects appears in Table 12.1.

The table highlights the difficulty of the connectome project, and how quantum methods might help. Even with modern technology, it took almost thirty years to progress from the worm (1992) to the fruit fly (2018) connectome. The mouse connectome is on the horizon, and the human connectome is more distant. The connectome challenge is reminiscent of the human genome project in the sense that the enormity of the project proved untenable with initial methods and inspired next-generation techniques to solve in reasonable time, much like the human connectome might prompt quantum models for its instantiation. The fly brain is already too large for conventional electron microscopy and custom high-throughput platform methods are required to obtain synaptic resolution. Being able to represent three-dimensional neural data directly in quantum computing models could obviate the need to convert and

Table 12.1. Whole-brain connectome projects.

| Organism | Neurons | Synapses | Ratio | Volume | Complete |
|---|---|---|---|---|---|
| Worm | 302 | 7,500 | 25 | $5 \times 10^4$ | 1992 |
| Fly | 100,000 | 10,000,000 | 100 | $5 \times 10^7$ | 2018 |
| Mouse | 71,000,000 | 100,000,000,000 | 1,408 | $5 \times 10^{11}$ | NA |
| Human | 86,000,000,000 | 242,000,000,000,000 | 2,814 | $5 \times 10^{14}$ | NA |

*Sources*: Abbott *et al.* (2020, p. 1373) with Zheng *et al.* (2018) for fly, Herculano-Houzel *et al.* (2006) for mouse, and Martins *et al.* (2019) for human. Brain volume: Cubic microns.

reconstruct datasets, in addition to providing vastly more computational capacity. The three-dimensional data inputs for quantum platforms could come from connectome tissue samples, or *in vivo* data acquired by noninvasive on-board neuronanorobots (Martins *et al.*, 2016).

Analogous to personalized genomics, the farther future might be one of personalized connectomics. As a start, over 50 individual human connectomes are available at the Virtual Brain (VirtualBrain.org) connectome-based brain simulation platform (Triebkorn *et al.*, 2020). These data could be used to develop healthy baseline and disease profiles for personalized pathology management based on the connectomics of brain disorders (Fornito *et al.*, 2015) and synaptome biomarkers (Cizeron *et al.*, 2020). Depending on the resolution, one estimate is that each human connectome would require one zettabyte (1,000 exabytes) of data, about 1,000-fold more than a rat cortex, which could require an exabyte of data (Lichtman *et al.*, 2014). This compares with IDC's forecast that worldwide data creation in 2020 was 59 zettabytes (Reinsel, 2020). The present goal of connectomics is to map the entire human brain. In the United States, the focus of this effort is the Human Connectome Project, sponsored by the National Institutes of Health (NIH). The program aims to build a network map of the human brain in healthy, living adults, through the Brain Initiative generally, and the Human Connectome Project specifically (van Essen *et al.*, 2013). Other efforts exist in Europe (the Blue Brain Project (Markram *et al.*, 2015)), China (the China Brain Project (Poo *et al.*, 2016)), and Japan (Japan's Brain/MINDS project (Okano *et al.*, 2015)).

## 12.2 Brain Imaging

Imaging is a central focus in neuroscience, particularly whole-brain imaging. Connectome projects have led to new methods in high-throughput imaging and recording techniques such that neuroscience data acquisition outpaces that of most other biomedical fields (Motta *et al.*, 2019). In high-throughput connectomics, ongoing work from the Allen Institute demonstrates terabyte-scale processing for contemporary neuron reconstruction (Wang *et al.*, 2019), and petabyte-scale next-generation dataset acquisition methods (Yin *et al.*, 2019). There are roughly two phases, capturing data and working with data in reconstruction, simulation, and structural-to-functional analysis. As in other fields, computational power is a key contributor to the kinds of techniques and resulting knowledge that is now possible. Notably, Graphics Processing Units (GPUs) have made a difference in neuroscience data acquisition processing times and analysis capabilities (Vescovi *et al.*, 2017). Neuroscience might continue to benefit from the computational chip progression suggested as CPU-GPU-TPU-QPU.

A notable advance is single-molecule scale resolution that captures synaptic proteins at dendritic spines, myelination along axons, and presynaptic densities at dopaminergic neurons with expansion light sheet microscopy (Gao *et al.*, 2019). The general research aim of whole-brain neuroscience is full-volume, three-dimensional, whole-brain analysis at multiple spatial and temporal scales. Efforts in whole-brain neuroscience imaging can be divided into three areas (Table 12.2). First is connectome parcellation methods in humans performed with data from electroencephalography (EEG), MEG, fMRI, and tractography techniques. Second is the high-throughput connectome imaging and volumetric reconstruction of preserved tissue samples with electron microscopy (the workhorse method) and light sheet microscopy (scanning excitation light in a volume). Third is high-throughput recording (recording action potential activation with chemical and genetically encoded fluorescent reporters) in behaving animals, with light field microscopy and calcium imaging, analyzed with simulation or brain network frameworks.

Table 12.2. Whole-brain imaging techniques.

| No. | Focus | Techniques | Focal Organism |
|---|---|---|---|
| 1 | Connectome parcellation | EEG, MEG, fMRI, Tractography | Human |
| 2 | High-throughput connectome imaging in preserved tissue samples | Electron microscopy<br>Light sheet microscopy<br>X-ray microtomography | Mouse |
| 3 | High-throughput recording in behaving organisms | Light field microscopy<br>Calcium imaging | Fruit fly zebrafish |

### 12.2.1 *Connectome parcellation*

One of the primary challenges for connectomics projects is determining the parcellations of the brain. Parcellation is the segmenting of the brain into functionally distinct parcels, regions with distinct architecture, connectivity, or topography (as opposed to other segmentation methods such as same-size segments). Glasser *et al.* (2016) conduct one the first whole-cortex parcellations of the human brain, finding 180 brain regions per hemisphere. Multimodal fMRI data are used ($n = 210$) to identify both functional and structural organization. The work extends previous parcellations which generally only covered a portion of the cortex and were based on only one neurobiological property (such as architecture, function, connectivity, or topography). A machine learning classifier was trained to recognize the multi-modal fingerprint of each cortical area, and was able to detect the presence of 96.6% of the cortical areas in new subjects, replicating the group parcellation, and correctly locating areas in individuals with atypical parcellations. The analysis highlights the point that spatially contiguous areas in the brain are anatomically and functionally distinct, and an understanding is sought for how these differences in microstructural architecture, functional specialization, connectivity with other areas, and topology are related. The whole-brain parcellation method attempts to bring together brain structure and function in a more complex and realistic way.

Neuroscientists use various noninvasive techniques to measure activity within the brain. On the one hand, EEG is one of the most commonly used methods. A network of electrodes is attached to the scalp and reveals the patterns of electrical activity occurring in brain tissue. EEG is good at revealing electrical activity across the surface of the scalp, but is less effective at linking the observed activity to specific locations in the brain. On the other hand, another widely used method is functional magnetic resonance imaging (fMRI). A subject lies inside a scanner containing a large magnet. The scanner tracks changes in the level of oxygen at different regions of the brain to provide a measure of how the activity of these regions changes over time. In contrast to EEG, fMRI is good at pinpointing the location of brain activity, but is only an indirect measure of brain activity as it depends on blood flow and several other factors. In terms of understanding how the brain works, EEG and fMRI thus provide different pieces of an incomplete puzzle. Also, there is no easy way to fit these pieces together. One method is not necessarily interrelating the two data streams together directly, but rather understanding them in the broader context of a brain network model with various data streams governed by neural dynamics (Breakspear, 2017).

Another project does try to integrate simultaneously collected EEG and fMRI data together into one coherent model. Schirner *et al.* (2018) propose a brain network framework for integrating the two data streams, and use empirical EEG data (structure) to generate predictions of fMRI response (function). The work results in a connectome-based brain network model that integrates structural and functional data with neural population dynamics and multiscale simulation. The simulations predicted resting-state fMRI time series and spatial network topologies for over twenty minutes of activity in subjects, which aligned with observations. The structural simulations also helped to reveal more about neurophysiological functional mechanisms that underlie empirical observations from different scales and modalities, including resting-state fMRI oscillations, excitation-inhibition balance, short and long-time scale spike-firing, fMRI power law scaling, and functional connectivity networks.

## 12.3 High-Throughput Connectome Imaging

### 12.3.1 *Electron microscopy*

Electron microscopy is the workhorse of neuroscience imaging, and substantial progress has been achieved in recent years in three-dimensional electron microscopy techniques (Eberle & Zeidler, 2018). Such advance applies to the life sciences in general, but neuroscience has been the main driver for developments regarding volumetric imaging. Scanning electron microscopy offers new insights into the organization of cells and tissues through volume-related imaging methods. In particular, multi-beam scanning electron microscope is optimized to the imaging of large sample areas. Complemented by the commercialization of automated sample preparation robots, the mapping of large tissue volumes (cubic millimeter size) at high-resolution takes time, but is undertaken routinely.

In a state-of-the-art microscopy-based connectomics effort, the Allen Institute develops a petabyte-scale automated imaging pipeline for mapping neuronal circuits with high-throughput transmission electron microscopy (Yin *et al.*, 2019). The project images a two-petabyte dataset of 26,500 images of a cubic millimeter of mouse visual cortex in just under six months with an array of six electron microscopes running autonomously 24/7. On the one hand, taking six months and requiring breakthrough microscopy techniques to image one cubic millimeter of cortex seems primitive. On the other hand, the project underlines the challenge of the accurate three-dimensional imaging of the brain. It took six months to produce images of 26,500 tissue sections (from a 1 $mm^3$ volume of mouse neocortex spanning four different visual areas) that comprise a two-petabyte dataset. A number of microscopy innovations are used, such as GridTape, an automated laser-milled tape that is drawn through the tunneling electron microscope grid structure (Graham *et al.*, 2019). Despite the novel design, the imaging array is cost-effective in the sense of using mainly off-the-shelf camera and microscopy components.

Earlier work also conducted a big data mouse brain volumetric reconstruction, on a smaller scale. The project collected 2,250 29-nm coronal brain slices (each section 1 $mm^2$ for a total volume 0.13 $mm^3$) from the somatosensory cortex of a young adult mouse. The work develops automated techniques to probe the structure of neural tissue at nanometer-scale resolution, and produces an annotated database of 1,700 synapses from the partial cortical reconstruction (Kasthuri *et al.*, 2015).

### 12.3.2 *Light sheet microscopy*

Light sheet microscopy is a high-speed optical method for reconstructing whole specimens in three dimensions (Keller *et al.*, 2008). In this method, the sample is prepared with fluorescent proteins and illuminated with a thin sheet of light. The fluorescence emission is collected along an axis perpendicular to the illumination plane. Only in-focus fluorophores are excited, and it is possible to achieve optical sectioning in a wide-field configuration with high frame rates. Specimens are prepared by a clearing and mounting procedure. A further advance, confocal light sheet microscopy, demonstrates the micron-scale reconstruction of entire mouse brains labeled with enhanced green fluorescent protein (Silvestri *et al.*, 2013). Combining light sheet illumination and confocal detection, confocal light sheet microscopy allows more extensive imaging within macroscopic cleared specimens with high contrast and speed.

### 12.3.3 *Expansion light sheet microscopy*

These ideas are extended by the Boyden laboratory to obtain single-molecule resolution. The work combines lattice light-sheet microscopy with expansion microscopy for terabyte-scale image processing (Gao *et al.*, 2019). The nanoscale lattice microscopy method is used to image the nanoscale spatial relationships between proteins across the thickness of the mouse cortex and the entire fruit fly brain. This includes synaptic proteins at dendritic spines, myelination along axons, and presynaptic densities at dopaminergic neurons, in every fruit fly brain region, with molecular contrast. The nanoscale lattice microscopy method solves the joint problem that optical microscopy offers insufficient resolution to reveal subcellular details, and electron microscopy lacks the throughput and molecular contrast to visualize specific molecular constituents. Molecular-level investigation is a substantial advance. A problem of interest, for example, is the interaction of the vast array of molecular species that contribute to neural communication by many mechanisms in addition to the synaptic connections determined by electron microscopy connectomics. The ability to probe molecular-level neural signaling at smaller-than-synapse resolution is striking. This capability is well beyond models that include electrical action potentials, and synaptic communication, reaching to single-molecule resolution.

Obtaining contrast is a significant challenge in microscopy. Electron microscopy was used to complete the fruit fly connectome, imaging down to the level of individual ion channels and synaptic vesicles across the ~0.03 $mm^3$ volume of the fruit fly brain (Zheng *et al.*, 2018). However, electron microscopy creates a grayscale image in which the segmentation of specific subcellular components and the tracing of the complete arborization of specific neurons remain difficult. As a result, specific proteins can rarely be identified unambiguously. The problems with previous methods are as follows. Optical microscopy combined with immunofluorescence and fluorescent proteins enables high sensitivity in the imaging of specific protein expression patterns in brain tissue, but has insufficient resolution for dense neural tracing or the precise localization of specific molecules within critical subcellular structures such as dendritic spines. A related method, diffraction-unlimited super-resolution fluorescence microscopy combines nanoscale resolution with protein-specific contrast, but bleaches fluorophores too quickly for large-volume imaging and, like electron microscopy, would require months to years to image a single fruit fly brain.

Instead, expansion light sheet microscopy is a combination of expansion microscopy, lattice light-sheet microscopy, and terabyte-scale image processing that achieves single-molecule sensitivity and ~$60 \times 60 \times 90$ $nm^3$ resolution at volumetric acquisition rates ~700× and 1200× faster than existing high-speed super-resolution (Tonnesen *et al.*, 2018) and electron microscopy (Zheng *et al.*, 2018) methods, respectively, at comparable or higher resolution. Expansion microscopy is an advance previously developed by the Boyden laboratory (Chen *et al.*, 2015). Expansion microscopy involves physically expanding a polymer network within a specimen to allow greater physical magnification. The method enables the ability to perform scalable super-resolution microscopy with diffraction-limited microscopes.

### 12.3.4 *X-ray microtomography*

Aside from the electron microscopy workhorse, and advances in light sheet microscopy, another innovative method for cortical imaging is X-ray microtomography (Bonse & Busch, 1996). The advantage of X-ray microtomography is being able to probe brain connectivity in a nondestructive manner. In contrast to optical three-dimensional techniques, X-ray microtomography does not require tissue slicing or clearing, and allows the investigation of several cells within the same three-dimensional region of the brain. Fonseca *et al.* (2018) present a method for imaging whole neurons in the brain, combining synchrotron-based X-ray microtomography with a Golgi-Cox mercury-based staining protocol. Visualization of the single-cell morphology of intact neuronal tissues with X-ray methods had not been achieved previously due to incomplete staining protocols and excessive sample artifacts. The Golgi-Cox method allows whole neurons to be defined clearly due to a continuous and homogeneous cell-staining procedure, which results in a reduced density of artifacts (scattered reflexive granules) that interfere with image segmentation. The whole neuron imaging method is demonstrated in mice, and suggested as a three-dimensional mapping technique suitable for both synchrotron and table-top tomograms.

Another team offers a technical improvement to the method, using a brighter X-ray source to record scans in minutes instead of hours (required by conventional X-ray tubes). In this work, Cole *et al.* (2018) note the problem that high-resolution microcomputed tomography with benchtop X-ray sources requires long scan times because of the heat load limitation on the anode. Instead, they present an alternative, a high-brightness plasma-based X-ray source that does not have this restriction. A demonstration of tomography of a centimeter-scale complex organism (mouse embryo) achieves equivalent quality to a commercial scanner. The implication is the possibility of recording such scans in minutes. The X-ray flux achievable with this approach scales with the laser repetition rate without compromising the source size, which allows the recording of high-resolution X-ray scans in minutes.

## 12.4 High-Throughput Recording

Optical techniques are central. Whereas light sheet microscopy is typically used to analyze nonliving samples, light field microscopy can be used to examine living tissue. Recording whole-brain activity in behaving organisms is a substantial research focus, primarily accomplished through light field microscopy and calcium imaging techniques.

### 12.4.1 *Light field microscopy*

*Light should be interpreted as a field*

— paraphrase of Michael Faraday (1846)

Light field microscopy is a scanning-free three-dimensional microscopic imaging method that treats light as a field. Such a light field is a vector function that describes the amount of light flowing in every direction through every point in space. The space of all possible light rays is given by a five-dimensional function (the plenoptic function), and the magnitude of each ray is given by the radiance. The measure for the amount of light traveling along a ray is radiance. The idea of the light field was proposed by Michael Faraday, that light too is a field, similar to the magnetic field. He supports a "view of the nature of matter which considers its ultimate atoms as centers of force", with "the lines of force as being perhaps the seat of vibrations of radiant phenomena" (Faraday, 1846).

Gershun introduces "the concept of the *light field*, as a part of space studied from the standpoint of transmission of radiant energy within that space" (Gershun, 1936, p. 56). Such a study of the light field consists of an investigation of the spatial distribution of luminous flux. The separate photons are disregarded and the assumption is made that radiant energy is continuous in time and space, and that the flux of the radiant energy varies continuously from point to point. Vector analysis is used to study the light field. Gershun notes that the light field is caused by electromagnetic phenomena, but is different from the electromagnetic field. On the one hand, the study of the electromagnetic field involves considering the electric and magnetic forces caused by an elementary emitter. On the other hand, the study of the light field means treating bodies of finite size consisting of a great number of elementary emitters. In contrast with the elementary electromagnetic field, in the light field theory, there is a macrocosm with respect to time as well as space (*Ibid.*).

In operation, light field microscopy is a scanning-free technique for the high-speed volumetric imaging of weakly scattering or fluorescent specimens using optical microscopy. The method employs an array of microlenses to capture a four-dimensional light field in a single photographic exposure without the need for scanning. The recorded light field can then be used to reconstruct a full volume computationally. The idea is that by inserting a microlens array into the light path of a conventional microscope, it is possible to image both the lateral and the angular distribution of light passing through the specimen volume in a single image (Levoy *et al.*, 2006). The raw spatio-angular data can be post-processed with software to produce a full three-dimensional reconstruction of the object. Since the light field is captured in snapshots, the implied speed of the method is the frame rate of the camera (Broxton *et al.*, 2013).

Light field microscopy allows the investigation of dynamic behavior in the brain. A key problem is understanding how sensory inputs are mapped dynamically to the functional activity of neuronal populations and how this processing leads to behavior. One team uses light field microscopy to perform the simultaneous whole-brain functional imaging of neuronal activity at single-neuron resolution for an entire worm, a larval zebrafish, and other organisms (Prevedel *et al.*, 2014). The technique captures the dynamics of spiking neurons in volumes of ~700 $\mu$m × 700 $\mu$m × 200 $\mu$m at 20 Hz. Measuring activity simultaneously in the whole-brain is important in understanding how different brain regions interact to process and control sensory inputs, internal states, and behavior. Whole-brain recordings reveal not only which regions are involved in which functions but also overall brain network dynamics.

#### 12.4.1.1 *Fruit fly grooming and walking*

Another team uses light field microscopy for the ultra-fast imaging of whole-brain activity (calcium and voltage) in behaving fruit flies (while walking, resting, or grooming) (Aimon *et al.*, 2019). The fly brain's fluorescence is imaged using light field microscopy as the fly is constrained in position but can rest, walk, and groom. Data collection volumes are reconstructed (about 600 × 300 × 200 $\mu m^3$ to encompass the whole-brain) using a known volumetric deconvolution method for light field microscopy. Unlike other microscopy techniques that are based on scanning (such as two-photon, confocal, or light-sheet microscopy), excitation light illuminates the entire brain continuously. All the photons emitted in the numerical aperture of the objective are used to reconstruct the image (minus approximately 40% loss through the objective, tube lens, microlens array, and relay lenses). This maximizes the number of photons collected (and thus the information about brain activity) per units of volume and time.

Whole-brain recordings provide a global perspective of the brain in action. This is already possible to some extent in humans, as fMRI allows the study of brain activity underlying behavior, but the technique has low spatial and temporal resolution. In animals, whole-brain imaging techniques have allowed recorded activity at much higher resolutions than fMRI imaging but are still orders-of-magnitude slower than real-life neuronal electrical activity. For example, scanning-based whole-brain imaging in zebrafish and fruit fly larvae had respective frame rates of 12 Hz and 5 Hz. By contrast, light field microscopy makes it possible to image large volumes of scattering brain tissue at more than 100 Hz. Aimon *et al.* (2019) leverage this technique to record large-scale activity in the brain of behaving adult fruit flies. The near-whole brain can be imaged with a 20× objective at a frame rate up to 200 Hz and fluorescence recorded from pan-neuronally expressed calcium (GCaMP6) or voltage (ArcLight) probes.

Brain activity data are analyzed in short and long timescales. First, activity is mapped for specific stimuli and behaviors with short timescales while the fly rests, walks, and grooms. One finding is that dopamine neurons, distributed over the whole-brain, have low activity during resting or grooming, but are strongly active during walking. Similarly, there is a global increase in overall neural activity when the fly is walking as compared to resting, but only a small local increase in neural activity when grooming over resting.

Second, a computational method (principal component analysis followed by independent component analysis) is applied to extract components representing spatially distinct sources of activity over longer timescales. Activity is extracted from small brain regions or specific neuron types, and identified with brain regions involved in behaviors such as turning left or right. Brain structures that respond to light and odor are consistent with previous reports, confirming the technique's validity. Certain global activity maps for other stimuli and behaviors are obtained for the first time. Spatiotemporal maps are extracted of spatially distinct sources of activity as well as their time series. Evaluating time series data at different scales (voxels, regions, and components) provides insight into the dynamics of the brain network. For example, the widespread activity patterns observed during walking suggest that greater coordination between different brain areas may be involved than was previously thought. The method is a step toward the understanding of large-scale brain states, brain networks, and the mechanisms underlying behavior.

### 12.4.2 *Calcium imaging*

Calcium imaging is a technique used to detect action potentials from calcium ion-based fluorescence transients, tracing calcium signals as they propagate through the brain over time to produce maps of neural signaling networks. The benefit is being able to trace activity across a large brain area in space and time. To enumerate such functional brain networks, Mann *et al.* (2017) measure the functional connectivity in the brain of the adult fruit fly with whole-brain calcium imaging. The work is among the first to combine anatomical atlas data with whole-brain calcium imaging by aligning imaging results to brain atlas regions. Calcium imaging and template registration are used to extract and compare calcium signals across individual animals and create a composite picture. A well-known calcium indicator (GCaMP6m) and a red fluorescent protein (tdTomato) are expressed and tracked pan-neuronally. After extracting calcium signals from each atlas region, time series data are correlated between each region for each fly, providing quantifications of overall functional connectivity. The calcium imaging and atlas registration technique has also been used to measure brain network activity at high spatial and temporal resolution in zebrafish and worms. The method confirms known relationships between brain regions and identifies previously unknown connections. Overall, measuring resting-state functional connectivity delivers an advance in mapping functional brain networks (including identifying correlations between midbrain and hindbrain) and in distinguishing normal neural activity from pathologies of disease and aging.

In other work, Lu *et al.* (2017) likewise capture calcium transients *in vivo*, by conducting video-rate (30 Hz) volumetric imaging through the creation of a Bessel beam. The problem with other methods is the limited brightness of calcium indicators and the inertia of laser scanning units. This makes it difficult to capture all available calcium transients in a volume at video rate while maintaining the ability to resolve synaptic structures such as dendritic spines and axonal boutons. One idea is to improve the method of focusing. Specifically in conventional methods, high-speed throughout is challenging for two-photon laser scanning microscopes because they depend on serial focal scanning and have limited indicator brightness. Instead, this work develops a Bessel focus scanning technique by building an additional optical module to the microscope. The new module uses a spatial light modulator to flexibly control the depths of field such that it can generate an axially elongated Bessel focus. The resulting Bessel foci are optimized for *in vivo* brain imaging. The result is that the Bessel beam scanning method allows high-speed volume imaging rates (30 Hz) in sparsely labeled samples, while maintaining the ability to resolve dendritic spines and axonal boutons. The Bessel focus scanning is applied to fly brains with the pan-neuronal expression of the calcium indicator GCaMP6f. The method is further used to illuminate the calcium dynamics of volumes of neurons and synapses in fruit flies, zebrafish larvae, mice, and ferrets that are imaged *in vivo*. Such video-rate methods might accelerate the capture of neural data.

## References

Abbott, L.F., Bock, D.D., Callaway, E.M. *et al.* (2020). The mind of a mouse. *Cell*. 182(6):1372–6.

Aimon, S., Katsuki, T., Jia, T. *et al.* (2019). Fast near-whole-brain imaging in adult Drosophila during responses to stimuli and behavior. *PLOS Biol.* 17(2):e2006732.

Bock, D.D., Lee, W.C., Kerlin, A.M. *et al.* (2011). Network anatomy and in vivo physiology of visual cortical neurons. *Nature*. 471(7337):177–82.

Bonse, U. & Busch, F. (1996). X-ray computed microtomography (microCT) using synchrotron radiation (SR). *Prog. Biophys. Mol. Biol.* 65:133–69.

Breakspear, M. (2017). Dynamic models of large-scale brain activity. *Nat. Neurosci*. 20:340–52.

Briggman, K.L., Helmstaedter, M. & Denk, W. (2011). Wiring specificity in the direction-selectivity circuit of the retina. *Nature*. 471(7337):183–8.

Broxton, M., Grosenick, L., Yang, S., *et al.* (2013). Wave optics theory and 3-D deconvolution for the light field microscope. *Opt. Express*. 21:25418–39.

Chen, F., Tillberg, P.W. & Boyden, E.S. (2015). Expansion microscopy. *Science*. 347:543–8.

Cizeron, M., Qiu, Z., Koniaris, B. *et al.* (2020). A brainwide atlas of synapses across the mouse life span. *Science*. 369:270–5.

Cole, J.M., Symes, D.R., Lopes, N.C. *et al.* (2018). High-resolution μCT of a mouse embryo using a compact laser-driven X-ray betatron source. *Proc. Natl. Acad. Sci.* 115(25):6335–40.

Eberle, A.L. & Zeidler, D. (2018). Multi-beam scanning electron microscopy for high-throughput imaging in connectomics research. *Front. Neuroanat.* 12(112):1–7.

Faraday, M. (1946). Thoughts on ray-vibrations. *The London, Edinburgh, and Dublin Philosophical Magazine and Journal of Science.* 3(28)N188: 345–50.

Fonseca, M.D.C., Araujo, B.H.S., Dias, C.S.B. *et al.* (2018). High-resolution synchrotron-based X-ray microtomography as a tool to unveil the three-dimensional neuronal architecture of the brain. *Sci. Rep.* 8(12074):1–13.

Fornito, A., Zalesky, A. & Breakspear, M. (2015). The connectomics of brain disorders. *Nat. Rev. Neurosci.* 16:159–72.

Gao, R., Asano, S.M., Upadhyayula, S. *et al.* (2019). Cortical column and whole-brain imaging with molecular contrast and nanoscale resolution. *Science.* 363(6424):eaau8302.

Gershun, A. (1936). The light field. Moscow. Translated by P. Moon & G. Timoshenko. *J. Math. and Physics.* 18(1939):51–151.

Glasser, M.F., Coalson, T.S., Robinson, E.C., *et al.* (2016). A multi-modal parcellation of human cerebral cortex. *Nature.* 536:171–81.

Graham, B.J., Hildebrand, D.G.C., Kuan, A.T. *et al.* (2019). High-throughput transmission electron microscopy with automated serial sectioning. bioRxiv: 657346.

Herculano-Houzel, S., Mota, B., Lent, R. (2006). Cellular scaling rules for rodent brains. *Proc. Natl. Acad. Sci.* 103(32):12138–143.

Kasthuri, N., Hayworth, K.J., Berger, D.R. *et al.* (2015). Saturated reconstruction of a volume of neocortex. *Cell.* 162(3):648–61.

Keller, P.J., Schmidt, A.D., Wittbrodt, J. & Stelzer, E.H.K. (2008). Reconstruction of zebrafish early embryonic development by scanned light sheet microscopy. *Science.* 322:1065–9.

Levoy, M., Ng, R., Adams, A. *et al.* (2006). Light field microscopy. *ACM Transactions on Graphics.* 25(3):924–34.

Lichtman, J.W., Pfister, H. & Shavit, N. (2014). The big data challenges of connectomics. *Nat. Neurosci.* 17(11):1448–54.

Lu, R., Sun, W., Liang, Y. *et al.* (2017). Video-rate volumetric functional imaging of the brain at synaptic resolution. *Nat. Neurosci.* 20:620–8.

Mann, K., Gallen, C.L. & Clandinin, T.R. (2017). Whole-brain calcium imaging reveals an intrinsic functional network in Drosophila. *Curr. Biol.* 27(e4):2389–96.

Markram, H., Muller, E., Ramaswamy, S. *et al.* (2015). Reconstruction and simulation of neocortical microcircuitry. *Cell.* 163:456–92.

Martins, N.R.B., Angelica, A., Chakravarthy, K. *et al.* (2019). Human brain/cloud interface. *Front. Neurosci.* 13(112):1–24.

Martins, N.R.B., Erlhagen, W. & Freitas, R.A. Jr. (2016). Human connectome mapping and monitoring using neuronanorobots. *J. Evol. Technol.* 26(1): 1–25.

Motta, A., Schurr, M., Staffler, B. & Helmstaedter, M. (2019). Big data in nanoscale connectomics, and the greed for training labels. *Curr. Opin. Neurobiol.* 55:180–7.

Okano, H., Miyawaki, A. & Kasai, K. (2015). Brain/MINDS: Brain-mapping project in Japan. *Philos. Trans. R. Soc. Lond. B. Biol. Sci.* 370(1668): 20140310.

Poo, M.-M., Du, J.-L., Ip. N.Y. *et al.* (2016). China brain project: Basic neuroscience, brain diseases, and brain-inspired computing. *Neuron.* 92:591–6.

Prevedel, R., Yoon, Y.-G., Hoffmann, M. *et al.* (2014). Simultaneous whole-animal 3D imaging of neuronal activity using light-field microscopy. *Nat. Methods.* 11:727–30.

Recanatesi, S., Ocker, G.K., Buice, M.A. & Shea-Brown, E. (2019). Dimensionality in recurrent spiking networks: Global trends in activity and local origins in connectivity. *PLoS Comput. Biol.* 15(7):e1006446.

Reinsel, D. (2020). IDC's Global DataSphere Forecast shows continued steady growth in the creation and consumption of data. *IDC Report: Worldwide Global DataSphere Forecast, 2020–2024: The COVID-19 Data Bump and the Future of Data Growth* (Doc #US44797920).

Scheffer, L.K., Xu, C.S., Januszewski, M. *et al.* (2020). A connectome and analysis of the adult Drosophila central brain. bioRxiv. 030213.

Schirner, M. McIntosh, A.R., Jirsa, V. *et al.* (2018). Inferring multi-scale neural mechanisms with brain network modeling. *eLife.* 7:e28927.

Silvestri, L., Bria, A., Costantini, I. *et al.* (2013). Micron-scale resolution optical tomography of entire mouse brains with confocal light sheet microscopy. *J. Vis. Exp.* 80:e50696.

Tonnesen, J., Inavalli, V.V.G.K. & Nagerl, U.V. (2018). Super-resolution imaging of the extracellular space in living brain tissue. *Cell.* 172:1108–21.

Triebkorn, P., Zimmermann, J., Stefanovski, L. *et al.* (2020). Identifying optimal working points of individual Virtual Brains: A large-scale brain network modelling study. BioRxiv: 009795.

van Essen, D.C., Smith, S.M., Barch, D.M. *et al.* (2013). The WU-Minn Human Connectome Project: An overview. *NeuroImage.* 80:62–79.

Vescovi, R.F.C., Cardoso, M.B. & Miqueles, E.X. (2017). Radiography registration for mosaic tomography. *J. Synchrotron Radiation.* 24:686–94.

Wang, Y., Li, Q., Liu, L. *et al.* (2019). TeraVR empowers precise reconstruction of complete 3-D neuronal morphology in the whole brain. *Nat. Comm.* 10(3474):1–9.

White, J.G., Southgate, E., Thomson, J.N. & Brenner, S. (1986). The structure of the nervous system of the nematode Caenorhabditis elegans. *Philos. Trans. R. Soc. Lond. B. Biol. Sci.* 314:1–340.

Yamamoto, W.S. & Achacoso, T.B. (1992). Scaling up the nervous system of Caenorhabditis elegans: Is one ape equal to 33 million worms? *Comput. Biom. Res.* 25(3):279–91.

Yin, W., Brittain, D., Borseth, J. *et al.* (2019). A petascale automated imaging pipeline for mapping neuronal circuits with high-throughput transmission electron microscopy. bioRxiv:791889.

Zheng, Z., Lauritzen, J.S., Perlman, E. *et al.* (2018). A complete electron microscopy volume of the brain of adult. *Drosophila melanogaster*. *Cell.* 174:730–43.e22.

# Chapter 13

# Brain Networks

*A neuron is a noise-limited device of restricted bandwidth*

— Laughlin and Sejnowski (2003, p. 5)

*Recent experimental advances are producing an avalanche of data on both neural connectivity and neural activity*

— Ocker *et al.* (2017, p. 1)

**Abstract**

This chapter discusses brain networks as having similar design principles to those seen in human-made electronic networks for computing devices and communications networks. Neural design principles are specified in the areas of wiring and circuit layout, connectivity, energy consumption, signal processing, signal-to-noise ratio, and network reconfiguration (synaptic plasticity). Seeing cortical relations as brain networks has led to the development of network neuroscience and facilitates the AdS/Brain multi-tier model of neural signaling.

## 13.1 Brain Networks' Approach

The brain has long been studied as a computational machine, and is also starting to be recognized as a sophisticated communications network.

As a communications network, the brain transfers large amounts of information between areas. Neurons can receive and deliver signals at perhaps as many as 10,000 synapses, and combine synaptic inputs, both linearly and nonlinearly, to implement a large repertoire of information processing operations (Koch, 1999). Sharpening the estimate, each neuron has about 7,000 axon terminals from other neurons, but there is substantial redundancy in the connectivity, so each neuron has effective connections from about 80 other neurons, mostly nearest neighbors (Cowan *et al.*, 2016, p. 2). Through synaptic plasticity, neurons can change their connections and vary their signaling properties according to a variety of rules and dynamical changes. This suggests that brain networks can adapt to circumstances and change their properties according to experience, thus creating a powerful and flexible local and long-distance communications network. Some of the statistics highlighted in the brain networks' approach appear in Table 13.1.

### 13.1.1 *The brain as a communications network*

The brain exhibits an economy of design principles that balance constraint with performance. Brains are remarkably efficient and operate according

Table 13.1. Summary of human brain statistics.

| No. | Brain Statistic |
|---|---|
| 1 | Weight of adult human brain: 1.2–1.4 kilograms (2.6–3.1 pounds); 2% body weight |
| 2 | Neurons: 86 billion, glia: 85 billion, synapses: 242 trillion (2,800 average/neuron) |
| 3 | Human firing rate estimate: 1 action potential per second per neuron (rat 5, cat 3–9, macaque 14–18 firing potentials per second) |
| 4 | Synaptic failure: 50–90%; only 10–20% of action potentials trigger release |
| 5 | Gray matter (outer layer) local area network and white matter (inner core processing layer) long-distance network, split in brain volume: 50/50 |
| 6 | Energy consumption of the brain 20% for adults and 60% for infants |
| 7 | Volume fraction of wiring in the brain: 40–60% versus classical CPUs: up to 90% |

*Sources*: (1): Bigos *et al.* (2015, p. 157); (2): Martins *et al.* (2019), von Bartheld *et al.* (2016); (3): Attwell and Laughlin (2001), Lennie (2003); Baddeley *et al.* (1997); (4): Atwell and Laughlin (2001), Sudhof (2004, p. 509); (5): Sampaio-Baptista and Johansen-Berg (2017); (6): Hofman (1983); (7): Laughlin and Sejnowski (2003, p. 2).

to a narrow set of geometric, biophysical, and energy-related constraints. The brain is expensive in terms of space and resource consumption, but has evolved to an optimal configuration in the sense that functionality would be diminished if any design parameter were to be substantially altered. Resource use is connected to performance.

Laughlin and Sejnowski (2003) argue that cortical networks have evolved according to design principles similar to those used in human-made electronic networks (computing devices and communications networks). Research suggests that the structure and function of neuronal networks are governed by the same basic principles of resource allocation and constraint minimization followed by human-made networks. Such discovery that neuronal networks follow simple design rules resembling those found in other networks is an interesting implication of universality in design principles. Simple design rules improve efficiency by minimizing the resources required to implement a given task. It is not surprising that brains have evolved to operate efficiently. Economy and efficiency are guiding principles that explain other biological mechanisms, for example, the way that the lungs, circulation, and mitochondria are constantly interacting and regulating the supply of oxygen and energy to muscles (Weibel, 2000). To identify and explain these principles, it is necessary to derive and apply the structural relationships that underlie effective resource use and contribute to performance. A summary of the brain network design principles is as follows:

1. *Wiring and Circuit Layout*: Geometrical wiring constraints make interconnects costly in circuit layout (volume) and use (energy consumption).
2. *Connectivity*: Sparse small-world connectivity in outermost gray matter as a local area network and innermost white matter as a long-distance network.
3. *Energy Consumption*: Signaling is expensive in energy consumption and constrains traffic volume; traffic volume and firing rate can be imputed from the energy required for signaling.
4. *Signal Processing*: Thresholding mechanism and high rate of synaptic failure (50–90%) (signal does not propagate) keeps the signaling energy budget low.

5. *Signal-to-Noise Ratio*: Nonlinear molecular channel noise and signal-to-noise ratio (square root of membrane ion channels) analysis suggests existing axonal diameter (0.3 $\mu$m) would have a lower size limit of 0.1 $\mu$m.
6. *Network Reconfiguration*: Synaptic plasticity allows the cortical network to reorganize signaling pathways in time and space including via local field potentials (extracellular electrical fields aggregating local synapse current).

The network configuration topics are geometrical wiring constraints, connectivity, energy consumption, signal processing, the signal-to-noise ratio, and network reconfiguration. The design principles are as follows. First, considering wiring and circuit layout, geometrical constraints on packing and wiring highlight that interconnects are costly in circuit layout (volume) and in use (energy consumption), and that the brain may be organized to reduce wiring costs. Second, regarding connectivity, the layout of cortical areas minimizes the total lengths of the axons needed to join them by instantiating the outer-layer gray matter as a local area network and the inner-layer white matter as a long-distance network with sparse small-world connectivity. As physicist Sean Carroll notes, the "small-world network" concept may describe "not only the spatial organization of the connectome", but also how temporal signals are hierarchically organized towards a "critical point" (Carroll, 2016, pp. 323–33). Third, energy consumption is a crucial constraint in brain network design. Signaling is expensive in terms of energy consumption and therefore constrains traffic volume. Traffic volume and neural firing rates can be imputed from the signaling energy required. A general heuristic is that the human neural firing rate is one action potential per second per neuron.

Fourth, in signal processing, the brain's high rate of synaptic failure (50–90%) and thresholding mechanism by which most incoming synaptic messages do not translate to an outbound signal serves to keep the overall energy budget for signaling low (half what it would be if more signals were propagated). Fifth, signal-to-noise ratio analysis (in a basic calculation as the square root of the number of membrane ion channels) suggests that the high degree of nonlinear molecular channel noise in neural signaling means that the axon diameter (currently only 0.3 $\mu$m on average) might be further optimized but would have a downside size limit of 0.1 $\mu$m. Finally, network reconfiguration by synaptic plasticity is an important design principle that gives the brain the ability to reorganize itself in time and space per dynamical change. A key influence on synaptic plasticity is local field potentials, a sort of brain network path integral of extracellular electric fields, which reflect the summed activity of local synaptic currents and ion channels.

## 13.2 Wiring and Circuit Layout

In any network, one of the first design considerations is wiring. Wiring involves the efficient spatial organization of the system components based on how they are going to communicate. Since the brain is a dense and complex organ, whatever design principles might govern its economical layout are of chief interest. In brain network components and connection wiring terms, this means the size of the neurons, and the layout of neurons so as to reduce the length of their connections.

### 13.2.1 *The brain is three-dimensional*

The brain makes good use of its three dimensionality. That the brain is three-dimensional further suggests quantum computing as both domains are three-dimensional and the brain can be represented directly without translating three-dimensional information into alternative formats. Just like the wires connecting components in electronic chips, the connections between neurons occupy a substantial fraction of the total volume, and the wires (axons and dendrites) are expensive to operate because they dissipate energy during signaling. Nature has an important benefit over electronic circuits because components are connected by wires in three-dimensional space, whereas even the most advanced classical microprocessor chips are only able to use a small number of layers of planar wiring. Quantum processing units more directly implement real-life nature in their three-dimensional accommodation.

The brain's three-dimensional wiring may explain why the volume fraction of wiring in the brain (40–60%) is much lower than that in classical chips (up to 90%) (Laughlin and Sejnowski, 2003, p. 2). In classical computer chips, the components are arranged to reduce the total length of the wiring. The brain's three-dimensional geometry provides a substantial wiring advantage. Such brain wiring efficiency has been confirmed in *C. elegans* (the nematode worm). The worm has 302 neurons arranged in eleven clusters of ganglia. An analysis of alternative ganglion placements shows that the observed layout of ganglia indeed minimizes wire length (Cherniak, 1994). Fruit fly, mouse, and human connectome (wiring diagram) projects may find the same kinds of efficient wiring layout principles at work.

#### 13.2.1.1 *Topographical projection*

Brain wiring, and also projection is topographically organized. Projection is the broadcast signaling by which the brain communicates. The brain's more recently evolved six-layer neocortex is able to target projection in a more efficient manner than the diffuse projection used by the older three-layer structures of the brain such as the olfactory cortex and the hippocampus. In the primary visual cortex, for example, input and processing are co-located. Input from the visual field is processed by neighboring neurons in the cortex. Connectivity is much higher between neurons separated by less than 1 mm than between neurons farther apart, reflecting the need for rapid, local processing within a cortical column (a stacked arrangement that minimizes wire length) (Markram, 2006). Since cortical neurons have elaborately branched dendritic trees (serving as input regions) and axonal trees (projecting the output to other neurons), it is possible to predict the best geometric patterns of connectivity.

#### 13.2.1.2 *Optimal ratios of axonal to dendritic arbor volumes*

Using the principle of wiring economy, Chklovskii (2000) proposes a rule to specify the sizes of axonal arbors of input neurons and dendritic arbors of output neurons in a topographic projection. A topographic projection between two neuronal layers with different densities of neurons is considered and a divergence-convergence ratio is calculated. Given the number of output neurons connected to each input neuron (divergence) and the number of input neurons synapsing on each output neuron (convergence), the widths of axonal and dendritic arbors which minimize the total volume of axons and dendrites is determined. Several projections between pairs of neuronal classes are considered, including for retinal, cerebellar, olfactory bulb, and neocortical neurons. The calculated ratio recapitulates known anatomical data, for example, in the case of cerebellar neurons, the theory predicts a ratio of dendritic and axonal arbor sizes of 58, and in the case of olfactory bulb neurons, the theory predicts the ratio of dendritic arbor diameters to be 10 (Chklovskii, 2000, p. 2117).

Economic principles are the basis for theory development. An assumption is made that space constraints require keeping the brain volume to a minimum. Since wiring (axons and dendrites) takes up a significant fraction of the volume, evolution may have optimized axonal and dendritic arbors in a way that minimizes their total volume. Therefore, one way to explain existing arbor sizes is as a result of wiring optimization.

The geometric analysis of dendritic arbors continues as an active research frontier. Cugno *et al.* (2019) investigate synaptic transmission as a function of dendritic size and geometry. A biophysics approach is used to model reaction-diffusion events within the dendritic spine. The results indicate that geometric features (ellipsoid shape curvature analogous to harmonic functions) show concentrations along the dendritic spine head that play an important role in the spatiotemporal dynamics of signaling. Further, substantial changes in dendritic spine shape are indicative of neuropathology development.

## 13.3 Connectivity

### 13.3.1 *Gray matter and white matter*

The cortex is composed of gray matter and white matter. The outer layer is gray matter, which contains the synapses, dendrites, cell bodies, and local axons of neurons that form the neural circuits that process information. The innermost layer is white matter, the deep subcortical regions of heavily myelinated axons that undertake the core processing of the brain. The gray and white matter each make up about half of the total brain

Table 13.2. Cortical gray matter and white matter.

| Brain Matter | Cortical Location | Prominent Communication | Brain Volume | Composition |
|---|---|---|---|---|
| Gray matter | Outermost layer | Short-distance communication in the local area | 50% | Axons, synapses, dendrites, cell bodies |
| White matter | Innermost core layer | Long-distance communication between cortical areas | 50% | Heavily myelinated axons |

volume (Sampaio-Baptista & Johansen-Berg, 2017) (Table 13.2). The gray matter is so-called as the area acquires a gray tone from the high concentration of neuronal cell bodies (Mercadante & Tadi, 2020).

#### 13.3.1.1 *Local gray matter and long-distance white matter*

The prominent communication within white matter (the central core of the brain network) is long-distance communication between cortical areas. The communication emphasis of gray matter is short-distance communication within the local area. Hence, by analogy to telecommunications networks, the gray matter is a local area network and the white matter is a long-distance network. This might seem counterintuitive until considering that communication comes at a premium, so to the extent that long-distance wiring connections can be minimized, the white matter represents an effective solution.

Research investigates the evolutionary relationship between gray and white matter in mammals (Zhang & Sejnowski, 2000). On the one hand, the thickness of gray matter, just a few millimeters, is nearly constant in species that range in brain volume over five orders of magnitude. On the other hand, the volume of the white matter scales approximately as the 4/3 power of the volume of the gray matter. This might be explained by the need to maintain a fixed bandwidth of long-distance communication capacity per unit area of the cortex. The point is that the thickness of gray matter is constant but the volume of white matter grows at a 4/3 ratio indicating that total brain volume increases.

The design principle that can be inferred from this analysis is that the layout of cortical areas minimizes the total lengths of the axons needed to join them. The prominent folds in the structure of the human cortex allow the large cortical area to be densely packed in the skull, but also allow cortical areas around the convolutions to minimize wire length. This trade-off appears to strike a balance between the two opposing tendencies of transmission speed and component density. Unlike the wires in chips, reducing the diameter of neural wires reduces the speed at which signals travel, prolonging delays. However, it also reduces axon volume, and this allows neurons to be packed closer together, thus shortening delays. Neural wire diameters are subject to different design concerns and trade-offs than those of less complex classical chips.

#### 13.3.1.2 *Sparse small-world connectivity*

The overall connectivity in the cortex is very sparse, which also helps in reducing the volume occupied by long-range connections. The cortical column demonstrates this principle. Even for neurons specifically organized in a vertical column (only 1 mm in diameter) for efficient communication, the probability of any two cortical neurons having a direct connection is quite low, about one in a hundred (1.0%). The probability declines significantly to one in a million (0.0001%) for distant neurons. Similarly, the distribution of wire lengths on chips follows an inverse power law, so that shorter wires also dominate. In a computational analysis of the brain, if a matrix were created with $10^{10}$ rows and columns to represent the connections between every pair of cortical neurons, it would have a relatively dense set of entries around the diagonal but only sparse entries outside the diagonal.

The sparse long-range connectivity of the cortex may offer some of the advantages of small-world connectivity. Small-world connectivity is a graph-theoretic principle of efficiency that means networks in which communications paths are shorter than would be random. Indeed, the brain's communications graph is extremely effective. Even though only a small fraction of neurons are connected to distant cortical areas, this is enough to produce activity coordinated in distant parts the brain, as reflected in the synchronous firing of action potentials in these areas.

Brain networks are found to have not only small-world connectivity but also that of rich-club hubs (Lynn & Bassett, 2019). A rich-club hub is a centralized hub that links otherwise distant regions of the network. Connectome analysis of empirical brain networks shows that there is a widespread shift away from the geometric center of the network toward more peripheral interconnected frameworks in each hemisphere (with discrete clusters persisting around the anterior insula, and the anterior and posterior midline regions of the cortex) (Roberts *et al.*, 2016). A relatively small number of strong interhemispheric connections assimilate these structures into a rich-club hub. The rich-club hub's connections are more heavily clustered locally as expected, but longer than would be predicted by geometry globally. The analysis highlights topological features that likely confer functional advantages but carry an additional metabolic cost.

## 13.4 Energy Consumption

In computer networks, as processor speeds increase, so too does energy dissipation, and thus cooling technology is critically important. Energy consumption also constrains neural processing. Nervous systems consume metabolic energy continuously at relatively high rates per gram, comparable to those of heart muscle. Consequently, powering a brain is a major drain on an organism's energy budget, typically consuming 2 to 10% of resting energy. In humans this proportion is 20% for adults and 60% for infants (Hofman, 1983).

A lot can be learned from the brain's different states such as cognition, rest, sleep, and seizure. For example, deep anesthesia blocks neural signaling and halves the brain's energy consumption. This is because anesthetics are thought to act through ion channel blockage and trigger changes in cellular membrane dynamics that lead to synaptic failure (Diao *et al.*, 2014). The ratio suggests that under anesthesia, while one half of the brain's overall energy budget is devoted to routing signals along axons and across synapses, the other half is supporting the maintenance of resting potentials and the passive functions of neurons and glia. The ratio may be quite different in awake signaling states. Specific to the signaling operation, the cortical gray matter may use more than 75% of the energy available for signaling due to the rich interconnections between axons and synapses (Aiello *et al.*, 2001).

### 13.4.1 *Imputing traffic volume from energy consumption*

An indirect analysis method imputes traffic volume from energy consumption (Attwell & Laughlin, 2001). Taking the amount of energy possibly used for neuronal signaling as an input, the analysis derives the maximum volume of signal traffic that could be supported by the brain's metabolic rate. For the cerebral cortex, the permissible traffic is less than one action potential per second for humans, and about five action potentials per second per neuron for rats (Laughlin & Sejnowksi, 2003, p. 9; Lennie, 2003). In other animal species, a study of the visual cortex found rates of neural firing averaging 3–4 spikes per second for cats and 14–18 spikes per second for macaques, and another study found 9 spikes per second for cats (Baddeley *et al.*, 1997).

Other work in the neocortical simulation efforts of the whole-brain emulation project notes the difficulty of estimating an average firing rate due to the non-linear behavior of one neuron triggering another (Gerstner *et al.*, 1997). Another variable in the firing rate of neural signaling is the necessary refractory period, which is a few milliseconds in humans (Nicholls *et al.*, 2012, p. 14). A general heuristic based on different analysis parameters estimates the human brain's firing rate at about a one action potential per second per neuron. However, there could be considerable variability based on the type of neuron and the firing situation, and the ability to confirm analysis results experimentally *in vivo*.

Irrespective of ascertaining an average human neural firing rate, the design point is that neurons are expensive. Since the brain responds quickly, and the permissible amount of traffic is remarkably low, metabolic limits may influence the way that information is processed. Research suggests that brains have countered metabolic constraint by adopting energy-efficient designs. These designs involve the miniaturization of components, the elimination of superfluous signals, and the representation of information with efficient coding schemes.

### 13.4.2 *Bandwidth*

One estimate for the overall potential bandwidth of all of the neurons in the human cortex is one terabit per second (Laughlin & Sejnowski, 2003, p. 3). This assumes a maximum rate of 100 bits per second for each axon in the white matter. The figure compares to the level of bandwidth in the total world backbone capacity of the internet in 2002 (*Ibid.*). However, in the brain, such a capacity of one terabit per second would never be achieved in practice since only a fraction of cortical neurons are firing at any time. As a reference, TeleGeography estimated the global internet capacity at 295 Tbps (terabits per second, $10^{12}$ bps) in 2017 (Rebatta, 2017).

## 13.5 Signal Processing

### 13.5.1 *Signal conversion*

Signal processing is a crucial task for any communications network to ensure that messages are sent and received with fidelity. Signals may be encoded for more efficient transfer. Telecommunications networks convert incoming electrical signals to optical signals for long-haul transfer, and then back to electrical signals for delivery at the destination. Brain networks too convert initially electrical signals from the axon's action potential into chemical signals that are sent across the synaptic channel by neurotransmitters. Then, neurotransmitter signals are converted back into electrical signals in the receiving dendrites in the postsynaptic density for

Table 13.3. Communications network signal conversion.

| Communications Network | Signal Ingress | Intermediate Transmission | Signal Egress |
|---|---|---|---|
| Telecommunications | Electrical | Optical | Electrical |
| Brain | Electrical (axon) | Chemical (synapse) | Electrical (dendrite) |

onward routing via dendritic spikes, possibly ultimately to the axon in the receiving neuron (Table 13.3).

Synaptic signals received by dendrites may be excitatory or inhibitory, which has the effect of increasing or decreasing the net voltage that reaches the soma (the cell body from which the axon potential begins). If an appropriate threshold is reached, the stimulus is sent down the axon as an electrical action potential. Reaching the signaling threshold is determined by the all-or-none character of action potential generation as follows. Neurons are electrically excitable, due to maintenance of voltage gradients across their membranes. If the voltage changes by a large enough amount over a short interval, the neuron generates an all-or-nothing electrochemical pulse called an action potential.

The action potential travels rapidly along the axon until it reaches the presynaptic terminal at the bouton (large-headed end of the neuron). In the presynaptic terminal, the action potential is converted from an electrical to chemical signal with the activity of calcium channel ions. The signal is then disgorged from the presynaptic terminal active zone and crosses the synaptic cleft as a chemical message in the form of neurotransmitters. In the postsynaptic terminal of the dendrites (postsynaptic density), the chemical signal is processed and converted back into an electrical signal with dendritic spiking per the same membrane-based potential-triggering mechanisms. The general form of neural signaling is through chemical synapses as described, but exclusively electrical synapses are used in high-stakes rapid-signaling applications such as in the heart and fight-or-flight escape reflexes.

#### 13.5.1.1 *Probabilistic signal transmission*

The brain regulates signal traffic at the level of the individual synaptic connections between neurons. A typical cortical neuron receives information from on the order of 10,000 synapses, but the probability that this information is converted to an action potential internally and ultimately passed on to other neurons by releasing neurotransmitter is very low, only 10 to 50% (50 to 90% synaptic failure (Sudhof, 2004, p. 509)). The all-or-none firing of action potentials means that a neuron rarely experiences the conditions of a large enough threshold of voltage changes over a short enough time interval to generate an action potential. Atwell and Laughlin

(2001) suggest that the high rate of synaptic failure might be an efficiency measure since the failure rate halves the energy consumption of gray matter. With so many neurons receiving synaptic inputs, there is no overall loss in information. Although information is not lost in healthy firing, the failure ratio degrades with the onset of pathology and is an early warning signal of deteriorating function (Budak & Michal Zochowski, 2019).

The mechanism for how the brain balances lossy signals against information loss is not well understood. The brain exhibits sparse encoding schemes in which only a small proportion of cells are signaling at any one time. This minimizes energy while maintaining a high representational capacity since there are many different ways in which a small number of signals can be distributed among a large number of neurons.

However, large populations of neurons are expensive to maintain, and if neurons rarely signal, they are redundant. The optimum proportion of active cells may depend on the ratio between the cost of maintaining a neuron at rest and the extra cost of sending a signal. When signals are relatively expensive, it is best to distribute a few of them among a large number of cells. When cells are expensive, it is more efficient to use a few of them and to have more or all of them signaling. Estimates of the ratio between the energy demands of signaling and maintenance suggest that, for maximum efficiency, between 1% and 16% of neurons should be active at any one time (Levy & Baxter, 1996). However, it is difficult to compare these predictions with experimental data.

Summarizing, the signal processing design problem is the situation of unreliable single neurons, noisy molecular signaling mechanisms, and redundant signal transmission, all toward the goal of reaching a relevant thresholding determination for signals to propagate. Levy and Baxter take an energy-efficiency view and argue that sparse coding improves energy efficiency and directs signaling. Baxter takes a statistical view and suggests that the brain economizes by sending impulses according to the statistical mean (calling the brain an "economy of impulses") (Barlow, 1972, p. 385). However, from a biophysics lens, it is not clear whether the process could be made more efficient. Considering a larger-scale perspective of fields and gradients, it is not "synaptic failure" as much as a simple "lack of thresholding" in constant ongoing operations. This suggests that the field gradient is an extremely effective means of signal construction and propagation.

# 13.6 Signal-to-Noise Ratio

## 13.6.1 *Ion channels*

The brain evolved to be efficient, and it may not be possible to improve on this design in other ways too. Noise makes it costly to transfer information along single neurons at high rates. Fundamentally, the neuron is a noise-limited device with restricted bandwidth. The brain's signal-to-noise ratio can be calculated to assess the effectiveness of the brain's network transmission activities. The signal-to-noise ratio measures the amount of effective signal propagation per the amount of noise in the communications channel. The signal-to-noise ratio is most readily calculated as the square root of the number of synapses, which might be interpreted as the square root of the number of ion channels in the membrane available for signal transfer (White *et al.*, 2000). The calculation takes a cue from diffusion, in that diffusive processes spread out by a factor of the square root of the relevant measure. The implication is that improving the information rate would require expensive changes. Doubling the signal-to-noise ratio would mean quadrupling the number of ion channels in the membrane, increasing the current flow, and using much more energy. With this implied relationship between noise and energy cost, an energy-efficient nervous system would be likely to divide information among a larger number of relatively noisy neurons of lower information capacity (as observed in the general splitting of retinal signals into "ON" and "OFF" pathways (von der Twer & MacLeod, 2001)), rather than a smaller number of high precision neurons.

### 13.6.1.1 *Molecular channel noise is nonlinear*

Continuing with the energy efficiency theme, one way to analyze the structural relationship between component miniaturization, energy consumption, and noise is based on component size and throughput. Even though the axon diameter is only 0.3 $\mu$m (on average), sending action potentials along these wires consumes more than one-third of the energy supplied to cortical gray matter (Attwell & Laughlin, 2001). Thus, as with computer chips, an efficient layout and a high component density are essential for energy efficiency, but, as is also true for chips, miniaturization raises problems about noise. In the brain, the signal-to-noise ratio worsens if a neuron's membrane area is reduced. The membrane is the number of molecular pores or ion channels available to carry electrical signals from one neuron to another.

The noise produced by ion channels, and by other molecular signaling mechanisms such as synaptic vesicles, is potentially damaging to signaling performance. However, the effects of noise are often difficult to determine because they depend on interactions between signaling molecules in signaling systems. The interactions are highly nonlinear and involve complicated spatial effects. On the one hand, the basic action potential itself is highly nonlinear as produced by the cycling behavior of voltage-dependent sodium and potassium ion channels. On the other hand, complicated spatial effects arise from the diffusion of chemical messengers between neurons and the transmission of electrical signals within neurons. It is difficult to assess the overall complexities of molecular noise and diffusion in neural signaling. However, considering miniaturization, simulations indicate that channel noise places a ceiling on the wiring density of the brain by setting a lower limit of about 0.1 $\mu$m on axon diameter (White *et al.*, 2000).

Some of the specific aspects and possibilities of measuring molecular channel noise have been analyzed in other research. Manwani *et al.* (1999) carry out a systematic investigation of the relationship between channel kinetics and the resulting membrane voltage noise using a stochastic Markov version of the Mainen–Sejnowski model of dendritic excitability in cortical neurons. They find that kinetic parameters which lead to an increase in membrane excitability (increasing channel densities and decreasing temperature) also lead to an increase in the magnitude of the sub-threshold voltage noise. Further, noise also increases as the membrane is depolarized from rest toward threshold. This suggests that channel fluctuations may interfere with a neuron's ability to function as an integrator of its synaptic inputs and may limit the reliability and precision of neural information processing.

#### 13.6.1.2 *Volumetric connectome data*

Ideally, volumetric analysis from connectome projects might be used to elucidate the potential trade-offs between component miniaturization, energy consumption, and noise. Braitenberg and Schutz (1998) made an early observation that (in 1 $mm^3$ of mouse cortex) distinguished 105 neurons, 108 synapses, and 4 km of axon. One conclusion from these data is that the brain may limit energy consumption by reducing the size and active area of components, a similar principle to that used in chip design. Braitenberg and Schutz's research found about 100 synapses per 1 $mm^3$ of volumetric brain tissue. A recent study reconstructing a sub-volume of mouse neocortex surprisingly reported in a particular sample, 1,700 synapses, at a density of one synapse per 1.13 $mm^3$ (Kasthuri *et al.*, 2015, p. 653). In another portion of the sample, the team found 193 dendrites and 1,407 unmyelinated axons (93% excitatory, 7% inhibitory).

In other work, the Allen Institute produced a petascale-dataset (2 petabytes) by imaging 26,500 tissue sections from a 1 $mm^3$ volume of mouse neocortex but did not comment on the composition (Yin *et al.*, 2019). The effort relied on an array of six electron microscopes operating continuously, and took six months. These various potentially conflicting, unreconciled, and unreplicated analyses highlight the point that quantitative metrics for the brain are not yet known, and further that the sought metrics may be incorrect for the underlying biological mechanisms. At minimum, given anatomical knowledge, the expectation would be many more synapses than axons in a given volume, and likewise, many more dendrites than axons in 1 $mm^3$ of volumetric brain tissue. Connectome efforts are important for obtaining the brain's wiring diagram, and other kinds of analytical progress are likely needed in accompaniment to elaborate how the brain actually works.

## 13.7 Network Rewiring: Synaptic Plasticity

The noise and variability observed among neurons is compensated by synaptic plasticity (the ability of neurons to modify their signaling properties). Telecommunications networks reconfigure signals in space and time (through space-division, time-division, and wave-division multiplexing) and the brain also has much more synaptic plasticity that was initially realized in distributing signals efficiently in space and time. Synaptic plasticity likewise seems to have the ability to direct scarce resources to where they will be of greatest benefit.

Synaptic plasticity enables the spatial relocation, and the short-term and long-term temporal reconfiguration of the brain. The cortical network is not a vast, fixed network whose connection strengths change slowly. Instead, cortical connectivity is highly dynamic, and changes on fast as well as slow timescales. This allows the cortex to be rapidly reconfigured to meet changing computational and communications needs. Whereas the initiation of action potentials takes place with millisecond precision, the throughput at cortical synapses is slower and probabilistic (Mainen & Sejnowski, 1995). On a short timescale of milliseconds to seconds, presynaptic mechanisms briefly increase or decrease the probability of transmission at cortical synapses, depending on the previous patterns of activity. On longer time scales, persistent correlated firing between the presynaptic and postsynaptic neurons can produce the long-term depression or long-term potentiation of the synaptic efficacy, depending on the relative timing of the spikes in the two neurons.

### 13.7.1 *Neural signaling path integral*

Local field potentials function as a path integral to describe neuronal firing. Local field potentials are extracellular electric fields that reflect the aggregate activity of local synaptic currents and ion channels on neurons and glia. The field potentials are generated by transient imbalances in ion concentrations in the intercellular space between neurons and glia due to cellular electrical activity. They are "local" because their main activity spreads out in a range of about a centimeter from their origin (in macaque) (Kajikawa & Schroeder, 2011). They are "potentials" because they are generated by the voltage that results from charge separation in the extracellular space. They are "fields" because the extracellular charge separations create a local electric field. Local field potentials are implicated in the dynamic flow of information across biological neural networks. Since local field potentials are extracellular, experimental data are available and more easily obtainable than for intracellular signaling.

A problem in systems neuroscience is that the function of neurons is often cast in terms of stimuli and response. However, empirical data such as recordings from the visual cortex in behaving animals shows that a large fraction of neural activity is not predictable from direct stimulus alone. Larger-scale network activity including local field potentials also plays a role. The local field potential is a composite signal that receives contributions from multiple neural sources. A key research finding suggests that the main factor that defines the amplitude of the local field potential is the geometry of the current sources (as opposed to the degree of synchronization of the signals or other explanations) (Herreras, 2016). Although the data may be more difficult to interpret than neural spikes due to the multiplicity of factors involved, a broader picture of neural signaling necessarily includes these influences (Einevoll *et al.*, 2013).

Local field potentials hint at how the larger-scale flow of information in cortical circuits may be regulated. Oscillations in the 20 to 80 Hertz range occur in local field potentials, leading to coherence between spikes and local field potential oscillations, that has been found to influence attention and working memory (Pesaran *et al.*, 2002).

#### 13.7.1.1 *Implications of brain networks' approach*

Seeing the brain as a local and long-distance communications network with design constraints, traffic management, and signal conversion (electrical-optical-electrical being similar to electrical-chemical-electrical) illuminates a new approach to add to the arsenal for tackling the dynamical complexity of the brain. Brain network trade-offs are indicated in the efficiency and performance of various communications network attributes (circuit wiring, connectivity, energy consumption, signal processing, signal-to-noise ratio, and network reconfiguration). The brain network description indicates how neurons, circuits, and signal transmission are designed to conserve space, materials, time, and energy, while delivering high performance and functionality.

## References

Aiello, L.C., Bates, N. & Joffe, T.H. (2001). In defense of the expensive tissue hypothesis. In *Evolutionary Anatomy of the Primate Cerebral Cortex*. Eds. Falk, D. & Gibson, K.R. Cambridge: Cambridge University Press, pp. 57–78.

Attwell, D. & Laughlin, S.B. (2001). An energy budget for signaling in the grey matter of the brain. *J. Cereb. Blood Flow Metab.* 21:1133–45.

Baddeley, R., Abbott, L.F., Booth, M.C. *et al.* (1997). Responses of neurons in primary and inferior temporal visual cortices to natural scenes. *Proc. Biol. Sci.* 264(1389):1775–83.

Barlow, H.B. (1972). Single units and sensation: A neuron doctrine for perceptual psychology? *Perception.* 1:371–94.

Bigos, K.L., Hariri, A. & Weinberger, D. (2015). *Neuroimaging Genetics: Principles and Practices*. Oxford: Oxford University Press.

Braitenberg, V. & Schutz, A. (1998). *Cortex: Statistics and Geometry of Neuronal Connectivity*. Vol. 2. Berlin: Springer.

Budak, M. and Michal Zochowski, M. (2019). Synaptic failure differentially affects pattern formation in heterogenous networks. *Front Neural Circuits.* 13(31):1–15.

Carroll, S. (2016). *The Big Picture*. New York: Dutton.

Cherniak, C. (1994). Communication in neuronal networks. *J. Neurosci.* 4:2408.

Chklovskii, D. (2000). Optimal sizes of dendritic and axonal arbors in a topographic projection. *J. Neurophysiol.* 83:2113–9.

Cowan, J.D., Neuman, J. & van Drongelen, W. (2016). Wilson-Cowan equations for neocortical dynamics. *J. Math. Neurosci.* 6(1):1–24.

Cugno, A., Bartol, T.M., Sejnowski, T.J. *et al.* (2019). Geometric principles of second messenger dynamics in dendritic spines. *Sci. Rep.* 9(1):11676.

Diao, S., Ni, J., Shi, X., Liu, P., and Xia, W. (2014). Mechanisms of action of general anesthetics. *Front Biosci.* 19:747–57.

Einevoll, G.T., Kayser, C., Logothetis, N.K. & Panzeri, S. (2013). Modelling and analysis of local field potentials for studying the function of cortical circuits. *Nat. Rev. Neurosci.* 14:770–85.

Gerstner, W., Kreiter, A.K., Markram, H. & Herz, A.V.M. (1997). Neural codes: Firing rates and beyond. *Proc. Natl. Acad. Sci.* 94(24):12740–1.

Herreras, O. (2016). Local field potentials: Myths and misunderstandings. *Front Neural. Circuits.* 10(101):1–16.

Hofman, M.A. (1983). Energy metabolism, brain size and longevity in mammals. *Q. Rev. Biol.* 58:495.

Kajikawa, Y. & Schroeder, C.E. (2011). How local is the local field potential? *Neuron.* 72(5):847–58.

Kasthuri, N., Hayworth, K.J., Berger, D.R. *et al.* (2015). Saturated reconstruction of a volume of neocortex. *Cell.* 162(3):648–61.

Koch, C. (1999). *Biophysics of Computation: Information Processing in Single Neurons*. Oxford: Oxford University Press.

Laughlin, S.B. & Sejnowski, T.J. (2003). Communication in neuronal networks. *Science*. 301(5641):1870–4.

Lennie, P. (2003). The cost of cortical computation. *Curr. Biol.* 13:493.

Levy, W.B. & Baxter, R.A. (1996). Energy efficient neural codes. *Neural. Comput.* 8:531.

Lynn, C.W. & Bassett, D.S. (2019). The physics of brain network structure, function and control. *Nat. Rev. Phys.* 1(5):318–32.

Mainen, Z.F. & Sejnowski, T.J. (1995). Reliability of spike timing in neocortical neurons. *Science.* 268(5216):1503–6.

Manwani, A., Steinmetz, P.N. & Koch, C. (1999). Channel noise in excitable neuronal membranes. *Adv. Neural. Info. Proc. Sys.* 12:143–9.

Markram, H. (2006). The Blue Brain Project. *Nat. Rev. Neurosci.* 7:153–60.

Martins, N.R.B., Angelica, A., Chakravarthy, K. *et al.* (2019). Human brain/cloud interface. *Front Neurosci.* 13(112):1–23.

Mercadante, A.A. & Tadi, P. (2020). *Neuroanatomy, Gray Matter.* NCBI Bookshelf. Treasure Island, FL: StatPearls Publishing.

Nicholls, J.G., Martin, A.R., Fuchs, P.A. *et al.* (2012). *From Neuron to Brain.* 5th Edition. Sunderland, MA: Sinauer Associates, Inc.

Ocker, G.K., Josic, K., Shea-Brown, E. & Buice, M.A. (2017). Linking structure and activity in nonlinear spiking networks. *PLOS Comput. Biol.* 13(6): 1–46.

Pesaran, B., Pezaris, J.S., Sahani, M. *et al.* (2002). Temporal structure in neuronal activity during working memory in macaque parietal cortex. *Nat. Neurosci.* 5:805.

Rebatta, A. (2017). 295 Tbps: Internet traffic and capacity in 2017. *TeleGeography.* https://blog.telegeography.com/295-tbps-internet-traffic-and-capacity-in-2017.

Roberts, J.A., Perry, A., Lord, A.R. *et al.* (2016). The contribution of geometry to the human connectome. *Neuroimage.* 124:379–93.

Sampaio-Baptista, C. & Johansen-Berg, H. (2017). White matter plasticity in the adult brain. *Neuron.* 96(6):1239–51.

Sudhof, T.C. (2004). The synaptic vesicle cycle. *Annu. Rev. Neurosci.* 27: 509–47.

TeleGeography. (2002). Global internet backbone growth slows dramatically. *TeleGeography.* https://www2.telegeography.com/telegeography-press.

von Bartheld, C.S., Bahney, J. & Herculano-Houzel, S. (2016). The search for true numbers of neurons and glial cells in the human brain: A review of 150 years of cell counting. *J. Comp. Neurol.* 524(18):3865–95.

von der Twer, T. & MacLeod, D.I. (2001). Optimal nonlinear codes for the perception of natural colors. *Network.* 12:395.

Weibel, E.R. (2000). *Symmorphosis: On Form and Function in Shaping Life*. Cambridge: Harvard University Press.

White, J.A., Rubinstein, J.T. & Kay, A.R. (2000). Channel noise in neurons. *Trends Neurosci.* 23:131–7.

Yin, W., Brittain, D., Borseth, J. *et al.* (2019). A petascale automated imaging pipeline for mapping neuronal circuits with high-throughput transmission electron microscopy. bioRxiv:791889.

Zhang, K. & Sejnowski, T.J. (2000). A universal scaling law between grey matter and white matter of cerebral cortex. *Proc. Natl. Acad. Sci.* 97:5621.

# Part 4

# System Evolution

# Chapter 14

# Quantum Dynamics

*[A]ll of the various conformations of the neuron and its various components are simply morphological adaptations governed by laws of conservation for time, space, and material*

— Ramon y Cajal (1995 (1894), p. 116)


## Abstract

This chapter discusses the foundational physics advances in the understanding of dynamics in quantum mechanical systems. Operator size and distribution growth are new levers for measuring the distribution of expectation values of operators acting on observables that produce dynamical behavior. Out-of-time-order correlation (OTOC) functions are applied to evolve thermofield double states (two entangled copies of a quantum state) back and forward in time to understand quantum information scrambling (diffusion). The holographic Sachdev–Ye–Kitaev (SYK) model interprets operator growth as a solvable SYK model in the boundary to calculate aspects of particle momentum in the bulk. Any system with time translation symmetry breaking can be interpreted as a time superfluid, and possibly as a spacetime crystal.

## 14.1 Dynamics of Quantum Systems

A contemporary topic in foundational physics research is predicting the dynamics of quantum system evolution over time. Quantum dynamics refers to the motion, energy, and momentum exchange of quantum mechanical systems. Quantum dynamics problems are nontrivial due to the $2^n$ problem, that quantum systems become exponentially larger and more complicated as they evolve from the initial state. As a simple instantiation of a black hole and minimal realization of the AdS/CFT duality, the Sachdev–Ye–Kitaev (SYK) model is used to examine various problems in quantum dynamics (Maldacena & Stanford, 2016). In a random matrix formulation of the SYK model, late-time chaotic dynamics are indicated (Cotler *et al.*, 2017). To understand a wider range of time scales and system evolution, operator-based formulations are employed.

Quantum systems are described by states and operators (mathematical functions) that act upon the states to describe the evolution of the system. Both states and operators grow and evolve over time. It is not possible to measure quantities directly in quantum mechanics without changing or destroying them. Instead, it is possible to measure the expectation values of operators acting on observable quantities, taking a distribution of many such expectation values to obtain an average, and this is how quantum systems are measured. The quantum state grows as the particle movements evolve from the initial $2^n$ states. The quantum operator grows since more complicated mathematical terms may need to be added to act on the system which has also grown in size and complexity.

Since quantum systems are measured by the distribution of expectation values of operators acting on observables, operator growth is a natural and accessible lever for studying quantum dynamics. A contemporary focus is investigating operator growth, meaning the size and distribution of operator growth as quantum systems evolve over time. Quantum states grow as a function of the operators that act upon them, so the central problem is crystallized as understanding operator behavior. In particular, the growth of operator size and distribution are being studied in the context of holography and quantum many-body problems.

## 14.2 Operator Size and Distribution Growth

Operators grow in size as time evolves. The growth (and distribution) of the size of an operator is a manifestation of many aspects related to the quantum dynamics of a system. The canonical way to calculate operator size and growth is with the Heisenberg equation of motion. However, the Heisenberg equation of motion is only a general approximation and does not include temperature, so other more fine-grained approaches are sought.

The term operator "size" is a flexible term used to mean various things, including the size of the underlying system or the size of the operator after it has evolved in time. In the most basic sense, size refers to the number of particles in the system. Roberts *et al.* (2018), for example, evaluate the size distribution for $N = 30$ elementary fermions. In this work, "size" means the size of the basis element (the number of elementary fermions that appear in the product of the equations) (Roberts *et al.*, 2018, p. 2). Likewise, Lin *et al.* (2019) indicate that the "size operator" counts the number of particles that are affected by applying the operator. In the more complex use of the term "size", it may refer to aspects of the operator or the system after the time evolution. Nahum *et al.* (2018, p. 2) discuss operator "size" as the size of the region in which a time-evolved operator fails to commute with local operators. In general, operator "size" may have different meanings related to the size of the system and the size of the operators. Also, the terms "size operator" and "operator size" are used interchangeably. Since quantum systems are not measured directly but with operators, operators are sometimes seen as being synonymous with the underlying system states (even though operators are mathematical functions that act on the system states). In other work, thermal scale quanta are the object with "size" to be analyzed (Sekino & Susskind, 2008, p. 2).

A quantum system typically has many operators and these operators interrelate. Further, there are different kinds of operator growth. For example, it has been elaborated that an operator might have both linear external spatial growth and exponential internal size growth (Qi & Streicher, 2019). In the simplest case, operators are assumed to be bosonic (force operators). However, if the operator of interest is fermionic (a matter operator), the bosonic operator is converted. Bosonic operators are converted to fermionic operators by being multiplied with an anti-commuting fermionic operator from an external system, for example.

Operator size and distribution growth are deployed as a standard tool to examine a number of more complex situations in quantum dynamics. Operator size is a key input to calculating out-of-time-order correlators (OTOCs) which are used to evolve quantum systems backward and forward in time. OTOCs are in turn linked to the chaos, thermalization, and information scrambling of quantum systems.

## 14.3 The Holographic SYK Model

### 14.3.1 *The Heisenberg uncertainty principle*

The Heisenberg uncertainty principle states that it is not possible to know the precise position and the momentum of a particle at the same time. The formula for the Heisenberg uncertainty principle is the product of two terms: Uncertainty about where the particle is (its location) multiplied by the uncertainty about how fast it is moving (its speed). The minimal value of the product of these two uncertainties is Planck's constant, a very small number referred to as "$h$" ($h = 6.626 \times 10^{-34}$ Joule-seconds). The Heisenberg uncertainty principle underlines two important aspects of quantum mechanics. First, there cannot be complete certainty about a particle's location or speed. Second, there is a trade-off about what can be measured. Knowing more about the particle's location means knowing less about its speed, and vice versa. Position-momentum (location-speed) are known as a conjugate pair. A conjugate pair is any pair of observable quantities of a particle or quantum system that obeys the Heisenberg uncertainty principle. These include position-momentum and energy-time. Their minimal uncertainty product is Planck's constant, in the trade-off between being able to know more about one and less about the other.

#### 14.3.1.1 *Size-momentum correspondence and holographic SYK*

One area of quantum dynamics research examines the relationship between size and momentum. Here, size means operator size and momentum means the speed of the particle. As the Heisenberg uncertainty principle indicates, a particle is determined by both its location and its momentum (speed). Operators describe how a quantum system evolves, and grow themselves as the system evolves. Therefore, the size of the operator might be related to the behavior of the particle. A relationship can be formalized between the particle speed and the rate of change of operator size. The particle momentum seems to be encoded in the operator by which it evolves. Lin *et al.* (2019) articulate the operator size-particle momentum relationship in the finding that "the time derivative of size is the same as the bulk momentum" (Lin *et al.*, 2019, p. 40). The time derivative of operator size is equivalent to the rate of growth of particle momentum.

The operator size-particle momentum relationship is interpreted through the AdS/CFT correspondence, in the flavor of AdS/SYK. The holographic SYK model interprets operator growth as a solvable SYK model in the boundary to calculate aspects of particle momentum as the bulk dual. Through the holographic SYK model, Lin *et al.* (2019) construct symmetry generator operators for operator-state mapping and temperature analysis between the bulk and the boundary domains. The work is a nice example of the SYK model in routine deployment. The correspondence is shown as a mathematically rigorous relationship that links a complicated domain to a simpler domain such that the one can be solved from the other (Table 14.1).

Using the holographic SYK model to examine the relationship between operator size growth in the boundary and particle momentum in

Table 14.1. AdS/SYK: Operator size-particle momentum.

| Domain | Bulk | Boundary |
|---|---|---|
| AdS/CFT | Quantum gravity | Quantum field theory |
| AdS/SYK | Near-extremal black hole ($AdS_2$) | SYK model |
| Model tractability | Not easily solvable | Solvable |
| Size-momentum | Particle momentum | Operator size growth |
| Black hole dynamics | Infalling gravitational attraction | Operator chaotic size |
| Size-momentum | Scrambling time | Chaotic operator growth |
| Black hole dynamics | Jackiw–Teitelboim gravity | SYK model |

the bulk is also of interest to the complexity debate. The complexity debate concerns the bulk-boundary relation of determining the computational complexity of preparing a quantum circuit in the boundary that corresponds to a bulk gravitational dual such as wormhole growth. The question centers around how the two domains (bulk and boundary) can have different growth rates yet somehow remain pegged in correspondence with each other. An early solution was a proposal that complexity = volume (maximizing bulk volume over all related boundary surfaces explains boundary complexity) (Susskind, 2016). The proposal was subsequently amended to complexity = action (evaluating the bulk gravitational action on a selected chunk of spacetime explains boundary complexity) (Brown *et al.*, 2016). The complexity debate intersects with the quantum dynamics OTOC investigation in that both approaches seek an understanding of operator size growth in the boundary.

The idea of momentum-dependent size is based on Feynman's parton theory that more and more "wee partons" appear as a particle's momentum increases (Susskind, 2018). The main idea is the phenomenon of the size of a relativistic string growing with momentum. In the holographic model, radial momentum in the bulk or infalling gravitational attraction is related to operator size growth on the boundary. A key application is diagnosing quantum chaos with the growth of operator size, through the formulation relating ordinary gravitational attraction in the bulk to the general properties of quantum chaos on the boundary (*Ibid.*).

Brown *et al.* (2018) extend the use of the size-momentum correspondence (operator size growth in the boundary and particle momentum or volume in the bulk) to examine charged black holes. The work finds that the scrambling time for a charged black hole (Reissner–Nordstrom) is smaller than might be expected because boundary operator size grows so rapidly at early times that it is already quite large when it starts a later exponential growth phase.

Other work from Susskind and Zhao (2020) examines the connection between operator size growth, complexity increase, and bulk radial momentum. A gluon splitting model is used to study operator growth and complexity increase in the case of a vacuum (empty regime). The work starts incorporates JT/SYK as one of the simplest possible implementations of the correspondence. The bulk is Jackiw–Teitelboim (JT) gravity, a simplified theory of gravitation with one space and one time dimension (much easier to compute than classical gravity with three space dimensions and one time dimension). The boundary is the usual solvable SYK model. Through the JT/SYK interpretation, the relation between complexity and momentum can be derived different ways, including from the symmetry generator operators proposed by Lin *et al.* (2019).

### 14.3.2 *Out-of-time-order correlators*

In the practical task of measuring operator growth, the standard method is computing OTOC functions (Swingle *et al.*, 2016). OTOC functions are operators used to evolve a quantum system back or forward through time so that a comparative measurement may be taken. In particular, OTOC functions are used to measure the scrambling time (how quickly information spreads out over the entire system such that a local measurement is not possible) (Hayden & Preskill, 2007). Black holes are found to be fast scramblers, meaning extremely efficient at spreading out information across the system (Sekino & Susskind, 2008). Further, many quantum systems display a chaotic dynamics, growing explosively, not even exponentially but ballistically, at early time (Shenker & Stanford, 2014). OTOC functions can be formulated for discrete or continuous variables (Zhuang *et al.*, 2019). In general, a theme is early exponential growth and then saturation (Table 14.2).

With these established methods of quantum system dynamics, the contemporary research targets the topics of chaos, thermalization, and information scrambling. Specific analysis is devoted to operator growth definitions, system expansion rates and bounds with the exponents defining system dynamics, differential growth rates of system attributes, and system characterization at early, intermediate, and late times.

Nahum *et al.* (2018) find that universal scaling forms of the OTOC can be obtained by using mappings to canonical problems in classical statistical mechanics such as the Ising model. The work shows that entanglement growth is generally smaller than operator growth, often by a ratio of one half (operator growth growing twice as fast as entanglement growth) (Nahum *et al.*, 2018, p. 19). Operator size growth is also deployed in the following sense. Under Heisenberg time evolution, an initial

Table 14.2. Quantum dynamics research advances.

| No. | Quantum Dynamics Research Advance | Reference |
|---|---|---|
| *Established methods* | | |
| 1 | Information scrambling in quantum systems | Hayden and Preskill (2007) |
| 2 | Black holes are fast scramblers | Sekino and Susskind (2008) |
| 3 | Chaotic dynamics and ballistic early time growth | Shenker and Stanford (2014) |
| 4 | Scrambling measurement with OTOCs | Swingle *et al.* (2016) |
| *Contemporary findings* | | |
| 5 | Entanglement growth is slower than operator growth | Nahum *et al.* (2018) |
| 6 | Early time OTOC grows exponentially then saturates | von Keyserlingk *et al.* (2018) |
| 7 | Operator size evolves to scrambling time and saturates | Qi and Streicher (2019) |
| 8 | Operator growth is slower than system growth | Lin *et al.* (2019) |
| 9 | Propose a universal form for the early growth region | Xu and Swingle (2020) |

operator (localized near the spatial origin, for example) evolves into a vastly more complicated operator. Hence, a relevant "operator size" measurement is the size of the region in which the time-evolved operator fails to commute with local operators (Nahum *et al.*, 2018, p. 2).

In the same research trajectory, von Keyserlingk *et al.* (2018) use operator growth to derive exact formulas for the OTOC and entanglement growth. The finding is that at early times (before the arrival of the main wavefront), the OTOC grows exponentially (with an exponent that increases with the initial separation of the two operators involved). At longer times (in the course of system evolution), the OTOC saturates to one.

Xu and Swingle (2020) propose a universal form for the early growth region of the squared commutator in the OTOC (assuming there is well-defined butterfly velocity). The work extends other work (Xu & Swingle, 2019) aiming to reconcile various analysis scenarios, including extending formulations to a broader range of physical systems (other than the most chaotic). The idea is to study intermediate time evolution, as to how early exponential system growth (described by the Lyapunov exponent) gives way to a diffusively broadened scrambling wavefront. Whereas a sharp wavefront picture holds for the most chaotic systems, the diffusively broadened wavefront picture is more accurate for physical systems with finite degrees of freedom. The overall finding is that the local operator growth wavefront broadens diffusively for generic Hamiltonians in finite local Hilbert space.

#### 14.3.2.1 *Quantum dynamics and temperature*

Qi and Streicher (2019) deploy a holographic SYK model that incorporates temperature to show how operator size evolves up to the scrambling time and then saturates. Notably, short-distance (UV) operators have the greatest effect, as opposed to bulk action, as previously thought. Temperature, though a crucial variable, has been difficult to include in quantum dynamics models. The traditional method is calculating the dynamics of the operator under Heisenberg system evolution, but this does not include temperature, so an improved model is needed. The work examines how operator size growth is related to OTOCs, chaos, and thermalization in a finite-temperature model. The result is the calculation of the full operator growth structure for the SYK model at all temperatures in fermionic systems.

#### 14.3.2.2 *The Heisenberg equation of motion*

The Heisenberg evolution model does not contain temperature. Therefore, any effect of temperature must be abstracted into the matrix elements of the operator. This has largely meant that investigating temperature in the context of operator size has not been probed. One target of interest is determining the natural finite-temperature generalization of operator size. By including temperature, Qi and Streicher (2019) are able to characterize not only the average size of an operator but its entire size distribution. The effective size distribution of an operator at finite-temperature is defined by the proportional relationship it has to the thermal density operator.

The Heisenberg equation of motion is applied to obtain the operator Hamiltonian. The operator's relationship to other operators can also be inferred from the Heisenberg equation. Operators grow as they evolve in time and become intertwined with other operators. As an operator evolves, it becomes supported along other operators of increasing size. In some sense, operator growth is a measure of how intertwined (entangled) it is with other operators (how much one operator cross supports another). Hence, operator size growth is calculated by taking the operator inner product (the Frobenius inner product in a finite-dimensional Hilbert space). Since the Heisenberg equation of motion does not include temperature, the process of system evolution needs to be supplemented to obtain a finer-grained measure of operator size distribution.

### 14.3.3 *Thermofield double state*

The aim is to understand the role of temperature in operator growth, as a next step in the quantum physics research agenda and since thermalization is an important property in real-life systems. Temperature can be introduced by considering an operator with a thermal state. A basic and computable thermal state for studying thermodynamic properties is the thermofield double, an entangled state between two copies of a state such that the reduced density matrix (purification) of each copy is thermal. The thermofield double state has a purification of thermal properties and a Hamiltonian that satisfies certain conditions. The operator and its average size can be measured directly by a finite-temperature four-point function.

To find the size distribution of a time-evolved thermal operator in general, a generating function is defined to describe the operator's different size moments. The generating function factorizes into a product of the generating function for the Gibbs state and a so-called connected piece. The connected piece is used to extract the size distribution of the thermal operator from the size distribution of the whole operator, and the operator's thermal size is thereby defined.

To calculate the full operator size distribution, other generating functions are constructed that include a weighting factor. First, the size distribution of the thermal operator is studied by setting up a generating function similar to a partition function. The generating function is defined for a certain size distribution based on a two-point function (with a twisted boundary condition) which determines the growth distribution. The two-point function with the twisted boundary condition is used to solve the ladder kernel, which allows the computation of four-point functions in the SYK model. The ladder kernel is part of an SYK model solution that involves constructing ladder diagrams that can be summed by defining a kernel in a structure that corresponds to adding rungs to a ladder (Maldacena & Stanford, 2016, p. 5). Second, the fractional distance to scrambling for the operator is investigated. On average, the size increase induced by a single fermion is given by the fractional scrambling distance.

#### 14.3.3.1 *Implications for the holographic SYK model*

The overall result is demonstrating how operator size evolves up to the scrambling time. In the model system, scrambling occurs when the average growth of the wavefunction reaches $N/2$ (the number of fermions in the system divided by two), a value which can be further fed into the full operator structure (Qi & Streicher, 2019, p. 20). Notably, the local interactions have the strongest effect. The short-range (UV) operators offer a better microscopic picture of operator growth and distribution in the SYK model. The short-range operators evaluate the fractional distance of the operator to scrambling, and the results suggest interpreting the scrambling distance in the context of finite-temperature thermalization.

The results also obtain a more generic bulk-boundary relation for the holographic SYK model. The analysis indicates that the full-size wavefunction of the SYK fermion (boundary) relates to the full momentum wavefunction of the infalling particle (bulk). The average growth at low temperatures is similar to that shown by Brown *et al.* (2018) to exactly match the classical momentum dynamics of a boundary particle falling into a near-extremal black hole. The average growth of an SYK fermion exactly matches the average momentum of an infalling particle in an $AdS_2$ black hole. The universal form of the operator growth distribution precisely gives the squared coefficients of the $AdS_2$ momentum bulk-to-boundary propagator. Future work could perform the same kind of analysis for different geometries. For example, it was found that adding the scrambling distance operator to the doubled SYK Hamiltonian causes the low-energy limit to eventually cross a Hawking-Page transition, forming a global $AdS_2$ geometry instead of the more limited geometry of an $AdS_2$ black hole in an eternal traversable wormhole (Maldacena & Qi, 2018).

## 14.4 Superconductivity and Spacetime Superfluids

### 14.4.1 *Time crystals*

Quantum dynamics and operator growth are further defined in the notion of time crystals. Central to quantum dynamics is understanding system criticality. Symmetry breaking is typically the key moment bringing about a phase transition in any physical system. Predicting phase transition is not just useful for managing quantum systems, but a feature that can be exploited, for example, in superconducting materials for QPU chips (quantum processing unit). An increasing range of physical behavior is being understood on the basis of symmetry breaking and phase transition including the Higgs boson (by which particles acquire mass), high-temperature superconductors, quantum liquids, and spatial crystals (Richerme, 2017). Although symmetry breaking is well understood in many domains, time-translation symmetry has been articulated more recently. So-called "time crystals" are systems which spontaneously break time-translation symmetry, by analogy to ordinary crystals, which break spatial translational symmetries (Wilczek, 2012).

Time crystals (whose regular pattern or lowest-energy configurations are periodic in time rather than space) exist in periodically driven systems that do not reach thermal equilibrium. They have been demonstrated experimentally in two systems, by the Monroe laboratory with trapped ions (Zhang *et al.*, 2016) and by the Lukin laboratory with nitrogen-vacancy centers (spin impurities) in diamond (Choi *et al.*, 2016). The usual inclination to describe symmetry breaking would be determining the expectation values of observables at thermal equilibrium. However, this is not possible in a system that does not exist at thermal equilibrium. Instead, it is necessary to look beyond thermal equilibrium to define a formulation for time crystal dynamics. Such periodically driven systems are characterized by the lifetime of a symmetry breaking state diverging as the system size grows such that (in the thermodynamic limit), the system never reaches thermal equilibrium. Else *et al.* (2016) propose a formulation incorporating these aspects in the notion of Floquet time crystals (using Floquet periodic linear differential equations). The model of time-translation symmetry breaking also invokes the point that oscillation under time evolution requires the superposition of states whose phases wind at different rates. For example, whereas in the Ising ferromagnet, two states are degenerate in the thermodynamic limit, in a time crystal, they would need to have different eigenvalues and different rates of operator winding (proceeding).

#### 14.4.1.1 *Spacetime superfluids and temperature*

Time crystals have a holographic correspondence-related interpretation. Lin *et al.* (2019) propose the notions of "time superfluid" and "spacetime superfluid" by analogy to superconductors. A basic definition of superconductors is that they break symmetry (by undergoing a phase transition at a critical temperature), and wormholes or thermofield double states also break symmetry. The setup of the two-sided wormhole experiment is a boundary with thermofield double states as ends of a wormhole that is connected through the bulk. The thermofield double states are two identical copies of a state that are initially entangled and then evolve on their own into nonidentical states. The wormhole or thermofield double state breaks time-translation symmetry in that the two sides of the system (effectively the right and left side of a partition) evolve separately (after having classical time dependence at the outset). Notably, any quantum state with an initial classical and then quantum time dependence may be a "time superfluid" in the sense that the time-translation symmetry is broken as the quantum system evolves over time.

The problem of interest is characterizing the distance between the two boundary regions connected by the wormhole. Both superconductors and two-sided wormholes break symmetry, have quantum and classical aspects, and have properties that are not defined for single particles but only emerge as collective macrostates when there are many particles.

In a specific example, the phase of a superconductor is a good classical variable in the large-$N$ limit, but is not well-defined for a small number of fermions. Lin *et al.* (2019) develop a model for calculating the distance between the two wormhole boundaries with a similar variable: The relative time shift between the two sides of the thermofield double (since the two sides have independent time evolution, inevitably, one side will be growing faster than the other). A similar approach can be used to measure superconductors as wormholes. As the superconductor is measured with fermion two-point functions, the two-sided wormhole's time shift variable is measured similarly with correlation functions. The wormhole case is even more distinct because time translation is also related to other symmetries. In particular, temperatures are also related between the two sides of an evolving system. Temperatures are connected by acting with an overall dilation to the system which makes the wormhole longer. Also, increasing the value of the time shift is essentially like adding a mass term. In the wormhole, both the time and space directions are related, so the state could be called a "spacetime superfluid" (Lin *et al.*, 2019, p. 45).

### 14.4.1.2 *UV–IR correlations: Order-disorder phase transition*

The repeating pattern of the crystal can be seen in time or space as the spatial crystal or the time crystal. Likewise, the UV–IR relationship of short-range and long-range correlations in quantum systems can be seen in time or space. In particular, when correlations are seen in time, they can be formatted in the scale of temperature, to indicate the critical temperature of the superconducting phase transition (Table 14.3). Further, UV–IR correlations can also be seen in the frame of the trade-off between ordered and disordered systems in the context of system phase transition,

Table 14.3. Time-energy conjugate pair formulations.

| No. | Time Term | Energy Term | Formulation |
|---|---|---|---|
| 1 | Time | Energy | Time = 1/energy |
| 2 | Time | Frequency | Time = 1/frequency |
| 3 | Time | Temperature | Energy ($k_B$) = Temperature ($k_B$); Time = 1/temperature |

as operator phase-winding occurs at different rates in the quantum system toward the critical temperature, causing a condensate to become superconducting (in the form of charged scalar hair on a toy model black hole) (Hartnoll *et al.*, 2020, p. 10).

## References

Brown, A.R., Gharibyan, H., Streicher, A. *et al.* (2018). Falling toward charged black holes. *Phys. Rev. D.* 98(12):126016.

Brown, A.R., Roberts, D.A., Susskind, L. *et al.* (2016). Holographic complexity equals bulk action? *Phys. Rev. Lett.* 116(19):191301.

Choi, S., Choi, J., Landig, R. *et al.* (2016). Observation of discrete time-crystalline order in a disordered dipolar many-body system. *Nature.* 543(7644):221–5.

Cotler, J.S., Gur-Ari, G., Hanada, M. *et al.* (2017). Black holes and random matrices. *J. High Energ. Phys.* 1705:118.

Else, D.V., Bauer, B. & Nayak, C. (2016). Floquet time crystals. *Phys. Rev. Lett.* 117(9):090402.

Hartnoll, S.A., Horowitz, G.T., Kruthoff, J. & Santos, J.E. (2020). Diving into a holographic superconductor. arXiv:2008.12786v2.

Hayden, P. & Preskill, J. (2007). Black holes as mirrors: Quantum information in random subsystems. *J. High Energ. Phys.* 0709:120.

Lin, H.W., Maldacena, J. & Zhao, Y. (2019). Symmetries near the Horizon. *J. High Energ. Phys.* 1908:049.

Maldacena, J. & Qi, X.-L. (2018). Eternal traversable wormhole. arXiv:1804.00491.

Maldacena, J. & Stanford, D. (2016). Comments on the Sachdev-Ye-Kitaev model. *Phys. Rev. D.* 94(10):106002.

Nahum, A., Vijay, S. & Haah, J. (2018). Operator spreading in random unitary circuits. *Phys. Rev. X.* 8(2):021014.

Qi, X.-L. & Streicher, A. (2019). Quantum epidemiology: Operator growth, thermal effects, and SYK. *J. High Energ. Phys.* 1908:012.

Ramon y Cajal, S. (1995, 1894). *Texture of the Nervous System of Man and the Vertebrates.* Volume I. Trans. Swanson, N. & Swanson, L.W. Oxford: Oxford University Press.

Richerme, P. (2017). How to create a time crystal. *Physics* (American Physical Society). 10(5):1–2.

Roberts, D.A., Stanford, D. & Streicher, A. (2018). Operator growth in the SYK model. *J. High Energ. Phys.* 1806(122).

Sachdev, S. (2010). Strange metals and the AdS/CFT correspondence. *J. Stat. Mech.* 1011:P11022.

Sekino, Y. & Susskind, L. (2008). Fast scramblers. *J. High Energ. Phys.* 0810:065.

Shenker, S.H. & Stanford, D. (2014). Black holes and the butterfly effect. *J. High Energ. Phys.* 1403:067.

Susskind, L. (2016). Computational complexity and black hole horizons. *Fortschr Physik.* 64(1):24–43.

Susskind, L. (2018). Why do things fall? arXiv:1802.01198.

Susskind, L. & Zhao, Y. (2020). Complexity and momentum. arXiv:2006.03019v1.

Swingle, B., Bentsen, G., Schleier-Smith, M. & Hayden, P. (2016). Measuring the scrambling of quantum information. *Phys. Rev. A.* 94(4):040302.

von Keyserlingk, C.W., Rakovszky, T., Pollmann, F. & Sondhi, S.L. (2018). Operator hydrodynamics, OTOCs, and entanglement growth in systems without conservation laws. *Phys. Rev. X.* 8(2):021013.

Wilczek, F. (2012). Quantum time crystals. *Phys. Rev. Lett.* 109(16):160401.

Xu, S. & Swingle, B. (2019). Locality, quantum fluctuations, and scrambling. *Phys. Rev. X.* 9(3):031048.

Xu, S. & Swingle, B. (2020). Accessing scrambling using matrix product operators. *Nat. Phys.* 16:199–204.

Zhang, J., Hess, P.W., Kyprianidis, A. *et al.* (2016). Observation of a discrete time crystal. *Nature.* 543:217–20.

Zhuang, Q., Schuster, T., Yoshida, B. & Yao, N.Y. (2019). Scrambling and complexity in phase space. *Phys. Rev. A.* 99(6):062334.

# Chapter 15

# Neural Dynamics

*The multiscale properties of spatiotemporal neural activity lead to mathematical challenges in both modeling strategies and analysis*

— Coombes (2005, p. 91)

**Abstract**

This chapter discusses multiscalar neural dynamics models. Large-scale models of brain behavior, including neural ensemble, neural mass, and neural field theories, populated with empirical data, have a strong need for more capacious computational platforms such as those offered by quantum computing. Probability distributions of large-scale neural signaling activity cannot be calculated with traditional reaction-diffusion methods applied with linear and nonlinear Fokker–Planck equations. In neural state dynamics, seizures indicate a straightforward chaotic dynamics, but resting states suggest a more complex mix of multistability and Hopf bifurcation, and active states in behaving brains are also likely to have complex dynamical behavior.

## 15.1 Multiscale Modeling

As the "Levels of Organization in the Brain" table in Chapter 1 indicates, the brain is a highly complex entity with behavior taking place on nine scale tiers across 12 orders of magnitude, from the smallest molecular transmission to an organism moving in the world. Each scale tier has its own spatial and temporal dynamics, thus suggesting multiscalar modeling approaches for the brain. Further, the differing dynamics at the various scale tiers need to be integrated into a common model.

Formulations of neural dynamics are typically considered at four different scales (Table 15.1). These are at the level of the single neuron, small ensembles of similar types of neurons, group populations of neurons, and whole-brain analysis. Different models of dynamics are proposed for each scale tier, but for anything larger than a single neuron, oscillatory behavior is often a central feature, as well as the concept of a network that connects individual nodes to overall behavior. At the single-neuron scale, the dynamics are determined by the models of basic biological neurons, such as Hodgkin–Huxley, integrate-and-fire, and theta neurons. At the ensemble level, there are dynamics models such as FitzHugh–Nagumo, Hindmarsh–Rose, and Morris–Lecor (Bassett *et al.*, 2018, p. 568). At the larger-scale of the population group, Wilson–Cowan mean-field equations, Jansen–Rit neural mass models, and tractography are used (Woolrich & Stephan, 2013). At the scale of the whole-brain, neural field models supply dynamics including bifurcation, multistability, and phase transition.

### 15.1.1 *Centrality of wavefunction modeling*

In neural dynamics, the first concern is wavefunction modeling. The brain is known for its "brain waves" both literally and figuratively. Some portion of neural activity is comprised of waves in the form of the EEG-detectable potentials given off by the scalp, and the action potentials that

Table 15.1. Neural dynamics formulations by scale.

| No. | Scale Focus | Dynamics Formulations |
|---|---|---|
| 1 | Single neuron | Hodgkin–Huxley, integrate-and-fire, theta neurons |
| 2 | Local ensemble | FitzHugh–Nagumo, Hindmarsh–Rose, Morris–Lecor |
| 3 | Population group (neural mass) | Neural mass models (Jansen–Rit), mean-field (Wilson–Cowan), tractography, oscillation, network models |
| 4 | Whole-brain (neural field) | Neural field models, Kuramoto oscillators, bifurcation, directed percolation phase transition, graph-based oscillation |

trigger neuronal firing. These are electrical waves, and chemical waves (calcium waves) too are involved in neural signaling.

EEG-detectable electrical waves have been studied for over a hundred years. These brain waves are not modeled with the standard quantum mechanical yet intractable Schrödinger wave equation, but with solvable effective nonlinear wave models (Nunez, 1974). Relating wave behavior between the local and global scale, by linking individually firing synapses to macroscale behavior such as movement and cognition, is an ongoing challenge in neuroscience. Although the electrical firing of neurons has been the predominant research focus, including because data are more readily available for this kind of activity, it is now appreciated that the fuller picture of brain behavior is more complex. Comprehensive neural signaling models would also need to incorporate the synaptic transfer of neurotransmitters (including via astrocyte calcium channel signaling), and the dendritic integration of incoming signals in the receiving neuron.

The centrality of wavefunction behavior in the brain's electrical and chemical signaling processes suggests quantum mechanical approaches. Wavefunction modeling is an important research area, with increasing sophistication in the treatment of wave-like behavior in both physics and neuroscience. The four main wavefunctions by which the brain propagates neural signals are action potentials, neurotransmitter activity, astrocyte calcium signaling, and dendritic spikes.

#### 15.1.1.1 *Practical perspective: Scale and model integration*

Wavefunction and multiscalar modeling are needed to investigate the brain at a wide range of levels since brain activity extends over many temporal and spatial scales. The scale tiers with the most data are single neurons, connectome tissue slices of partial brain volumes, and local field potentials. Data are collected from imaging modalities such as electroencephalography (EEG), magnetoencephalography (MEG), and functional magnetic resonance imaging (fMRI) which are able to detect signals resulting from the aggregate activity of large numbers of neurons. In imaging, a key challenge is integrating electric potentials at different scales, such as EEG (large-scale) and local field potentials (medium-scale), and then further relating these to functional imaging techniques such as fMRI. Another challenge is not only integrating scales but also models, for example, how biophysical models are represented in computational models and further connected to neuropathology disease and treatment models.

Computational neuroscience is partly driven by the demand for next-generation multiscalar models to support experimental findings. Theoretical and empirical models evolve in lockstep. Several factors in particular are influencing the need for models that more rigorously consider multiple temporal and spatial scales. First, data are often simultaneously acquired from EEG and fMRI, which requires the integration of structural and functional information. The problem arises acutely in connectome projects, in the attempt to identify function from structure. Second, data are available for multiple modes of brain activity including rest, sleep, cognition, and seizure. There is a need to examine not only pathology, but also the healthy brain as a baseline norm. Third, there is a need for greater sophistication in the modeling of synaptic interactions with neurotransmitters, to understand among other aspects, their pharmacological impact.

#### 15.1.1.2 *Nonlinear dynamical systems approach*

Although the causes of single neuron spikes are well understood, the processes that determine collective neural behavior in cortical circuits across the large-scale systems of the brain are not. A systems biology approach using nonlinear dynamical systems theory is required. Models of nonlinear dynamics are likely to be implicated in explaining adaptive cortical activity and the aberrant processes that underlie a number of brain disorders. Dynamic models of large-scale brain activity are needed in the experimental context of brain imaging linked to pathology resolution. Macroscopic imaging data (from fMRI, EEG, and MEG) reflect the collective activity of thousands of neurons. However, what is lacking is a broadly accepted mathematical theory (or theories) for the collective activity of neuronal populations. Without such organizing principles, the analysis of cognitive and functional neuroimaging data largely proceeds without formal biophysical models of the underlying large-scale neuronal activity (Breakspear, 2017, p. 340).

## 15.2 Approaches to Collective Neural Behavior

In the theoretical and experimental literature, the main approaches to the modeling of large-scale collective neural behavior are neural ensemble, neural mass, and neural field models (Table 15.2). Neural ensemble models consider groups of individual neurons whose states are assumed to be uncorrelated. Neural mass models consider a local population of neurons interacting together as a group. Neural field models consider large-scale neural models that treat the entire cortex as a continuous sheet of signaling activity.

### 15.2.1 *Nonlinear dynamical systems*

A variety of methods are used in the study of nonlinear dynamical systems. An ongoing challenge is the problem of modeling three-body systems. Newton and Leibniz invented the calculus in the 1600s in response to the need for a dynamical systems theory to study celestial mechanics. Surprisingly, although the differential equations for the motion of two planetary bodies can be solved analytically, the motion of three bodies is exceedingly complex, and the resulting dynamical system is chaotic for most initial conditions and generally intractable. Hence, a "many-body problem" refers to a system with three or more entities. The complexity only grows in greater than three-body systems, especially in those involving millions of quantum mechanical particles or the brain with 86 million neurons and each neuron having on average 2,800 (Martins *et al.*, 2019) or in an earlier estimate, as many as 10,000 synaptic connections (Koch, 1999).

Table 15.2. Approaches to collective neural behavior.

| No. | Approach | Description |
|---|---|---|
| 1 | Neural ensemble models | Groups of individual neurons whose states are not correlated |
| 2 | Neural mass models | Local populations of neurons interacting together as a group |
| 3 | Neural field models | The entire cortex as a continuous sheet of signaling activity |

#### 15.2.1.1 *Stochastic calculus and diffusion*

Stochastic calculus, the calculus of random processes, is central to modeling many-body problems. Integrals of stochastic processes are defined to model systems that behave randomly. A key process of concern is Brownian motion (the quantum mechanical "jiggling" of particles in constant motion) and its relation to diffusion. The problem is describing how particles in motion react to system changes. Diffusion is the physical process of spreading out from higher to lower concentration, temperature, or pressure. Such diffusive processes apply to a wide range of areas in physical science and social science (the same mathematics may describe the diffusion of water and the diffusion of stock prices). Diffusion can be random or constant. An important influencing factor is the gradient, which is the change in one variable per the change in another (for example, the change in temperature with respect to a change in distance). The notion of a random walk (although not truly random in a multi-particle system due to collisions with other particles) is important in describing diffusion. Random walk theory suggests that a particle is governed by the overall kinetic energy in the system as a global variable that is influenced by changes in the diffusion variables (e.g. concentration, pressure, temperature). Stochastic calculus is widely used to model Brownian motion and diffusion, and the concept of diffusion is often applied to any complex system that involves large ensembles of individual elements.

### 15.2.2 *Neural dynamics in large-scale models*

Since stochastic calculus is used to model complex systems with large numbers of particle-many elements and random behavior that is not fully understood, these methods are often applied to large-scale brain dynamics modeling. The aim is to establish a neural dynamics model that reproduces the overall system behavior (the collective large-scale behavior of the brain). The approaches to large-scale neural modeling have different dynamics formulations, influenced by their statistical distributions (Table 15.3). In the three model types, the statistical distributions of collective neural spiking are different. Empirical evidence supporting neural ensemble methods suggests that they are either normally distributed or are non-normally distributed but still have a recognized distribution (such as

Table 15.3. Collective neural behavior: Statistical distributions.

| No. | Approach | Description | Statistical Distribution |
|---|---|---|---|
| 1 | Neural ensemble models | Groups of individual neurons with uncorrelated states | Normal (Gaussian), non-Gaussian but known (e.g. power law) |
| 2 | Neural mass models | Local population groups of interacting neurons | Unrecognized |
| 3 | Neural field models | The cortex as a continuous sheet | Unrecognized |

bimodal or power law). The larger-scale models, neural mass and neural field, do not indicate a recognized statistical distribution to explain collective neural firing behavior. Research questions thus target the problem that collective neural behavior generates unrecognized statistical distributions.

## 15.3 Neural Ensemble Models

The neural ensemble approach considers groups of individual neurons (a patch of cortex) whose states are assumed to be uncorrelated. Single-neuron spikes are highly nonlinear. However, it is not clear how to incorporate such nonlinear microscale behavior of neurons into graduated tiers of macroscopic activity, and how different dynamics models might translate across system scales. In neural ensemble modeling, differential equations are used to model pools of spiking neurons according to two key elements. There is a coupling term that represents synaptic interactions between neurons and promotes synchronization within the ensemble, and there is a stochastic term that disrupts this effect. The resulting ensemble dynamics reflect this mix of interneural coupling and nonlinear neural dynamics, and also include noise. Notably, this structure of linear synchronization followed by nonlinear activation is the same that is used in the general model of machine learning.

In neural ensemble modeling, the assumption is made that the states of the neurons in the ensemble are not correlated. The impetus for this is the central limit theorem, in which the sum of uncorrelated random processes converges to a Gaussian probability distribution, even if the individual processes are highly non-Gaussian. The result is the so-called "diffusion approximation" as a *de facto* standard arising in neural ensemble modeling based on the assumption that whatever the underlying individual nonlinearities, they can be averaged into system-level measures that are normally distributed and obey Gaussian statistics.

Applying the notion of "diffusion approximation", the activity of the neural ensemble, consisting of nonlinear but uncorrelated spikes, can be reduced to a standard normal probability distribution described by simple linear statistics. The implication is that the activity of such an ensemble of neurons can be described by the mean and the variance of the firing rate. The mean firing rate reflects the response of the population to its total synaptic inputs and the variance reflects the dispersion of stochastic effects. The point is that the activity of an ensemble of neurons can be described by the mean and variance of the firing rate.

### 15.3.1 *Fokker–Planck dynamics for normal distributions*

The activity of the neural ensemble is captured by the mean and variance of the firing rate, and the dynamics are articulated by the Fokker–Planck equation. The Fokker–Planck equation is typically used to describe the dynamics of a linear, normally distributed ensemble because it estimates system change per evolution in time. In statistical physics, the Fokker–Planck equation is a partial differential equation that describes the time evolution of the probability density function of particle velocity under the influence of drag forces, as in Brownian motion. The same equation can be generalized to other systems and different observables.

For a neural ensemble, a Fokker–Planck equation can be derived from a basic integrate-and-fire single-neuron model, together with the diffusion approximation (El Boustani & Destexhe, 2009). The Fokker–Planck equation captures the collective response of a neural population to a stimulus. Each neuron consolidates its own inputs and effectively submits an independent vote to the collective. The mean firing rate is a passive summation of the individual neuron responses and encodes the average (most likely) population-based representation of received inputs. The Fokker–Planck equation also describes the dynamics of the population variance. As the inputs to the ensemble change, the Fokker–Planck equation captures the drift (of the mean) and the diffusion (change in the variance) of the ensemble activity.

The Fokker–Planck equation is an analytically achievable model suggesting how local neuron populations may represent their inputs collectively. Using the Fokker–Planck equation reduces the thousands of degrees of freedom of a large-scale model of spiking neurons to a picture of neural dynamics that is driven by just two variables (the mean activity and the dispersion around the mean). Such dimensionality reduction is crucial to efforts to move beyond brute-force accounts of the brain (Huys *et al.*, 2016). The Gaussian distribution maximizes the ratio of the entropy (information diversity) to the variance of the distribution.

#### 15.3.1.1 *Heavy tail distributions*

To the extent that the statistics of a local ensemble are Gaussian, the standard (linear) Fokker–Planck equation may provide an accurate description of neural dynamics. However, converging evidence from a variety of neuronal recording modalities suggests that the statistics of neural population activity are often heavy-tailed and non-Gaussian (Breakspear, 2017, p. 344).

A heavy-tailed distribution has tails that are heavier than an exponential distribution (Bryson, 1974). The tails are heavier, with the greater bulk indicating that the probability of extreme events is higher than normal. Sometimes "heavy tail" and "fat tail" are used to mean the same thing, for example, in finance with the black swan effect that high-magnitude events occur more frequently than expected (Taleb, 2007). However, "fat tail" refers to a specific subclass of heavy-tailed distributions that exhibit power law decay behavior as well as infinite variance. Every fat-tailed distribution is heavy-tailed, but not every heavy-tailed distribution is fat-tailed.

In neural signaling, heavy-tailed distributions are typically those in which the right tail is larger or heavier than that of an exponential distribution, closely following a Fisher–Tippett (double-exponential) distribution. This means that large-amplitude events occur by chance more often than expected for an exponential distribution because they are drawn from a heavier right-hand tail (Roberts *et al.*, 2015). In the neural context, the heavy tails mean the occurrence of synchronized bursts of activity that violate the diffusion approximation. The synchronized activity consists of erratic bursts of correlated states from the microscale to the macroscale that cause non-Gaussian fluctuations.

The heavy tails arise from fluctuations that are larger and more frequent than those permitted under the diffusion approximation and correspond to the formation of correlations among distant neurons. Correlations among neurons appear to arise from synchronization either in their firing or in the modulations of their firing rates. It seems that long-range correlations occur when the underlying tendency for coupled dynamical systems to synchronize overwhelms the disruptive effects of the noise within the ensemble. The implication is that neurons do not simply filter their inputs and passively contribute to the ensemble mean, but synchronize themselves according to dynamic feedback from the mean in an active real-time feedback loop which acts to increase firing coherence. This is evidence of active behavior in synaptic integration.

The traditional (linear) Fokker–Planck equation depends on the diffusion approximation, namely, that the activity of neurons or groups of neurons is not correlated when measured at different points in the system of interest. However, real-life neuronal behavior is correlated. The Fokker–Planck equation is limited in that while it can accommodate local spike correlations among neurons within small circuits, on a larger-scale, it requires that correlations between more distant neurons are weak, and disappear at the scale level of the entire system. The Fokker–Planck model therefore does not support long-range correlations. The correlation length in the model is considerably shorter than the spatial scale of the system. The reality exceeds the model.

### 15.3.2 *Beyond linear Fokker–Planck equations*

Breakspear (2017) is in some sense the Taleb of neural dynamics modeling in drawing attention to the fact that large-scale statistical activity in the brain is not normally distributed and that heavy tails are more prevalent than might be thought, just as the black swan effect indicates that high-magnitude events happen more frequently in real-life than might be thought (Taleb, 2007). Since the traditional neural ensemble method based on the diffusion approximation does not explain large-scale neural signaling behavior, alternative models are needed to describe the short-distance (UV) and long-distance (IR) correlations that are observed in neural imaging data. Two directions are taken, adjusted Fokker–Planck equations if the statistical distributions are nonlinear but still recognized (e.g. bimodal or power law), or various oscillation-based and other models when the statistical distributions are unrecognized.

#### 15.3.2.1 *Recognized nonlinear probability distributions*

In the case that collective neural firing statistics conform to other known probability distributions, they can be modeled with nonlinear or fractional variations of the Fokker–Planck equation. Of these, nonlinear Fokker–Planck equations accommodate higher order interactions between the mean and noise terms. The result is that a system (such as a financial market) that becomes more volatile during high throughput (such as high-volume trading) can be modeled with a nonlinear Fokker–Planck equation. Another variation, fractional Fokker–Planck equations, is based on a generalization of the calculus to model stochastic systems with persistent long-range correlations, as widely observed in neuroscience.

Longer-range correlations typically have slower timescales than shorter-range behavior. In an example of fractional calculus neuroscience research, Lundstrom *et al.* (2008) investigate how stimuli with complex temporal dynamics influence the dynamics of system adaptation and the resulting firing rate. The finding is that rodent neocortical pyramidal neurons adapt with a time scale that depends on the time scale of changes in the stimulus statistics. The time scale adaptation is consistent with fractional order differentiation, such that the neuron's firing rate is a fractional derivative of stimulus parameters that vary more slowly.

The two non-standard Fokker–Planck equations (nonlinear and fractional) are part of the broader domain of random field theory methods which can be adapted to non-Gaussian yet well-behaved scenarios. Random field theory is an emerging area of mathematics which defines results for smooth statistical maps. An assumption is made that values in a random field nevertheless have some degree of spatial correlation (Adler & Taylor, 2007). AdS/Mathematics approaches might apply.

#### 15.3.2.2 *Unknown probability distributions*

In the case that collective neural firing statistics do not obey recognized probability distributions, there are two proposals for their modeling: neural mass and neural field models. Neural mass models consider a local population of interacting neurons together as a group. Neural field models treat the cortex as a continuous sheet. Analyzing unrecognized probability distributions in dynamical systems is a research frontier, and while an active area in theoretical physics, is not as well explored in neuroscience.

The brain modeling exercise undergoes a conceptual shift in transitioning from small ensembles of neurons to the large-scale behavior of population groups (neural mass models) and whole-brain analysis (neural field theories). Probability distributions are no longer the main framework for analysis but rather networks of connected nodes. There may not be a significant distinction in methods between the two scale tiers, as both neural mass and neural field models draw from the same basic principles and neural mass models are themselves the building blocks of neural field models (Coombes & Byrne, 2019). The three approaches to collective neural behavior modeling (neural ensembles, neural mass, and neural field theories) appear in Table 15.4 along with their statistical distribution status and neural dynamics models.

Table 15.4. Collective neural behavior: Neural dynamics.

| No. | Level | Description | Statistical Distribution | Neural Dynamics |
|---|---|---|---|---|
| 1 | Neural ensemble models | Small groups of neurons, uncorrelated states | Normal (Gaussian) | Linear Fokker–Planck equation (FPE) |
| 2 | Neural ensemble models | Small groups of neurons, correlated states | Non-Gaussian but known (e.g. power law) | Nonlinear FPE, Fractional FPE |
| 3 | Neural mass models | Large-scale populations of interacting neurons | Unrecognized | Wilson–Cowan, Jansen–Rit, Floquet model, Glass networks, ODE |
| 4 | Neural field models | Entire cortex as a continuous sheet | Unrecognized | Wavefunction, PDE, Oscillation analysis |

### 15.3.3 *Neural signaling: Orbits and bifurcation*

The large-scale brain modeling of collective neural firing is generally based on a model of the interaction between some parts of the system that are stable and others that are unstable, and how they influence each other. The two central aspects may be orbits and activations. Activation or firing is modeled through bifurcation. A bifurcation is an instability, an attractor (organizing parameter) that changes dramatically, such as transitioning from a resting state to a firing state. A resting-to-firing bifurcation is triggered by the coordination of information signals. Signaling information occurring around system critical points is modeled as orbits (just as those of a particle or astronomical bodies) which in general may be regular and periodic, but have corrections and influencing effects. Dynamical instability is implicated in the formation of disease and assessed in biomedical modeling (Swan, 1984).

System critical points are related to stability. The basic model is the Turing instability, a violation of the Turing pattern. The Turing pattern is a reaction-diffusion model showing that two diffusible substances are likely to interact with each other to form a spatially periodic pattern irrespective of diverse initial circumstances (Turing, 1952). However, the Turing model is known to be insufficient at fully explaining nonlinear behavior in complex systems (Ermentrout & Cowan, 1979). Beyond-Turing instability models are needed to account for the more complex nonlinearity observed in neural signaling behavior (Coombes, 2005). For signaling activation, many models assess the Hopf bifurcation (Gardiner, 2009), a system critical point at which a periodic orbit appears or disappears due to a local change in stability (Byrne *et al.*, 2019). A more advanced model is the Bogdanov–Takens bifurcation, which is codimensional, as opposed to Hopf bifurcations and saddle-node bifurcations which have a codimensionality of one (Cowan *et al.*, 2016). The codimension is the difference between the dimension of an object and the dimension of a smaller object contained within it.

#### 15.3.3.1 *Empirical data and oscillatory neural dynamics*

These models could persist in the further attempt to study new kinds of whole-brain data as they become available. Empirical data (EEG) and computational modeling (null hypothesis testing) support the oscillatory models of neural dynamics used in neural mass models and neural field theories. Such research models of observational data (applying the Hopf bifurcation) indicate multistability in healthy brain resting states, and bifurcation to a chaotic attractor in brains undergoing seizure (Breakspear, 2017, p. 346). Multistability occurs in dynamical systems when system noise causes the states to jump erratically between two or more co-occurring phase-space attractors, each with their own basin of attraction, essentially as a noise-driven switch between multiple weakly stable states. In healthy brain resting states, an analysis finds the multistability of cortical activity to switch between a high-amplitude, nonlinear 10 Hz oscillation (alpha rhythm) and low-amplitude filtered noise (Freyer *et al.*, 2012). This is not unusual as other multistable neural patterns exist such as binocular rivalry and certain sensorimotor system behaviors. In the case of seizure, onset is found to correspond to the appearance of sustained high-amplitude nonlinear oscillations, suggesting a bifurcation from the resting state to a limit cycle or chaotic attractor (Altenburg *et al.*, 2003).

## 15.4 Neural Mass Models

### 15.4.1 *Brain networks approach*

Neural mass models consider the mass action of a local population of neurons interacting together as a group. The method attempts to reduce dimensionality while incorporating short-distance (UV) and long-distance (IR) correlations within a network structure. The idea is that "Each center is a pool of neurons acting in parallel with each other, and the action of each center is considered to be the sum of the actions of its neurons" (Freeman, 1975, p. 4). Neural mass models are widely used in large-scale brain modeling. At the individual node level, they are written in terms of a set of ordinary differential equations with a nonlinearity (spiking activation) that is typically a sigmoidal shape. Using structural data from brain atlases, neural mass models are connected in a network structure to investigate the emergence of functional dynamic states such as synchronous firing. Neural mass models are used in connectome projects and are empirically informed by tractography (a three-dimensional modeling technique used to visually represent nerve tract data collected by diffusion MRI). A network framework is used to explicitly analyze transitions between the individual node level and the network level.

The coupling of neural mass models into a larger brain network structure is accomplished through the growing knowledge of anatomical connectivity. Connectome data is helping to elucidate short-distance and long-distance correlations in the brain. One finding is that although long-distance correlations play a role, the main form of collective neural activity is dense short-range connections that quickly (exponentially) diminish with distance (Horvat *et al.*, 2016). As compared with other species (rodent and primate), the human brain has weaker long-distance connections, which could explain why humans are subject to disconnection-related pathologies such as Alzheimer's disease. Connectomics and tractography are good sources of accurate human anatomical information that facilitate this kind of study.

### 15.4.2 *Technical aspects of neural mass methods*

The statistical basis for neural mass models is investigating how an overall population of neurons behaves, as opposed to whether individual neuron states are correlated or not (as in neural ensemble models). Neural mass models are based on the assumption that the coherence between neurons in a population is so strong that the overall dynamics of a population of neurons resembles that of each single neuron. Accordingly, the overall population activity is modeled with the same conductance-based model as used in single-neuron models. The assumption is relaxed somewhat by replacing the all-or-nothing firing of individual neurons with a sigmoid-shaped activation function that maps the average membrane potential to the mean firing rate. The breadth of the sigmoid function incorporates the variance of individual neural thresholds (Breakspear, 2017). An important difference between modeling projects using neural mass models and Fokker–Planck equations is that the variance is constant in neural mass models whereas it varies in Fokker–Planck equation-based methods. Neural mass models often consist of a conductance-based spiking excitatory neuron pool coupled to a passive local inhibitory pool and can exhibit steady state, periodic, or chaotic oscillations such as through the mixing of fast and slow timescales.

In terms of dimensionality reduction, since there is a strong presence of coherence (indicated by signaling synchronization), a further assumption is made that the ensemble activity is sufficiently close to the mean that the variance can be discarded. This reduces the number of dimensions to one and allows multiple interacting local populations, such as excitatory and inhibitory neurons in different layers of the cortex, to be modeled by a small number of equations, each describing the mean activity of a neural population (Breakspear, 2017). The conductance-based models that describe the behavior of individual neurons can be translated into signals that comprise an equivalent neural mass, applied at the population level (Woolrich & Stephan, 2013, p. 332). The point is that the dynamics within each network node incorporate both activity from the local population, and influences from farther regions in the form of stochastic fluctuations (correlations), elements which have been difficult to combine in one model. Such large-scale brain network models produce a multiscale ensemble-of-ensembles with distinct principles of organization operating at different scales (Breakspear & Stam, 2005). Neural mass models could be the start towards a set of universal principles for bridging scales and connecting a local patch of the cortex to the overall brain.

#### 15.4.2.1 *Oscillatory dynamics: Jansen–Rit neural mass model*

A well-known neural mass model developed from empirical data is the Jansen–Rit model (1975). The model recapitulates a large variety of observed EEG-like waveforms and rhythms. The structure is the coupling of two models, with delays in the interconnections to simulate the synaptic connections within and between cortical areas. The delayed interconnection of the two models makes it possible to replicate the spatial distribution of alpha and beta wave activity. Electrical potentials are simulated by presenting pulses to the input of the coupled models. The simulations suggest that real-life scalp-recorded electrical potential is at least partially due to a phase reordering of the ongoing activity. Such Jansen–Rit structures of delay-coupled subsystems are one standard model of neural dynamics.

Forrester *et al.* (2020) employ a network approach to find that local oscillatory dynamics can have a substantial role in shaping the large-scale functional connectivity patterns in the brain. The work uses data from the Human Connectome Project (van Essen *et al.*, 2013) to develop a tractography-based network of structural connectivity. Within this network connectivity structure, the research considers synchrony between neural subunits whose dynamics are described by a Jansen–Rit model. Specifically, connected pyramidal populations are analyzed, encoded in a connectivity matrix with elements describing both structural and functional connectivity. The key finding is that structural connectivity heavily influences functional connectivity in certain structural cases, and otherwise only has a weak influence. Functional connectivity is inherited robustly from structure when node dynamics are poised near a Hopf bifurcation, while structure only weakly influences functional connectivity near false bifurcations. Neural dynamics can be complicated to model as both global and local patterns of oscillation arising from structural connections appear to impact the brain.

#### 15.4.2.2 *Non-smooth dynamics and the Floquet model*

Coombes *et al.* (2018) extend the Wilson–Cowan mean-field model with Floquet (periodic) methods, to propose networks of piecewise intervals to study non-smooth dynamical systems. Neural models have mainly examined smooth dynamical systems (via low-dimensional coupled ordinary differential equations within a smooth sigmoidal firing rate nonlinearity), but might be improved by an understanding of non-smooth dynamical behavior. In both physics (Colombo *et al.*, 2012) and neuroscience, there is an impetus to investigate non-smooth dynamical systems.

The main aim of neural mass models is elaborating the interrelation of individual nodes within the overall network. A key problem of interest is understanding stable periodic network states that nevertheless give way to discontinuous firing behavior. Coombes *et al.* (2018) proceed by replacing the smooth sigmoidal nonlinearities in neural mass models with more tractable functions as a piecewise linear alternative. Floquet theory (treating periodicity) is applied at both the node and the network level as a stability calculation measure, to assess spatiotemporal patterns arising from instability (firing). Stability analysis is more complicated at the network level and a model of Glass networks is incorporated to model the stability of periodic network states in neural mass models with discontinuous interactions. Glass networks are used to study periodic and aperiodic switch-like behavior in biochemical networks (Glass & Kauffman, 1971). The result of the work is extending neural mass models to the network level by articulating the construction of periodic orbits, and completing an analysis of network states of discontinuous firing rates.

Floquet theory is the class of solutions to periodic linear differential equations in which there is a piecewise continuous periodic function. Piecewise functions are defined by multiple sub-functions applying to different intervals in the domain. Non-smooth dynamical models might apply to neural signaling because piecewise functions are consistent with other neural systems such as the human visual system.

## 15.5 Neural Field Models

*Cortical neural tissues can be regarded mathematically as neural fields which form and propagate interacting patterns of excitation*

— Amari (1977, p. 77)

For the robust treatment of the whole brain, neural field models are employed which consider the cortex as a continuous sheet. Transmitting information between brain regions produces waves of activity that fan out across the entire brain. Such brain waves are readily observed using noninvasive techniques such as EEG and MEG, and also appear in brain slices (Byrne *et al.*, 2019). Both experimental and theoretical research indicates that EEG/MEG recordings and evoked potentials exhibit traveling and standing waves (Nunez & Srinivasan, 2006). Neural field models are thus developed based on the needs of empirical science to describe wave states in the brain (Nunez, 1974). The word "field" denotes a continuous mathematical function in time and space, in the neural context, to relate the number densities of active excitatory and inhibitory synapses in each cortical tissue mass. EEG activity seems to be generated by synaptic current sources that can be characterized as "global fields of synaptic action" (Nunez & Srinivasan, 2006, p. 2424). Such synaptic action fields are short-time modulations in the number densities of active excitatory and inhibitory synapses.

Neural field models have long been used as models of large-scale pattern formation in the cortex (Bressloff, 2012; Coombes, 2005). These models are typically structured as a system of nonlocal partial differential equations which describes the spatiotemporal evolution of coarse-grained population variables, such as the firing rate of a neuronal population, the average synaptic current, and the mean membrane potential (Coombes *et al.*, 2014). Nonlocality arises via spatial integrals that are meant to represent the influence of neurons at many different spatial locations onto the dynamics of a specific location. In the laboratory setting, neural field models are essentially nonlinear wave models. Neural field theories attempt to account for a broad spectrum of empirically obtained wave-like data, such as the propagating fronts of oscillatory activity observed in sensory and motor cortices (Muller *et al.*, 2014). The local connectivity footprint can be written as a wave equation, in the form of a partial differential equation with temporal and spatial derivatives (Jirsa & Haken, 1996). Neural field models have been successful in describing neurophysiological phenomena such as EEG/MEG rhythms, working memory, binocular rivalry, and orientation tuning in the visual cortex (Byrne *et al.*, 2019).

### 15.5.1 *Statistical theory of neuron dynamics*

Realizing the need to formulate a statistical theory of neuronal dynamics, the first neural field models focused on the description of excitatory spike activation and the propagation of large-scale brain activity (Beurle, 1956). Wilson and Cowan developed these ideas into a mean-field theory model that includes a second inhibitory layer and refractory behavior (accommodating the three quiescent, active, and refractory neuronal states) (Wilson & Cowan, 1972, 1973). Mean-field theory is a renormalization method in which the mean value of a field is taken as a solvable value that approximates a generally intractable system of underlying complexity by averaging over its degrees of freedom. Applications include recasting a wavefunction or lattice-based problem into the solvable model of a mean-field theory.

In the brain, connectivity patterns in the neocortex appear to follow a laminar arrangement, with strong vertical coupling between layers. Thus, cortical activity in models is often considered as occurring on a two-dimensional plane, with the coupling between layers providing for near instantaneous vertical propagation. Synaptic input current is modeled as a function of the presynaptic firing rate function. The Wilson–Cowan mean-field theory is aimed at describing spatially localized bumps (concentrated clusters of observed behavior) and confirmed with computer-simulated experiments that indicate recurring patterns of dynamics. Amari further develops the "standard neural field model" into a single equation (Amari, 1975, 1977). Introducing a Mexican hat-type coupling function (local excitation coupled with long-range inhibition), the model is reduced to a single equation with a mix of excitatory and inhibitory connections that accurately computes spatially localized patterns. Subsequent work extends these ideas into a statistical neural field theory (Buice & Cowan, 2009) which considers system criticality by using path integral methods to make corrections to the mean-field theory approach. Adaptations to neural field theory methods persist, for example, in the investigation of criticality in models with very large deviations (Bressloff, 2015).

#### 15.5.1.1 *Oscillatory neural dynamics*

Neural dynamics are elaborated in the Amari model (1977) via oscillatory behavior. The dynamics of patterns in the neural field play an essential role in cortical information processing. An excitatory-inhibitory oscillation model is proposed in the form of a two-layer network. In the model, a field's dynamics depend on the mutual connections (entropy, correlations) within the field and the level of homogeneous stimulus the field receives. The neural field theory is an example of how nonhomogeneous pattern formation can occur in a homogeneous field. The problem of nonhomogeneous pattern formation from homogeneous fields has been studied extensively using the reaction-diffusion model, starting with Turing (1952) in the context of morphogenesis. The structure of Amari's theory, which has an alternating linear (input function) and nonlinear (output function) structure, lends itself to the similar alternating linear-nonlinear structures of tensor networks (disentanglers and isometries (Vidal, 2008)) and machine learning (max pooling, and convolutions-activations (LeCun *et al.*, 2015)). The problem frame of homogeneous fields giving rise to non-homogeneous pattern formation identified by Amari (1977) is similar to that of understanding stable periodic network states that nevertheless give way to discontinuous firing behavior (Coombes *et al.*, 2018).

## 15.5.2 *Neural field theory in practice*

### 15.5.2.1 *Multiscale models*

In the empirical setting, Nunez *et al.* (2019) develop a biophysical framework for the interpretation of electrophysiological data recorded at multiple spatial scales of brain tissue. Microscale current sources at membrane surfaces produce local field potentials, electrocorticography, and EEG data that need to be understood together in an overall macroscale model. The team conducts a columnar analysis to connect microscale current sources to the macroscale. Microscale current source properties are determined by brain dynamics and the columnar structure of cortical tissue. Specifically, macroscale current sources are defined at the macrocolumn scale (mm) and depend on several features of the microscale current source properties, such as magnitude, micro synchrony within columns, and distribution through the cortical depths. The proposed theoretical framework informs studies of EEG source localization and characterization, and could facilitate interpretations of brain dynamics including synchrony, functional connections between cortical locations, and other aspects of brain complexity.

### 15.5.2.2 *Synchrony: Simultaneous arrival of signals*

In other work, Nunez *et al.* (2015) investigate axon propagation speeds. Synaptic signals must have different speeds because they arrive simultaneously at the postsynaptic neuron despite having widely varying path lengths (Fields, 2013). Such synchrony appears to be achieved by farther away axons having higher propagation speeds, and nearby axons having slower speeds (an interesting puzzle given the relative basis of "near" and "far"). For example, axons from peripheral retinal regions conduct faster than axons from neurons at the center of the retina to ensure the simultaneous arrival of impulses in the brain (Stanford, 1987). Myelination is also implicated as myelin-deficient rats showed that myelination was the primary factor producing uniform propagation latency despite variation in axon length (Lang & Rosenbluth, 2003).

Hence, myelination is known to be a factor in an axon's potential speed. Propagation speed varies among different types of axons, and many axons are slowly conducting and unmyelinated. The human corpus callosum is unmyelinated at birth, and about 30% of the fibers remain unmyelinated in adults. The propagation time between the hemispheres was found to be 30 milliseconds through myelinated callosal fibers and 150–300 milliseconds through unmyelinated fibers (Fields, 2008). Demyelination pathologies severely limit signal conductance, and thus having higher-resolution tools to measure such degradation is of interest. To better assess the conduction time through axons from presynaptic neurons, Nunez *et al.* (2015) propose a closer analytical relationship between EEG functional connectivity measures. The specific recommendation is to examine the relation of narrow band (1 Hz) alpha and theta wave coherence to axon propagation.

#### 15.5.2.3 *Neural field theory simulation and filtering*

Contemporary research often starts with traditional neural field theories as a base and adds new features. The mean-field model developed by Wilson and Cowan (1972) and the two-layer excitatory-inhibitory network model developed by Amari (1977) are the basic neural field models. Although there are many software tools for modeling single neurons and neuronal networks (such as NEURON, GENESIS, BRIAN, and NeoCortical Simulator), there have not been many options for larger-scale neuronal models. Sanz-Leon *et al.* (2018) present a user-ready software package, *NFTsim*, to facilitate the numerical simulation of a wide range of brain systems using continuum neural field modeling. The package code is written in C++ and bundled with Matlab routines for the rapid quantitative analysis and visualization of the outputs. *NFTsim* is at the scale of the whole brain, in particular incorporating long-range pathways such as thalamocortical projections when generating macroscopic activity fields.

The multiscale nature of the model allows various neuroimaging techniques (EEG, MEG, fMRI) to be integrated with neural field analysis.

Janvier and Robinson (2018) extend ongoing neural field theory work to model corticothalamic responses to visual stimuli. The result is transfer functions that embody key features in common with those of engineering control systems, which enables the interpretation of brain dynamics in terms of data filters. Corticothalamic dynamics are shown to be analogous to the classical proportional-integral-derivative (PID) filters that are widely used in engineering. The work concludes that neural dynamics can be interpreted within a control systems framework. This suggests the further application of engineering concepts in filtering (such as gain tuning) to neural field theories. The method surpasses other control systems methods used to analyze neural dynamics such as Kalman filtering (Rao & Ballard, 1999), which become reduced or constrained forms of Bayesian learning under optimal estimation theory. Optimal control has been demonstrated as an important method of biomedical modeling in drug delivery as disease states may be manifestations of unstable control loops (Swan, 1984, p. 47; Moore, 2018), and is now being extended to quantum optical control (Boscain *et al.*, 2020).

### 15.5.2.4 *Firing synchrony within populations of neurons*

Establishing models of firing synchronization within populations of neurons is an important research topic in neural field theory. EEG scalp electrodes typically capture the activity of about 109 cortical pyramidal cells and can only detect an electric field if all of the individual cell dipoles add coherently (da Silva & Rotterdam, 2005). Only being able to capture fully coherent synchronizations (looking for keys under the light) may ignore other more subtle synchronization and desynchronization processes operating within a population of neurons. These kinds of subtleties are also observed, as an increase and decrease of power in certain EEG/MEG frequency bands. The temporal variations are thought to be the result of changes in synchrony within the neural tissue. Consequently, neural field models need to incorporate dynamic within-population synchrony processes to more accurately describe the evolution of large-scale spatio-temporal brain rhythms.

The usual method for modeling within-population synchronization is a spiking neural network model, a network-based on standard biological neuron models such as theta neurons or integrate-and-fire neurons. Sometimes these models are too high-dimensional for the problem and need to be reduced. For example, spiking neural network models may admit an exact mean-field description, but without a spatial component. It is important, however, to localize population signaling activity and synchronization in space and time. Byrne *et al.* (2019) construct a more precise and reduced neural field model based on spatially distributed theta neurons that incorporates within-population synchrony and synaptic coupling. The model recapitulates patterns seen in networks of spiking neurons such as bumps (spatially localized increases in population firing), breathers (stable breathing-type rhythms), and waves. The work provides a general mathematical procedure for linking microscopic dynamics to macroscopic dynamics. In addition, a beyond-Turing instability analysis is given for spatially and temporally periodic patterns in neural behavior.

Byrne *et al.*'s (2019) model describes novel synchronization behavior, namely, exotic states (spatiotemporal patterns), which might further explain within-population synchronization processes. Applying instability analysis to articulate transitions from resting to signaling behavior, the finding is that Turing and Hopf unstable modes compete, resulting in a characteristically complex spatiotemporal pattern, in which temporal oscillations develop within each bump of a Turing pattern. The intersection point of the Turing and Hopf curves and the exotic spatiotemporal patterns are robust to changes in parameters. The surprise is that the Hopf bifurcation creates regional bistability in some cases, such that the signaling network supports both local oscillations and dynamic global patterns. Such exotic state patterns have both a spatial and a temporal period. In this way, the brain is like a superconducting spacetime crystal, namely, becoming superconducting in the sense of undergoing a phase transition (from resting to signaling) based on periodic spatial and temporal behavior (Lin *et al.*, 2019), which might possibly be further described by a Floquet (periodic) model (Else *et al.*, 2016).

In the same research trajectory, Laing likewise develops a network of spatially extended theta neurons to demonstrate how large networks of spiking neurons might self-organize in time in both synaptic (2015) and gap junction coupled systems (2016). Montbrio *et al.* (2015) also employ a spatially extended approach, in a reduced network based on quadratic integrate-and-fire neurons instead of theta neurons. The work indicates that spike generation in individual neurons introduces an effective coupling between two biophysically relevant macroscopic quantities, the firing rate and the mean membrane potential, which together govern the evolution of the network. Further, a conformal mapping is used to relate the firing rate description to a low-dimensional description of the Kuramoto oscillation order parameter. This suggests a prototypical AdS/Brain application in the sense of a mapping between higher and lower-dimensional regimes.

The central idea is studying brain-wide signaling as a field theory. The flexibility of neural field models indicates their potential adaptability to more extensive physics-based modeling and quantum computational platforms. For example, it is possible to choose the model of space, and of time (Laing, 2016). It is also possible to choose and interchange coordinate systems, between quadratic integrate-and-fire biological neuron model and theta neurons, for example (Byrne *et al.*, 2019). Given the computational requirements of calculating the partial differential equations that define neural field theories, quantum computing platforms might be of aid. Greater computational capacity could allow more biologically realistic features to be incorporated into the models such as dendritic integration. Numerical advances have already enabled more complicated large-scale neural firing behavior to be described that is inaccessible to earlier methods (such as getting beyond the Heaviside firing rate function limit in the Amari equation, and beyond-Turing instability analysis with more sophisticated spatial and temporal periodicity models). Overall, neural field theories, and all models of neural dynamics, could see further development on quantum platforms.

### 15.5.3 *Statistical neural field theory*

Statistical neural field theory is a method developed by Cowan to extend the mean-field Wilson–Cowan equations to situations of criticality and to include fluctuation and correlation effects (Ohira & Cowan, 1993;

Buice & Cowan, 2009). The method includes many foundational physics formulations that extend traditional neuroscience models. Neural signaling is modeled as a Markov process of Gaussian random walks consolidated into random fields with path integrals, structured as a diffusion equation. The solution to the diffusion equation is a Gaussian propagator or Green's function. The Green's function plays the role of propagators that refer to two-point correlation functions (amplitudes or expectation values). From the Markov model, the master equation describing the overall system is written, through which further derivations include neural field equations, the neural spike Hamiltonian, and the renormalized action.

The neural dynamics are based on a random graph process, called directed percolation, which results in phase transition. Notably, Fokker–Planck equations are not used to model the dynamics, but rather a tripartite model of $3 \times 3$ matrices in the SU(3) Lie algebra group that better corresponds to the three states of neurons (quiescent, active, refractory). These dynamics lead to a nonlinear system whose renormalized action is that of Reggeon field theory (an early model of strong force scattering amplitudes). The result is that the transition from spontaneous neocortical activity around a critical point to large-scale activity can be modeled as a nonequilibrium phase transition, in the same universality class as directed percolation, which describes the observed neural behavior of branching-aggregating neurons in random walks (Hinrichsen, 2000). The implication is that such a phase transition has a known mathematical signature characterized by certain critical exponents, and can be readily recognized in real-life experimental data (Buice & Cowan, 2009, p. 83).

State transitions are managed by ladder operators, a quantum mechanical method by which first an annihilation operator (lowering operator) is applied to remove a particle from the initial state, and then a creation operator (raising operator) is applied to add a particle to the final (new) state. The ladder operators act on combinations of the tripartite matrices to produce system state transitions. The mathematical benefit is that the master equation for the system can be written algebraically in terms of easy-to-manipulate ladder operators. Coherent states (oscillatory quantum states), used to represent statistics in quantum field theory, are used to interpret the Markov random fields. The neural action (equations of motion) is based on a Poisson initial state distribution and then a coherent state (oscillatory) Hamiltonian (Buice & Cowan, 2009, p. 63).

The neurons themselves are structured as a $d$-dimensional lattice. The neural state vector describes the possible configurations of the network. A probability is assigned to each possible configuration, and the weighted probability configurations are summed over with a path integral to obtain the probability state vector of the system. Number density operators are used to count the number of neurons in the three different states, and also the electric current (excitation) coming onto the network. The influx of excitation is computed by weighting the number density of active states by the weighting function of each active neuron. The result is that the master equation is written as an evolution operator that counts all the possible state transitions in and out of the system states, in terms of space and time, and is equal to the total energy of the system.

The statistical neural field theory, especially the dynamics structure of the directed percolation phase transition, has implications for further extension to time symmetry and superconducting models. An intrinsic property of the directed percolation phase transition is that it exhibits time-reversal symmetry (Buice & Cowan, 2009, p. 81), and thus might be modeled with out-of-time-order correlation functions (Swingle *et al.*, 2016), spacetime crystals (Lin *et al.*, 2019), or at minimum Floquet periodicity (Else *et al.*, 2016). The link to superconducting is also through the phase transition structure as materials become superconducting when they reach a critical temperature and undergo a phase transition. The directed percolation phase transition has an upper critical dimension governing the transition from the critical point to a nonequilibrium phase transition. The critical exponent of four (Buice & Cowan, 2009, p. 83) may be interpreted in the context of the Ginzburg criterion for phase transition to superconductivity based on an expression involving $4\pi$ for the upper limit to the density of atomic vortices in material in the Landau–Ginzburg theory of superconducting (Hartnoll *et al.*, 2018, p. 130).

### 15.5.4 *Quantum neural field theory*

Contemporary neural field theories fall into four classes, each with various models of neural dynamics (Table 15.5). These include empirically driven models (with dynamics described by multistability, Hopf bifurcation, oscillation, and synchrony), theoretically driven models (with dynamics articulated by Floquet models and Hopf bifurcation), foundational physics-driven statistical neural field theory (with directed percolation phase transition dynamics), and network neuroscience models (with oscillatory graph-based dynamics).

In the empirical setting, neural field theories are proving successful in the interpretation of neuroimaging data, as indicated by Nunez *et al.* (2019), Breakspear (2017), and Valdes-Sosa *et al.* (2009), particularly using the mean-field theories of Jansen and Rit (1995) and Liley *et al.* (2002). These models could persist in the further attempt to study new kinds of whole-brain data as they become available. In theoretically driven approaches, promising expansions in mathematical analysis are suggested by Coombes *et al.* (2018) and Laing (2016) in the use of Floquet theory and Hopf bifurcation to develop beyond-Turing instabilities to characterize stable periodic network states that produce discontinuous firing behavior. With its foundational physics-based roots, Cowan's statistical neural field theory could be central to the implementation of neural field theories on quantum platforms (Swan *et al.*, 2020). The neural field theory is structured as a master equation with Markov processes expressed as a solvable path integral. Bressloff (2015) and Chow and Buice (2015) have further adapted path integral methods to the specialized context of large-scale

Table 15.5. Neural field theory classes.

| No. | Focus | Neural Dynamics |
|---|---|---|
| 1 | Empirically driven | Multistability, Hopf bifurcation, oscillation, synchrony |
| 2 | Theoretically driven | Floquet theory, Hopf bifurcation, beyond-Turing instability |
| 3 | Foundational physics-based | Directed percolation on random graphs |
| 4 | Network-based | Graph-based oscillation |

neural modeling. Finally, network neuroscience models with a conducive format of graph-based oscillatory structures of neural dynamics might be the most readily implemented neural field theories on quantum platforms (Bassett *et al.*, 2018; Papadopoulos *et al.*, 2020).

Neural field theories and other models of neural dynamics and large-scale brain behavior highlight the relevance of physics-based neuroscience approaches. The possibility of instantiating neural models on quantum computing platforms, together with the influx of greater stores of real-life whole-brain data, could greatly extend the reach, explanatory capability, and further innovation of these models. The physics-based underpinnings of neural field theories suggest their well-formedness for quantum implementation to target the bulk properties of the brain at relevant scales and dynamics, including for projects that are difficult to manage at present such as dendritic integration.

## References

Adler, R.J. & Taylor, J. (2007). *Random Fields and Geometry*. London: Springer.

Altenburg, J., Vermeulen, R.J., Strijers, R.L. *et al.* (2003). Seizure detection in the neonatal EEG with synchronization likelihood. *Clin. Neurophysiol.* 114:50–5.

Amari, S. (1975). Homogeneous nets of neuron-like elements. *Biol. Cybern.* 17:211–20.

Amari, S. (1977). Dynamics of pattern formation in lateral-inhibition type neural fields. *Biol. Cybern.* 27:77–87.

Bassett, D.S., Zurn, P. & Gold, J.I. (2018). On the nature and use of models in network neuroscience. *Nat. Rev. Neurosci.* 19(9):566–78.

Beurle, R.L. (1956). Properties of a mass of cells capable of regenerating pulses. *Trans Roy. Soc. London B*. 240:55–94.

Boscain, U., Sigalotti, M. & Sugny D. (2020). Introduction to the foundations of quantum optimal control. arXiv:2010.09368v1.

Breakspear, M. (2017). Dynamic models of large-scale brain activity. *Nat. Neurosci.* 20:340–52.

Breakspear, M. & Stam, C.J. (2005). Dynamics of a neural system with a multiscale architecture. *Phil. Trans. R. Soc. Lond. B*. 360:1051–74.

Bressloff, P.C. (2012). Spatiotemporal dynamics of continuum neural fields. *J. Phys. A: Math. Theor.* 45(3):033001.

Bressloff, P.C. (2015). Path-integral methods for analyzing the effects of fluctuations in stochastic hybrid neural networks. *J. Math. Neurosci.* 5(4):1–33.

Bryson, M. (1974). Heavy-tailed distributions: Properties and tests. *Technometrics.* 16(1):61–68.

Buice, M.A. & Cowan, J.D. (2009). Statistical mechanics of the neocortex. *Prog. Biophys. Mol. Biol.* 99:53–86.

Byrne, A., Avitabile, D. & Coombes, S. (2019). A next generation neural field model. *Phys. Rev. E.* 99(1):012313.

Chow, C.C. & Buice, M.A. (2015). Path integral methods for stochastic differential equations. *J. Math. Neurosci.* 5(8):1–35.

Colombo, A., di Bernardo, M., Hogan, S.J. & Jeffrey, M.R. (2012). Bifurcations of piecewise smooth flows: Perspectives, methodologies and open problems. *Physica D.* 241:1845–60.

Coombes, S. (2005). Waves, bumps, and patterns in neural field theories. *Biol. Cybern.* 93(2):91–108.

Coombes, S. & Byrne, A. (2019). Next generation neural mass models. In *Lecture Notes Nonlinear Dynamics in Computational Neuroscience: From Physics and Biology to ICT.* Eds. Torcini, A. & Corinto, F. London: Springer, pp. 1–16.

Coombes, S., Graben, P.P.B., Potthast, R. & Wright, J. (2014). *Neural Fields: Theory and Applications*. London: Springer.

Coombes, S., Lai, Y.M., Sayli, M. & Thul, R. (2018). Networks of piecewise linear neural mass models. *Eur. J. Appl. Math.* 29(5):869–90.

Cowan, J.D., Neuman, J. & van Drongelen, W. (2016). Wilson-Cowan equations for neocortical dynamics. *J. Math. Neurosci.* 6(1):1–24.

da Silva, F.L. & Rotterdam, A.V. (2005). Biophysical aspects of EEG and magnetoencephalogram generation. In *Electroencephalography: Basic Principles, Clinical Applications and Related Fields.* Eds. Niedermeyer, E. & da Silva, F.L. London: Lippincott, Williams & Wilkins, pp. 107–26.

El Boustani, S. & Destexhe, A. (2009). A master equation formalism for macroscopic modeling of asynchronous irregular activity states. *Neural Comput.* 21:46–100.

Else, D.V., Bauer, B. & Nayak, C. (2016). Floquet time crystals. *Phys. Rev. Lett.* 117(9):090402.

Ermentrout, G.B. & Cowan, J.D. (1979). A mathematical theory of visual hallucination patterns. *Biol. Cybern.* 34:137–50.

Fields, R.D. (2008). White matter in learning, cognition and psychiatric disorders. *Trends Neurosci.* 31:361–70.

Fields, RD. (2013). Regulation of myelination by functional activity. In *Neuroglia*. Ed. Kettenmann, R., 3rd Edition. Oxford: Oxford University Press, pp. 573–85.

Forrester, M. Crofts, J.J., Sotiropoulos, S.N. *et al.* (2020). The role of node dynamics in shaping emergent functional connectivity patterns in the brain. *Network Neuroscience*. 4(2):467–83.

Freeman, W.J. (1975). *Mass Action in the Nervous System: Examination of the Neurophysiological Basis of Adaptive Behavior through the EEG.* London: Academic Press.

Freyer, F., Roberts, J.A., Ritter, P. & Breakspear, M. (2012). A canonical model of multistability and scale-invariance in biological systems. *PLoS Comput. Biol.* 8:e1002634.

Gardiner, C.W. (2009). *Stochastic Methods: A Handbook for the Natural and Social Sciences*. Berlin: Springer.

Glass, L. & Kauffman, S.A. (1971). The logical analysis of continuous non-linear biochemical control networks. *Journal of Theoretical Biology*. 39:103–29.

Hartnoll, S.A., Lucas, A. & Sachdev, S. (2018). *Holographic Quantum Matter*. Cambridge: MIT Press.

Hinrichsen, H. (2000). Non-equilibrium critical phenomena and phase transitions into absorbing states. *Adv. Phys*. 49:815–958.

Horvat, S., Gamanut, R., Ercsey-Ravasz, M. *et al.* (2016). Spatial embedding and wiring cost constrain the functional layout of the cortical network of rodents and primates. *PLoS Biol.* 14:e1002512.

Huys, Q.J., Maia, T.V. & Frank, M.J. (2016). Computational psychiatry as a bridge from neuroscience to clinical applications. *Nat. Neurosci.* 19:404–13.

Jansen, B.H. & Rit, V.G. (1995). Electroencephalogram and visual evoked potential generation in a mathematical model of coupled cortical columns. *Biol. Cybern.* 73:357–66.

Janvier, T.B. & Robinson, P.A. (2018). Neural field theory of corticothalamic prediction with control systems analysis. *Front. Hum. Neurosci.* 12:334.

Jirsa, V.K. & Haken, H. (1996). Field theory of electromagnetic brain activity. *Phys. Rev. Lett.* 77(5):960–63.

Koch, C. (1999). *Biophysics of Computation: Information Processing in Single Neurons*. Oxford: Oxford University Press.

Laing, C.R. (2015). Exact neural fields incorporating gap junctions. *SIAM Journal on Applied Dynamical Systems*. 14:1899–929.

Laing, C.R. (2016). Phase oscillator network models of brain dynamics. *Computational Models of Brain and Behavior*. London: Wiley-Blackwell.

Lang, E.J. & Rosenbluth, J. (2003). Role of myelination in the development of a uniform olivocerebellar conduction time. *J. Neurophysiol.* 89:2259–70.

LeCun, Y., Bengio, Y. & Hinton, G. (2015). Deep learning. *Nature.* 521(7553): 436–44.

Liley, D.T.J., Cadusch, P.J. & Dafilis, M.P. (2002). A spatially continuous mean field theory of electrocortical activity. *Network.* 13:67–113.

Lin, H.W., Maldacena, J. & Zhao, Y. (2019). Symmetries near the horizon. *J. High Energ. Phys.* 1908:049.

Lundstrom, B.N., Higgs, M.H., Spain, W.J. & Fairhall, A.L. (2008). Fractional differentiation by neocortical pyramidal neurons. *Nat. Neurosci.* 11:1335–42.

Martins, N.R.B., Angelica, A., Chakravarthy, K. *et al.* (2019). Human brain/cloud interface. *Front. Neurosci.* 13(112):1–24.

Montbrio, E., Pazo, D. & Roxin, A. (2015). Macroscopic description for networks of spiking neurons. *Phys. Rev. X.* 5(2):021028.

Moore, H. (2018). How to mathematically optimize drug regimens using optimal control. *J. Pharmacokinet Phar.* 45(1):127–37.

Muller, L., Reynaud, A., Chavane, F. & Destexhe, A. (2014). The stimulus-evoked population response in visual cortex of awake monkey is a propagating wave. *Nat. Commun.* 5:3675.

Nunez, P.L. (1974). The brain wave equation: A model for the EEG. *Math. Biosci.* 21:279–97.

Nunez, P.L., Nunez, M.D. & Srinivasan, R. (2019). Multi-scale neural sources of EEG: Genuine, equivalent, and representative. A tutorial review. *Brain Topogr.* 32(2):193–214.

Nunez, P.L. & Srinivasan, R. (2006). A theoretical basis for standing and traveling brain waves measured with human EEG with implications for an integrated consciousness. *Clin. Neurophysiol.* 117(11):2424–35.

Nunez, P.L., Srinivasan, R. & Fields, R.D. (2015). EEG functional connectivity, axon delays and white matter disease. *Clin. Neurophysiol.* 126(1):110–20.

Ohira, T. & Cowan, J.D. (1993). Master-equation approach to stochastic neurodynamics. *Phys. Rev. E.* 48:2259–66.

Papadopoulos, L., Lynn, C.W., Battaglia, D. & Bassett, D.S. (2020). Relations between large-scale brain connectivity and effects of regional stimulation depend on collective dynamical state. *PLoS Comput. Biol.* 16(9):e1008144.

Rao, R.P.N. & Ballard, D.H. (1999). Predictive coding in the visual cortex: A functional interpretation of some extra-classical receptive-field effects. *Nat. Neurosci.* 2:79–87.

Roberts, J.A., Boonstra, T.W. & Breakspear, M. (2015). The heavy tail of the human brain. *Curr. Opin. Neurobiol.* 31:164–72.

Sanz-Leon, P., Robinson, P.A., Knock, S.A. *et al.* (2018). NFTsim: Theory and simulation of multiscale neural field dynamics. *PLoS Comput. Biol.* 14(8):e1006387.

Stanford, L.R. (1987). Conduction velocity variations minimize conduction time differences among retinal ganglion cell axons. *Science.* 238:358–60.

Swan, G.W. (1984). *Applications of Optimal Control Theory in Biomedicine.* New York: Marcel Dekker, Inc.

Swan, M., dos Santos, R.P. & Witte, F. (2020). *Quantum Computing: Physics, Blockchains, and Deep Learning Smart Networks.* London: World Scientific.

Swingle, B., Bentsen, G., Schleier-Smith, M. & Hayden, P. (2016). Measuring the scrambling of quantum information. *Phys. Rev. A.* 94(4):040302.

Taleb, N.N. (2007). *The Black Swan: The Impact of the Highly Improbable.* New York: Random House.

Turing, A. (1952). The chemical basis of morphogenesis. *Phil. Trans. Roy. Soc. London B.* 237:32–72.

Valdes-Sosa, P.A., Sanchez-Bornot, J.M., Sotero, R.C. *et al.* (2009). Model driven EEG/fMRI fusion of brain oscillations. *Human Brain Mapping.* 30:2701–21.

van Essen, D.C., Smith, S.M., Barch, D.M. *et al.* (2013). The WU-Minn Human Connectome Project: An overview. *NeuroImage.* 80:62–79.

Vidal, G. (2008). Class of quantum many-body states that can be efficiently simulated. *Phys. Rev. Lett.* 101(11):110501.

Wilson, H.R. & Cowan, J.D. (1972). Excitatory and inhibitory interactions in local populations of model neurons. *Biophysical J.* 12:1–24.

Wilson, H.R. & Cowan, J.D. (1973). A mathematical theory of the functional dynamics of cortical and thalamic nervous tissue. *Kybernetik.* 13:55–80.

Woolrich, M.W. & Stephan, K.E. (2013). Biophysical network models and the human connectome. *Neuroimage.* 80:330–38.

# Part 5

# Modeling Toolkit

# Chapter 16

# Quantum Machine Learning

*The wave function is the fundamental object in quantum physics and possibly the hardest to grasp in a classical world ... the systematic machine learning of the wave function can reduce this complexity to a tractable computational form*

— Carleo and Troyer (2017, p. 602)

**Abstract**

This chapter discusses quantum machine learning as one of the first mainstream applications of quantum computing. Modeling classical data as quantum wavefunction states allows hidden information in the underlying system to be accessed through wavefunction amplitude. A greater amount of information can be incorporated in the compact and complex format by encoding an exponentially large number of values into a set of qubits. Wavefunction approximation and quantum state simulation (with transformer neural networks) are central applications in using machine learning to study problems in quantum mechanics (ML/Q).

## 16.1 Machine Learning-Physics Collaboration

Quantum machine learning first and most basically means running machine learning algorithms on a quantum computer (ML/QC). The emblematic examples (discussed in the Quantum Computing 101 chapter) are Farhi and Neven's (2018) quantum neural networks and Grant *et al.*'s (2018) quantum tensor networks. Some of the first real-life quantum platform demonstrations are Grant *et al.* (2018) on the IBM QX4 and Benedetti *et al.* (2019) with an ion trap platform. Quantum machine learning also means applying machine learning techniques to quantum mechanical problems and data (ML/Q), and the converse, applying quantum mechanical ideas and methods to improve machine learning techniques (Q/ML) (Table 16.1). The last two may be run on quantum or classical computers. The term "machine learning" is used generically in this work, although in practice is often synonymous with "deep learning" (networks with hidden layers that operate to find higher-order relationships in input data) (Schulte & Lee, 2019). Machine learning is deployed in different forms such as kernel learning, neural networks, and tensor networks. ML/Q is discussed here and Q/ML in Chapter 17.

A further means of distinguishing Quantum Machine Learning is by which parts of a system (data, algorithms, and platforms) are classical or quantum (Table 16.2). The first level is data, which classically might

Table 16.1. Quantum machine learning terminology.

| Abbr. | Definition | Sample Reference |
|---|---|---|
| ML/QC | Running machine learning algorithms on a quantum computer | Farhi and Neven (2018); Grant *et al.* (2018) |
| ML/Q | Applying machine learning to quantum mechanical problems and data | Carleo and Troyer (2017) |
| Q/ML | Using quantum mechanical approaches to improve machine learning techniques | Stoudenmire and Schwab (2017) |

Table 16.2. Quantum data, algorithm, and platform.

| Topic | Classical | Quantum |
|---|---|---|
| Data | Facial recognition images | Meson spectral data |
| Algorithm | Loss function | VQE, QAOA |
| Platform | Desktop computer | NISQ devices |

*Notes*: VQE: Variational quantum eigensolvers; QAOA: Quantum approximate optimization algorithm; NISQ: Commercially available noisy intermediate-scale quantum devices.

involve facial recognition images, and in the quantum sense, meson spectral output from the Large Hadron Collider. Second is the algorithms deployed in the computation, whether classical algorithms such as a loss function, or quantum algorithms that have been designed specifically to operate on quantum data or run on a quantum platform. Third is the computational platform, which could be a classical computer such as a desktop or cloud computing environment, or in the quantum domain, a NISQ device (currently available quantum computer with 50–100 qubits that does not require error correction). There could be different permutations such as running classical data on a quantum platform, or simulating quantum systems with a classical computer.

A key focus is developing quantum algorithms and quantum circuits. Quantum algorithms mean writing new algorithms and adapting classical algorithms to the quantum environment, particularly to take advantage of quantum speedups in linear algebra and vector-based calculations. Quantum circuits entail mapping quantum algorithms to a computable gate logic structure to run on quantum computers or on classical computers simulating quantum computers. There are many resources available such as Google's TensorFlow Quantum as a software framework for quantum machine learning that includes quantum optimization, thermal state sampling, and Hamiltonian learning algorithms (Broughton *et al.*, 2020).

Quantum machine learning has important practical applications in many areas such as quantum circuit design, quantum chemistry (molecular simulation and drug discovery), and quantum physics. There are also several theoretical formulations. For example, in an advanced application of holographic quantum machine learning (AdS/QML), Cottrell *et al.* (2019) suggest how machine learning might be used to learn the operator mappings between the left and right system evolutions in the thermofield double state. In other efforts, the Olshausen laboratory develops a body of theoretical work using machine learning for novel quantum formulations of renormalization group flow and entropy minimization (Hu *et al.*, 2020).

### 16.1.1 *Quantum machine learning overview*

Quantum machine learning is addressed in different chapters based on the application class (Table 16.3). In the first application of running machine

Table 16.3. Approaches to quantum machine learning.

| No. | Class | Approach | Reference | Chapter |
|---|---|---|---|---|
| 1 | ML/QC | Quantum neural networks | Farhi and Nevin (2018) | 7 |
| 2 | ML/QC | Quantum tensor networks | Grant *et al.* (2018) | 7 |
| 3 | ML/Q | Restricted Boltzmann machine | Carleo and Troyer (2017) | 16 |
| 4 | ML/Q | Quantum transformer networks | Carrasquilla *et al.* (2019) | 16 |
| 5 | Q/ML | Born machine | Cheng *et al.* (2018) | 17 |
| 6 | Q/ML | Reduced density matrix | Bradley *et al.* (2019) | 17 |
| 7 | Q/ML | Pixel = spin (qubit) | Stoudenmire and Schwab (2017) | 17 |
| 8 | Q/ML | Wavelet = spin (qubit) | Reyes and Stoudenmire (2020) | 17 |
| 9 | Q/ML | Quantum kernel methods | Schuld and Killoran (2019) | 18 |
| 10 | Q/ML | Entanglement system design | Martyn *et al.* (2020) | 18 |

learning algorithms on quantum computers (ML/QC), demonstrations of quantum neural networks (Farhi & Neven, 2018) and quantum tensor networks (Grant *et al.*, 2018) are discussed in Quantum Computing 101 (Chapter 7). The second application class is machine learning techniques applied to quantum mechanical problems (ML/Q), typified by approximating wavefunctions and energy levels with a restricted Boltzmann machine (Carleo and Troyer, 2017) and simulating quantum states on classical computers with a transformer neural network implementation (Carrasquilla *et al.*, 2019). These are discussed in Chapter 16. The third application class is quantum mechanical ideas and methods applied to improving machine learning techniques (Q/ML), elaborated in Chapters 17 and 18.

The persistent theme of Q/ML is quantum probabilistic methods. This means probability directed toward the identification of the emergent collective behavior of complex systems with a large number of degrees of freedom, renormalization across system scales from the microscale to the macroscale, and the management of high dimensionality. A notable conceptual development is the idea of writing classical probability distributions as quantum states. Two methods for this are becoming standard, the Born machine and the reduced density matrix. The Born machine, introduced by Cheng *et al.* (2018), is used to interpret machine learning probability outputs according to the Born rule as opposed to the Boltzmann distribution and energy-based functions used in the classical Boltzmann machine. The reduced density matrix formulation is the quantum version of the classical marginal probability distribution, which notably elicits entanglement in classical systems by preserving system correlations as described by Bradley *et al.* (2019).

Another important conceptual advance is the idea that "pixel = spin" and "wavelet = spin". This insight recognizes the machine learning image pixel as a quantum mechanical spin (and thus qubit) (Stoudenmire & Schwab, 2017). Likewise, a wavelet in machine learning sequential data is recognized as a quantum mechanical spin and qubit (Reyes & Stoudenmire, 2020). Advanced applications of Q/ML are presented in Chapter 18, quantum kernel methods (Schuld & Killoran, 2019) and the idea of using entanglement as a design principle (Martyn *et al.*, 2020).

In other notable work establishing standardized tools, Huggins *et al.* (2019) introduce a framework for quantum machine learning using tensor networks. The research proposes a tensor network framework for both discriminative and generative learning (supervised and unsupervised learning) which is based in tree tensor networks and matrix product state tensor networks, for use with both classical and quantum data with NISQ devices, demonstrated with a numerical experiment on MNIST data. A similar example of quantum machine learning using tensor networks is offered by Liu *et al.* (2019). In this work, classical images are transformed to vectors in a $d^n$-dimensional Hilbert space, and the vectors (vectorized images) are mapped to a tree tensor network to predict the classes as outputs. The algorithm is tested on both the MNIST (handwriting recognition) and CIFAR (image recognition) databases.

Another tool is matrix quantum mechanics, a specialized version of quantum mechanics in which squared harmonic oscillators are written in the form of a large-$N$ matrix (Han *et al.*, 2020). The trace structure of the matrix allows the oscillators (matrix elements) to be coupled and interactions to be defined between them, and the trace structure also gives rise to an emergent dimension of space (Han & Hartnoll, 2020).

### 16.1.2 *Structural similarities*

A key motivation for quantum machine learning is that much more is understood about why certain methods work in addressing quantum mechanical problems than in machine learning problems (Martyn *et al.*, 2020). Machine learning is a notorious "black box" technology in that results are obtained (accurately classifying images, for example), but it is not understood precisely how. Quantum mechanical methods are much more transparent. The lack of understanding in machine learning hampers the ability to apply these methods to new classes of more complicated problems (Hassabis *et al.*, 2017), even with recent tools such as transformer networks (Vaswani *et al.*, 2017). A parallel is drawn between the two fields, arguing that the success in machine learning can be explained by the properties of fundamental physics. One suggestion of a dictionary is mapped between the two areas (Table 16.4).

Approaches to quantum machine learning start to articulate more specifically how the two domains are related. Structurally, quantum mechanics and machine learning are large-scale systems with high-dimensional problem spaces, too large and unwieldy for anything other than statistical methods, and whose central task is finding a function that approximates

Table 16.4. Physics-machine learning dictionary.

| No. | Physics | Machine Learning |
|---|---|---|
| 1 | Hamiltonian | Surprisal — ln probability |
| 2 | Simple Hamiltonian | Cheap learning (few layers) |
| 3 | Quadratic Hamiltonian | Gaussian probability |
| 4 | Locality | Sparsity |
| 5 | Symmetric Hamiltonian | Convnet (convolutional networks) |
| 6 | Probability via Hamiltonian | Softmaxing (scaling to sum to one) |
| 7 | Spin | Bit |
| 8 | Free energy difference | Kullback–Leibler divergence (relative entropy) |
| 9 | Effective theory | Nearly lossless data distillation |
| 10 | Irrelevant operator | Noise |
| 11 | Relevant operator | Failure |

*Source*: Adapted from Lin *et al.* (2017, p. 3).

data. Both systems operate in a vast possibility space yet try to quickly truncate it to a relevant subset. Machine learning operates in the space of all equations, but expediently tries to find equations to describe a particular dataset. In natural language processing, for example, only a fraction of all grammatically correct phrases have meaning. Similarly, quantum states are not simply random vectors in the high-dimensional possibility space of all vectors, but have some sort of identifiable patterns based on direction and movement. The interest is only in a local Hamiltonian, not in the entire Hilbert space. Both systems are multiscalar, operating at multiple scales at different tiers with different dynamics.

The field of quantum machine learning is thus inspired by quantum mechanics and machine learning being naturally aligned in the way that the problems are set up as probabilistic movements through a larger possibility space of high-dimensional complexity and necessarily solved with indirect methods. These structural similarities suggest that quantum states can be represented with a neural network. It is not a stretch to see that the brain is a domain in which many of these properties also hold (a large-scale high-dimensional possibility space with multiple dynamical levels which can be truncated to a subsystem of interest described by a wavefunction), and further the possibilities of quantum machine learning as a lens for studying the brain. Arguably, entire classes of recent findings in neuroscience with whole-brain modeling, big data acquisition, imaging, and multiscale models are only just beginning to be incorporated into machine learning models.

### 16.1.3 *Problems in quantum mechanics*

Some of the primary applications at which quantum machine learning is targeted are wavefunction approximation and quantum state simulation. In the application of machine learning to the study of quantum mechanical problems (ML/Q), the question arises as to exactly which problems might be most conducive to resolution (Table 16.5). The primary problem in quantum mechanics is wavefunction approximation. The Schrödinger equation describes wavefunctions mathematically, but is intractable to solve and so other methods that approximate wavefunctions are sought. The insight to use machine learning is motivated by the fact that neural

Table 16.5. Quantum mechanical problems for machine learning.

| No. | Quantum Mechanical Problem | Reference |
|---|---|---|
| *Approximation* | | |
| 1 | Wavefunction approximation (amplitude and phase) | Carleo and Troyer (2017) |
| 2 | Ground state and excited energy levels: Exact ground state properties of strongly interacting fermions | Stokes *et al.* (2020) |
| 3 | Quantum system dynamics and time evolution: Dynamical properties of high-dimensional systems | Eisert *et al.* (2015) |
| 4 | Criticality and nonequilibrium dynamics: Quantum system phase transition | Freericks *et al.* (2014) |
| *Simulation* | | |
| 5 | Quantum state measurement (tomography): Reconstruct quantum states | Paris and Rehacek (2004) |
| 6 | Quantum state simulation of GHZ states with a transformer neural network | Carrasquilla *et al.* (2019); Cha *et al.* (2020) |

networks are function approximators, which is precisely what is needed for the quantum mechanical wavefunction. The generic task in machine learning is finding the best function to fit input data. Similarly, in quantum machine learning, the idea is to take particle spins and other quantum mechanical state data as input, and output a wavefunction. Also in the general class of approximation applications are finding the ground state and excited energy levels of a system, and specifying quantum system dynamics and time evolution behavior, including nonequilibrium dynamics at system criticality. The other main application class is simulating and benchmarking quantum systems. Quantum machine learning applied to problems of approximation and simulation are discussed in the next sections.

#### 16.1.3.1 *Variational methods: The method of varying*

Variational methods refer to a specific quantum mechanical technique for approximating wavefunctions. The term "variational methods" means using variation as a method, in the sense of varying trial-and-error guesses to determine a value. The method is variation — it is not that the methods vary. The variational method is applied by choosing a trial wavefunction that depends on one or more parameters, and solving for the values of the parameters for which the system energy is the lowest. The process is repeated several times to provide an overall profile for the wavefunction at the lowest energy values of the system.

The insight is that a lot of structural information is already known about quantum systems ahead of time (Montorsi, 1992). There are scale tiers of allowable energies in any quantum system. Since quantum systems are organized in discrete tiers of allowable energies, the idea is that to some extent, it may be possible to guess the scale tiers in a system. Further, a quantum system is bounded in important ways. First, the lower energy bound is zero. Second, energy tiers scale up from low to high. This governs the range of energies at any scale tier which limits the variational guessing activity to a more finitely solvable problem. Third, modern trial-and-error guesses are performed by computer which means the process iterations can be essentially unlimited.

The variational method may target the lowest energy eigenstate or ground state of a system, or any higher-level excited states. For quantum machine learning, the problem is either taken directly as a quantum system wavefunction approximation problem, or written in terms of an energy optimization problem. Conceptually in quantum machine learning, the variational method is seen as an efficient algorithm to find salient signals in a large possibility space, and can be implemented as a statistical sampling method. However, one of the drawbacks of all variational methods is that since they select a random spot and start guessing and bootstrapping from there, they can get stuck in a local minimum and obtaining a global minimum is not guaranteed.

## 16.2 Wavefunction Approximation

### 16.2.1 *Quantum state neural networks*

Carleo and Troyer (2017) demonstrate the use of machine learning to solve quantum many-body problems, first examining basic quantum systems with interacting spins and then strongly coupled fermionic systems. The computational challenge of quantum many-body problems is the difficulty of describing the correlations encoded in the exponential complexity of the many-body wavefunction. However, the idea is that the systematic machine learning of the wavefunction might reduce the complexity to a tractable computational form, at least for certain physical systems. Generically, the machine learning model takes data as input and outputs a function that describes the data. The input data in this case are quantum states of a physical system, which are generated by a variational method, and the neural network is tasked with inferring the wavefunction that best describes the data. The goal is finding the ground state energy in a basic interacting spin system and recapitulating the unitary time evolution of a complex interacting system. The approach achieves high accuracy in the description of equilibrium and dynamical properties of prototypical interacting spins models in both one and two dimensions. Overall, the demonstration offers a new computational tool for solving quantum many-body problems. The basic input–output framework of the quantum state neural network appears in Table 16.6.

#### 16.2.1.1 *Traditional approaches to wavefunction modeling*

The wavefunction is the fundamental object in quantum physics. It is a mathematical quantity containing all of the information about a quantum state, whether a single particle or complex molecules. In principle, an exponential amount of information is needed to fully encode a generic many-body quantum state (due to the $2^n$ problem). However, a wavefunction can often be characterized by a much smaller amount of information than the maximum capacity of the corresponding Hilbert space would indicate. A small number of physical states, together with entanglement properties, are the building blocks used by modern approaches to solve the many-body Schrödinger equation with a limited amount of classical resources.

Table 16.6. Quantum state neural network framework.

| Focus | Input | Output |
|---|---|---|
| Generic | Quantum state data | Wavefunction |
| Specific | Correlated quantum state data produced by variational methods | Ground state and time-dependent physical states of a quantum system |

The traditional methods of wavefunction modeling are stochastic approaches and compression approaches (Table 16.7). Each treats complexity in a different way. Stochastic approaches sample a finite number of physically relevant configurations. Compression approaches compress the information content of the quantum state. Stochastic approaches include techniques such as quantum Monte Carlo methods, which rely on probabilistic frameworks and typically require a positive-semidefinite wavefunction. Compression approaches, instead use efficient representations of the wavefunction, most notably tensor networks (via matrix product states or other general representations). However, these complexity management techniques are limited, in particular by the sign problem (phase problem) in quantum Monte Carlo, and the ability to address high-dimensional systems in early tensor network models. Different or improved methods may be needed to target new classes of open problems such as fundamental questions ranging from the dynamical properties of high-dimensional systems to the exact ground state properties of strongly interacting fermions.

### 16.2.1.2 *Motivation for machine learning*

A theoretical problem lies at the heart of wavefunction modeling. This is a lack of understanding of the foundational physics involved in terms of finding a general strategy to reduce the exponential complexity of the full many-body wavefunction to its most essential features (Freericks *et al.*, 2014). The problem can be cast as one of dimension reduction and feature extraction at which machine learning excels. Machine learning has demonstrated success in attacking these kinds of problems, for example, in image and speech recognition, and game playing. As an example, some of

Table 16.7. Wavefunction modeling: Complexity reduction.

| Approach Class | Focus | Method | Limitation |
|---|---|---|---|
| Stochastic approaches | Probabilistic frameworks | Quantum Monte Carlo | Sign problem |
| Compression approaches | Efficient wavefunction representation | Tensor networks | High dimensionality |

the first applications of neural networks to physics have been used to study physical phenomena such as the phases of quantum matter (Carrasquilla & Melko, 2017). So far, these approaches have focused on the classification of complex phases of matter in which exact sampling of configurations from these phases is known, and thus it is possible to confirm the results. The challenging goal of solving a quantum many-body problem without prior knowledge of exact samples is an open problem for machine learning. Thus, it is of fundamental and practical interest to understand whether an artificial neural network can modify and adapt itself to describe and analyze a quantum system. This ability could be used to address quantum many-body problems in regimes that have been inaccessible to existing approaches.

#### 16.2.1.3 *Machine learning approach to wavefunction modeling*

Carleo and Troyer (2017) introduce a representation of the wavefunction in terms of artificial neural networks specified by a set of internal parameters. A stochastic framework is presented for the reinforcement learning of the parameters to determine the best possible representation of both ground state and time-dependent physical states of a given quantum Hamiltonian. The parameters of the neural network are then optimized (trained), either by static variational Monte Carlo sampling, or by time-dependent variational Monte Carlo sampling if dynamical properties are of interest. The accuracy of the approach is validated by studying the Ising and Heisenberg models in both one and two-dimensions. The quantum state neural network is demonstrated by obtaining state-of-the-art accuracy in both ground state and out-of-equilibrium dynamics. The time-dependent approach effectively solves the sign problem that traditionally affects stochastic quantum Monte Carlo approaches.

#### 16.2.1.4 *Encoding quantum states*

A key question is how quantum states are to be encoded for neural network representation. A quantum system can be characterized as having $N$ discrete-valued degrees of freedom (parameters), which may be spins, bosonic occupation numbers, or similar measures. The many-body wavefunction is a mapping of the $N$-dimensional set of parameters to exponentially many complex numbers which fully specify the amplitude and the phase of a quantum state. The wavefunction is a computational black box such that when given a quantum state (as many-body configuration parameters), it returns an amplitude and phase according a certain wavefunction of the parameters. The aim of quantum machine learning is to approximate the computational black box with a neural network, trained to best represent the wavefunction given the many-body quantum state inputs. In this example, the neural network encodes a many-body quantum state of $N$ spins. For each value of the many-body spin configuration received as input, the artificial neural network computes the value of the wavefunction.

There can be different choices of neural network architecture based on the task at hand. A straightforward choice in classical machine learning is a restricted Boltzmann machine with reinforcement learning. The restricted Boltzmann machine is selected as it has a standard neural network structure with hidden layers which can be used to find unseen correlations in the data. A reinforcement learning model is used because supervised learning with labeled data is not an option as samples for the exact wavefunction are unknown. The neural network is used to describe a standard quantum system (a spin ½ (fermionic) quantum system).

The restricted Boltzmann machine neural network is constituted by one visible layer of $N$ nodes, corresponding to the physical spin variables in a chosen basis, and a single hidden layer of auxiliary (hidden) spin variables. In this restricted Boltzmann machine configuration, there is a single hidden layer of auxiliary spin variables (later, in running the neural network, the hidden variables density is set to four). This network description corresponds to a variational expression for the quantum states. The hidden spin variables and the parameter weights fully specify the response of the network to a given input state and are used to determine the wavefunction. The network weights are necessarily complex-valued in order to provide a complete description of the amplitude and phase of the wavefunctions. The input to the neural network is a quantum state and the output (response) is a specific amplitude and phase for a wavefunction that describes that quantum state at that moment. In the restricted Boltzmann machine, the first layer of the neural network receives the inputs. Coefficients (weights) are attached to these inputs and a linear combination of the weighted inputs are passed (fed forward) to the hidden layer. The quantum machine learning steps are listed in Table 16.8.

#### 16.2.1.5 *Neural network mathematics*

Representation theory provides the mathematical justification for the neural network's ability to represent quantum states that describe intricate many-body wavefunctions. Established representability theorems suggest valid network approximations of high-dimensional functions, provided a sufficient level of smoothness and regularity is met in the function to be approximated (Le Roux & Bengio, 2008). In most physically relevant situations, the many-body wavefunction reasonably satisfies these requirements. Therefore, a neural network representation of quantum states should be broadly applicable.

One of the advantages of the neural network quantum states representation is that the quality of the network can be systematically improved upon by increasing the number of hidden variables. The correlations induced by the hidden units are intrinsically non-local in space and are therefore well suited to describe quantum systems in arbitrary dimension.

Table 16.8. Implementations steps: Quantum state neural network.

| | |
|---|---|
| 1 | Describe quantum system with $N$ discrete-valued degrees of freedom (e.g. spin) |
| 2 | Encode quantum states based on this description to use in variational methods |
| 3 | Choose machine learning architecture: Restricted Boltzmann machine (hidden layers) with reinforcement learning (unlabeled data) |
| 4 | Obtain data: Apply variational methods to encoded quantum states to guess possible wavefunction amplitudes and phases to use as neural network input |
| 5 | Obtain algorithm: Write an expression for the quantum many-body state with neural network theorems |
| 6 | Run the neural network to solve specific problems such as ground state energy |
| 6a | Static case: Recapitulate known spin models: The transverse-field Ising model and the antiferromagnetic Heisenberg model |
| 6b | Time-dependent case: Recapitulate quantum quenches in the coupling constants of two spin models (spin polarization and nearest-neighbor correlations) |

The number of hidden variables in neural network models plays a role analogous to the bond dimension in tensor networks. Another benefit of the neural network quantum states representation is that it can be formulated in a symmetry-conserving fashion. For example, lattice translation symmetry can be used to reduce the number of variational parameters in the quantum state ansatz in the neural network. An architecture using stacks of convolutional restricted Boltzmann machines for shift-invariant feature learning has demonstrated this possibility.

From this theoretical background, neural network theorems are used to write a machine learning algorithm that provides the general expression for the quantum many-body state. The algorithm is implemented with the neural network and used to solve specific quantum many-body problems based on the machine learning of the network parameters (quantum state information). In the most interesting applications, the exact many-body state is unknown, and it is traditionally found by solving the static or time-dependent Schrödinger equation for a given Hamiltonian. In such a case without samples for the exact wavefunction, it is not possible to find it with supervised learning. Therefore, a reinforcement learning approach is used in which the wavefunction is learned on the basis of feedback from variational principles.

#### 16.2.1.6 *Demonstration: Quantum spin systems' ground states*

To demonstrate the accuracy of the neural network quantum states representation in the description of complex many-body quantum states, the work first focuses on the goal of finding the best neural network representation of the unknown ground state of a given Hamiltonian. A reinforcement learning model is implemented to minimize the expectation value of the energy with respect to the network weights. This is achieved with an iterative scheme. At each iteration, a Monte Carlo sampling is taken for a given set of parameters. At the same time, stochastic estimates of the energy gradient are obtained. The energy gradient estimates are used to propose the next set of weights for an improved gradient descent optimization. The overall computational cost of this approach is comparable to that of standard ground state quantum Monte Carlo simulations. The iterative variational method means that it is not necessary to know a network weight at the outset. The method is to start by picking any possibly relevant weight, determine if a rational energy calculation is obtained, and use that for the next iteration to see if the result is any better than the others, meanwhile building the gradient as a grid of the guesses.

The quantum state neural network method is validated in the test problem of finding the ground states in two prototypical known spin models, the transverse-field Ising model and the antiferromagnetic Heisenberg model. The Ising and Heisenberg models are considered in the case of both one-dimensional and two-dimensional lattices with periodic boundary conditions. The optimal neural network structure is obtained for the ground states of the two spin models for a neural network hidden variables density of four and with imposed translational symmetries. The finding is that each filter (layer) learns specific correlation features emerging in the ground state wavefunction. For example, in the two-dimensional case, the neural network learns patterns corresponding to anti-ferromagnetic correlations. The general behavior of the quantum state neural network is analogous to that observed in convolutional neural networks (CNNs), in which different layers similarly learn specific structures of the input data. In the quantum state neural network, feature maps act as effective filters on the spin configurations, to capture the most important quantum correlations.

#### 16.2.1.7 *Neural network-tensor network comparison*

Machine learning algorithms can be implemented with different structural platforms (namely, kernel learning, neural networks, and tensor networks). The neural network approach used here is compared with tensor networks. The number of hidden variables in a neural network is analogous to the bond dimension in a tensor network. Both mean the degree of precision in the network needed to achieve accuracy. The antiferromagnetic Heisenberg model is compared in two cases. First considering the antiferromagnetic Heisenberg model (one-dimensional lattice) with periodic boundary conditions, the finding is that a standard tensor network implementation (DMRG: density matrix renormalization group) would need a bond dimension of 160 to reach the same level of accuracy obtained with a hidden variables density of four in the neural network model. This suggests that a more compact representation of quantum many-body states might be available with neural networks, in particular requiring three orders of magnitude fewer variational parameters than the corresponding matrix product state ansatz in tensor networks.

Second, the antiferromagnetic Heisenberg model is considered on a two-dimensional square lattice. The finding is that the neural network algorithm with the low hidden unit density (four) compares favorably with more sophisticated tensor network models (EPS and PEPS: entangled pair states and projected entangled pair states) used for finite cluster analysis. A further result is that increasing the hidden unit density leads to a sizable improvement and consequently yields the best variational results reported so far for the two-dimensional antiferromagnetic Heisenberg model on finite lattices. Overall, when compared with tensor networks, the quantum state neural network allows intrinsically nonlocal correlations which might lead to more compact representations of many-body quantum states.

#### 16.2.1.8 *Demonstration: Time-dependent quantum dynamics*

Having initiated the quantum state neural network to solve unknown ground state problems, it is next applied to the more complicated time-dependent Schrödinger equation, in problems with known results. In this case, complex-valued and time-dependent network weights are defined which are trained to best reproduce the quantum dynamics at each moment in time. The Dirac–Frenkel time-dependent variational principle is used. The variational residuals are the objective functions to be minimized as a function of the time derivatives of the weights. In the stochastic framework, this is achieved by a time-dependent variational Monte Carlo method which samples at each time and provides the best stochastic estimate of the weights that minimize the function and computational cost. The time derivatives are used to obtain the structure of the complete time evolution of the quantum system.

To demonstrate the effectiveness of the quantum state neural network in the dynamical context, the unitary dynamics induced by quantum quenches in the coupling constants of the two different spin models are considered. In the transverse-field Ising model, nontrivial quantum dynamics are introduced by means of an instantaneous change in the transverse-field. The system is initially prepared in the ground state of the transverse-field Ising model for some transverse-field, and then let to evolve under the action of the Hamiltonian. The results are compared with the analytical solution obtained from the fermionization of the transverse-field Ising model for a one-dimensional chain with periodic boundary conditions. The quantum state neural network results recapitulate the known exact results for time-dependent transverse spin polarization. An alternative approach is used to assess system dynamics via quantum quenching in the antiferromagnetic Heisenberg model. In this case, quantum quenches in the longitudinal coupling are noted while monitoring the time evolution of nearest-neighbor correlations. Again, the results for the time evolution compare favorably with known numerically exact dynamics (produced with matrix product states) for a system with open boundaries (Vidal, 2004).

#### 16.2.1.9 *Implications of quantum state neural networks*

The quantum state neural network demonstrated in this work suggests that variational quantum states based on neural networks can be used to efficiently capture the complexity of entangled many-body systems both in one and two dimensions. The restricted Boltzmann machines used here are relatively simple (with a hidden variables density of four and imposed translational symmetries), yet produce accurate results for both ground state and dynamical properties of prototypical spin models. The high accuracy obtained for the unitary dynamics confirms that neural network-based approaches can be used to solve quantum many-body problems for both ground state properties and excited quantum states. These problems have been traditionally inaccessible to quantum Monte Carlo methods. However, the neural network representation allows for an effective solution of the sign problem that has hampered these kinds of stochastic schemes based on Feynman path integrals. In later work, the quantum state neural network approach is extended beyond interacting spin systems to study strongly coupled fermionic systems on a lattice (Stokes *et al.*, 2020). The ground state of spinless fermions on a square lattice is approximated with nearest-neighbor interactions. The neural network approach compares favorably with exact diagonalization results for energy-based and correlation functions in small systems.

## 16.3 Quantum Transformer Neural Networks

Aside from the approximation of wavefunctions and energy levels, the other main class of quantum machine learning applications applied to quantum mechanical problems is simulation and benchmarking. The characterization and validation of quantum systems is crucial for establishing the capability of quantum computing. Methods typically proceed by reconstructing the density matrix of quantum states. The density matrix is a matrix representation of the statistical state of a quantum system, as the (more complicated) quantum version of the classical probability distribution.

Quantum states can be measured with tomography or simulated with classical systems, including with machine learning methods. In quantum state tomography, the density matrix is reconstructed from projective measurements on identically prepared copies of the quantum state (Paris & Rehacek, 2004). However, tomography is limited in technical capacity for examining the exponential Hilbert space of many-body states. Exact tomography techniques (such as maximum likelihood estimation) are slow and costly, and thus many experiments rely on indirect methods for error determination, and use randomized benchmarking. Instead, simulating quantum states on classical computers with machine learning techniques is a promising alternative, and suggests the expedient processing of density matrix reconstruction and analysis.

These kinds of machine learning approaches, namely, deep neural networks and generative models, have been suggested for overcoming the curse of dimensionality in quantum state analysis. As discussed, Carleo and Troyer (2017) set the foundation for this approach by training a restricted Boltzmann machine to represent complex quantum many-body states. However, the expressibility of restricted Boltzmann machines and the scalability of training are often restricted to pure, positive quantum states and small mixed states, which limits their applicability at the scale of modern noisy quantum computers.

To support NISQ device analysis, Carrasquilla *et al.* (2019) implement a transformer neural network-based model to generate and simulate quantum state data, and extend the model to analyze real-life quantum state data (3-qubit GHZ state data) published by IBMQ (Cha *et al.*, 2020). The latter work proposes attention-based quantum tomography which adopts elements of the transformer neural network, a generative deep neural network for natural language processing, to the task of quantum state tomography. The attention-based quantum tomography approach reconstructs a 6-qubit GHZ state and tests up to 90-qubit systems, indicating agreement with the traditional measurement of maximum likelihood estimation. GHZ states (Greenberg–Horne–Zeilinger) are entangled quantum states involving at least three subsystems (particle states, or qubits) that are used to encode quantum information. Platform agnostic, the team also proposes a tensor network-based model for quantum state tomography (Torlai *et al.*, 2020).

### 16.3.1 *Transformer attention mechanism*

The transformer neural network is a novel form of neural network used in natural language processing (Vaswani *et al.*, 2017). Transformer-based natural language models such as GPT-3 (Generative Pre-trained Transformer 3) are autoregressive language models that use deep learning to produce human-like text that is nearly indistinguishable from human-written examples, the risks of which are debated (Brown *et al.*, 2020). In the less controversial domain of quantum state analysis, the same probability features that are commonly used in language modeling and translation prove equally conducive to the study of quantum mechanics.

The transformer neural network is based on a deep learning model, but uses a probability-based attention mechanism as opposed to convolution or recurrence as in the traditional models of neural networks (CNNs) and recurrent neural networks (RNNs)). Sequence transduction in the usual RNN-based processing of natural language is a sequentially constrained memory function that is restricted to short-range correlations in the input data. Instead, the transformer neural network uses an attention-based mechanism to study the correlations between all words in a sentence simultaneously. The method is able to learn which long-range correlations between words are important to the overall meaning of the sentence, and effectively has access to both short-range and long-range correlations in the underlying data. The method is called "attention" because the algorithm determines which elements are important to pay attention to in attributing meaning. For each input read into the encoding block of the transformer neural network, the attention-based mechanism takes into account several inputs simultaneously and decides which ones are important by attributing different weights to them.

#### 16.3.1.1 *Transformer neural networks and quantum states*

The transformer neural network is a useful format for quantum state analysis for several reasons. First is the ability to model long-range correlations (often suppressed in other quantum state models for sequential analysis). Second is the autoregressive nature of the model which is good at managing series data by modeling the current values of a series as a function of past values, and has a finite dynamic response to time series input. Third is the attention-based mechanism which allows a high degree of parallelization for the required computations. Fourth is that information about the spatial structure of the problem can be encoded which was not possible in other models.

Cha *et al.* (2020) consider prototypical autoregressive models commonly used in neural machine translation and language modeling based on transformer encoder blocks. The central element in the transformer architecture is the attention-based mechanism. The attention-based mechanism takes an embedding of the measurement outcomes, and computes an auto-correlation matrix in which the different measurement outcomes across the different qubits form the columns and rows. The embedding is a linear transformation performed on the original input. The attention-based mechanism and its correlation matrix are used to introduce correlations between qubits separated at any distance in the quantum system. This is analogous to a two-body Jastrow factor which likewise introduces pairwise long-distance correlations between the degrees of freedom (i.e. spins, qubits, electrons) in a wavefunction. In contrast to traditional sequential models based on RNNs (which suppress correlations beyond a certain length), attention-based networks are able to model systems exhibiting power-law correlations present in natural sequences as well as physical systems exhibiting (classical or quantum) critical behavior.

As in the main transformer neural network formulation, the attention-based mechanism is executed as a map between a query array, a key array and a value, and an output vector. The input is a query, weighted by some key-value. The query, keys, and values are linear transformations of the input vectors. The linear transformations give a dimensional embedding of the measurement outcomes at the different qubits as a parameter of the model. Analogously, the values and queries are calculated as a parameterized linear transformation on the embedding. The primary attention mechanism used is in the form of a scaled dot-product. The input consists of queries, dimensional keys, and dimensional values, and the output is computed with a softmax (rescaling) function. The softmax function acts on the vector results of softmax-related matrix operations. The argument of the softmax function induces pairwise, all-to-all correlations between the qubits in the system. This resembles a Jastrow factor (a factor used for factorizing or simplifying quantum mechanical calculations). An efficient sampling scheme is used to update the transformer neural network after each gate application within the quantum circuit. The sampling scheme works well for a large number of qubits simulations with up to 90-qubit systems demonstrated.

Other aspects specific to the quantum state simulation network include a multi-head attention mechanism (with eight attention heads) so that instead of computing a single attention function, the queries, keys and values are projected multiple times with different, learned linear projections. Each projection is followed by the attention function in parallel. The network architecture is a fully connected position-wise feed-forward network. The general layer structure is two linear transformations with a ReLU (rectified linear unit; square-shaped not s-shaped) activation in between. Each sublayer (which consists of the attention-based mechanism and the position-wise feed-forward mechanism) is followed by a layer normalization step. Since the transformer neural network model does not contain recurrence or convolutions, an enhancement is made to include information about the spatial ordering of the qubits by adding enhanced positional encodings to the input embeddings. The last element of the transformer neural network is a linear layer followed by a softmax activation that outputs the conditional distribution. Several transformer neural network layers can be used together to improve the expressiveness of the model, however, the one-layer transformer encoder architecture is sufficient for modeling the relevant distributions in the test cases. The model is trained using the Adam Optimizer in Pytorch.

#### 16.3.1.2 *The attention mechanism*

The network architecture of the transformer neural network is as follows. As in other neural sequence transduction models, there is an encoder-decoder structure. The encoder maps an input sequence of symbol representations to a sequence of continuous representations. The decoder generates an output sequence of symbols one element at a time. At each step, the model is autoregressive in the sense of consuming the previously generated symbols as additional input when generating the next input. The transformer neural network follows this general architecture using stacked attention-based mechanisms and point-wise fully connected layers for both the encoder and decoder.

The attention function is defined as mapping a query and a set of key-value pairs to an output, in which the query, keys, values, and output are all vectors. The output is computed as a weighted sum of the values, in which the weight assigned to each value is computed by a compatibility function of the query with the corresponding key.

The two most commonly used attention functions are additive attention and dot-product (multiplicative) attention. In a scaled dot-product attention function, the input consists of queries, keys, and values (Vaswani *et al.*, 2017, p. 3). The dot products of the query with all keys are computed and a softmax function is applied to obtain the weights on the values. Softmax is a function frequently used in machine learning that exponentiates and rescales a set of numbers so that they sum to one. The attention function is then computed on a set of queries simultaneously, packed together into a matrix. The keys and values are also packed together into matrices. The overall attention value is computed as the weighted average of the softmax applied to an expression of the query, key, and value matrices. A multi-head attention function can be used to compute the attention function in parallel, rather than the network being limited to performing a single attention function at a time.

## References

Benedetti, M., Garcia-Pintos, D., Perdomo, O. *et al.* (2019). A generative modeling approach for benchmarking and training shallow quantum circuits. *NPJ Quantum Inf.* 5(45):1–9.

Bradley, T.-D., Stoudenmire, E.M. & Terilla, J. (2019). Modeling sequences with quantum states: A look under the hood. *Mach. Learn.: Sci. Technol.* 1:035008.

Broughton, M., Verdon, G., McCourt, T. *et al.* (2020). TensorFlow quantum: A software framework for quantum machine learning. arXiv:2003.02989v1.

Brown, T.B., Mann, B., Ryder, N. *et al.* (2020). Language models are few-shot learners. arXiv:2005.14165.

Carleo, G. & Troyer, M. (2017). Solving the quantum many-body problem with artificial neural networks. *Science.* 355(6325):602–26.

Carrasquilla, J. & Melko, R.G. (2017). Machine learning phases of matter. *Nat. Phys.* 13(5):431–4.

Carrasquilla, J., Torlai, G., Melko, R.G. & Aolita, L. (2019). Reconstructing quantum states with generative models. *Nat. Mach. Intel.* 1:155–61.

Cha, P., Ginsparg, P., Wu, F. *et al.* (2020). Attention-based quantum tomography. arXiv:2006.12469.

Cheng, S., Chen, J. & Wang L. (2018). Information perspective to probabilistic modeling: Boltzmann machines versus Born machines. *Entropy.* 20(8):583.

Cottrell, W., Freivogel, B., Hofman, D.M. & Lokhande, S.F. (2019). How to build the thermofield double state. *J. High Energ. Phys.* 1902:058.

Eisert, J., Friesdorf, M. & Gogolin, C. (2015). Quantum many-body systems out of equilibrium. *Nat. Phys.* 11:124–30.

Farhi, E. & Neven, H. (2018). Classification with quantum neural networks on near term processors. arXiv:1802.06002. MIT-CTP/4985.

Freericks, J.K., Nikolic, B.K. & Frieder, O. (2014). The nonequilibrium quantum many-body problem as a paradigm for extreme data science. *Int. J. Mod. Phys. B.* 28:1430021.

Grant, E., Benedetti, M., Cao, S., *et al.* (2018). Hierarchical quantum classifiers. *NPJ Quantum Inf.* 4(65):1–8.

Han, X. & Hartnoll, S.A. (2020). Deep quantum geometry of matrices. *Phys. Rev. X.* 10(011069).

Han, X., Hartnoll, S.A. & Kruthoff, J. (2020). Bootstrapping matrix quantum mechanics. *Phys. Rev. Lett.* 125(041601).

Hassabis, D., Kumaran, D., Summerfield, C. & Botvinick, M. (2017). Neuroscience-inspired artificial intelligence. *Neuron.* 95:245–58.

Hu, H.-Y., Wu, D., You, Y.-Z. *et al.* (2020). RG-Flow: A hierarchical and explainable flow model based on renormalization group and sparse prior. arXiv: 2010.00029.

Huggins, W., Patel, P., Mitchell, B., *et al.* (2019). Towards quantum machine learning with tensor networks. *Quantum Sci. Technol.* 4(2):024001.

Le Roux, N. & Bengio, Y. (2008). Representational power of restricted Boltzmann machines and deep belief networks. *Neural. Comput.* 20:1631–49.

Lin, H.W., Tegmark, M. & Rolnick, D. (2017). Why does deep and cheap learning work so well? *J. Stat. Phys.* 168(6):1223–47.

Liu, D., Ran, S.-J., Wittek, P. *et al.* (2019). Machine learning by unitary tensor network of hierarchical tree structure. arXiv:1710.04833v4.

Martyn, J., Vidal, G., Roberts, C. & Leichenauer, S. (2020). Entanglement and tensor networks for supervised image classification. arXiv:2007.06082v1.

Montorsi, A. (1992). *The Hubbard Model: A Collection of Reprints*. London: World Scientific.

Paris, M. & Rehacek, J. (2004). *Quantum State Estimation*. Vol. 649. London: Springer Science & Business Media.

Reyes, J. & Stoudenmire, E.M. (2020). A multi-scale tensor network architecture for classification and regression. arXiv:2001.08286v1.

Schuld, M. & Killoran, N. (2019). Quantum machine learning in feature Hilbert spaces. *Phys. Rev. Lett.* 122(4):040504.

Schulte, P. & Lee, D.K.C. (2019). *AI & Quantum Computing for Finance & Insurance: Fortunes and Challenges for China and America*. Singapore: World Scientific.

Stokes, J., Moreno, J.R., Pnevmatikakis, E.A. *et al.* (2020). Phases of two-dimensional spinless lattice fermions with first-quantized deep neural-network quantum states. arXiv:2008.00118v1.

Stoudenmire, E.M. & Schwab, D.J. (2017). Supervised learning with quantum inspired tensor networks. *Adv. Neural. Info. Proc. Sys.* 29:4799.

Torlai, G., Wood, C.J., Acharya, A. *et al.* (2020). Quantum process tomography with unsupervised learning and tensor networks. arXiv:2006.02424.

Vaswani, A., Shazeer, N., Parmar, N. *et al.* (2017). Attention is all you need. In *NIPS'17: Proceedings of the 31st International Conference on Neural Information Processing Systems (NIPS 2017)*, Long Beach, CA, USA, December 4–9, 2017, pp. 6000–10.

Vidal, G. (2004). Efficient simulation of one-dimensional quantum many-body systems. *Phys. Rev. Lett.* 93(4):040502.

# Chapter 17

# Born Machine and Pixel = Qubit

*Born machines acknowledge the probabilistic interpretation of quantum mechanics*

— Cheng *et al.* (2018, p. 1)

**Abstract**

This chapter discusses probabilistic methods for quantum machine learning. One model is the Born machine which employs the Born rule to determine output probabilities (as opposed to the Boltzmann distribution-based energy function traditionally used in machine learning). Born machines are relevant to generative unsupervised (unlabeled data) learning, extending discriminative supervised learning approaches. Discriminative algorithms learn directly from data, but generative algorithms learn the distribution of the data to produce new samples. Reduced density matrices are used to rewrite classical probability distributions in quantum terms. A key insight is that pixel = spin (qubit) for point data, and wavelet = spin (qubit) for sequential data; an image pixel or wavelet equates to a spin value in a quantum system (qubit).

## 17.1 The Born Machine

Probability is central to machine learning. The chief aim of a machine learning algorithm is to learn the probability distribution of a dataset and write a function that describes these data such that it can make accurate guesses about unseen data. The canonical machine learning approach is the Boltzmann machine (Ackley *et al.*, 1985) which uses a probability model based on the Boltzmann distribution. The Born machine (Cheng *et al.*, 2018) is an alternative probabilistic model for machine learning that is based on the Born rule. Using the Born rule to determine output probabilities (rather than a Boltzmann distribution-based energy function) is proving successful in quantum machine learning, particularly to enable unsupervised generative learning models.

The Born machine reflects the contemporary awareness of the benefit of performing probabilistic modeling tasks with quantum-based methods, in particular by using the Born rule to find wavefunction probabilities. The Boltzmann machine and other machine learning approaches also use probability in many ways, including to assess the neural network performance with an energy-related measure based on the Boltzmann distribution. What is new is the idea of using quantum-based methods (the Born rule) to perform probability-related tasks. The instantiation of this idea is a new class of machine learning methods collectively called Born machines.

The Born machine incorporates the Born rule which is a solvable probabilistic formulation of quantum mechanics. The Born rule gives the probability that a measurement of a quantum system will have a certain result. Specifically, the rule is that the probability density of finding a particle at a given point is proportional to the square of the magnitude of the particle's wavefunction at that point (Born, 1926). The probabilistic interpretation of quantum mechanics naturally suggests modeling data distributions with a quantum state.

The advantages are that the Born machine is more quantum-compatible and more flexible than existing machine learning probability functions which are largely based on the Boltzmann distribution. The Born machine can operate on either classical or quantum data. The method translates input data into the form of a quantum state which the Born rule takes as input. A clear benefit of the Born machine is that it is by definition structured in a quantum mechanical format that is conducive to quantum computing implementation.

In general, a machine learning model is tasked with learning the probability distribution of input data. A probability equation is the functional form of the machine learning algorithm. In the Boltzmann machine (or traditional machine learning methods more generally), the probability distribution is modeled using an energy function. In the Born machine, the probability distribution is modeled using a quantum state. In the Boltzmann machine, the probability function equals the weighted sum of the observation values of the input data. In the Born machine, the probability function equals the weighted sum of the observation values of a quantum state (the expectation values of the observables that comprise a quantum state). Although structurally similar, the Born machine is able to treat quantum phenomena.

The Born machine is one of the latest proposals in wavefunction ansatz (guessing) methods. Various ansatz methods have been developed to express quantum states including variational Monte Carlo (random sampling), tensor network states, and artificial neural networks (Carleo & Troyer, 2017, discussed in the other chapter). In the Born rule, the wavefunction probability distributions are given by their squared norm. This eliminates the sign problem that makes other wavefunction ansatz such as Monte Carlo methods difficult to calculate.

Some of the research developments regarding Born machines are listed in Table 17.1. In terms of platform, Born machines are typically deployed on tensor networks (a quantum-compatible format) or directly onto quantum circuits. Subsequent work from the team proposing the Born machine discusses how to map a restricted Boltzmann machine to a tensor network to implement the Born machine (Chen *et al.*, 2018). Other work proposes a tensor network-based formulation of the Born machine for unsupervised generative learning (Han *et al.*, 2018) and a generic quantum circuit formulation of the Born machine (Liu & Wang, 2018).

Benedetti *et al.* (2018) propose a model of quantum circuit Born machines obtained by learning a GHZ (Greenberger–Horne–Zeilinger) state preparation process which could be deployed on NISQ devices such as an ion trap quantum computer. Glasser *et al.* (2019) propose a quantum circuit Born machine preparation based on factorization in which the network demonstrates better expressive power in the probabilistic

Table 17.1. Born machine research advances.

| No. | Research Advance | Reference |
|---|---|---|
| 1 | Introduce the Born machine | Cheng *et al.* (2018) |
| 2 | Map Boltzmann machine to Born machine | Chen *et al.* (2018) |
| 3 | Tensor network Born machines | Han *et al.* (2018) |
| 4 | Quantum circuit Born machines: Generic | Liu and Wang (2018) |
| 5 | Quantum circuit Born machines: GHZ state preparation | Benedetti *et al.* (2019) |
| 6 | Quantum circuit Born machines: Locally purified states | Glasser *et al.* (2019) |
| 7 | Quantum finance: Ion trap demonstration | Alcazar *et al.* (2020) |

interpretation of local quantum circuits. Alcazar *et al.* (2020) implement a generic quantum circuit Born machine for quantum finance, aimed at constructing portfolio optimization scenarios by using time series pricing data from the S&P500 stock market index.

### 17.1.1 *Boltzmann machine versus born machine*

The Boltzmann machine and the Born machine are two approaches to probabilistic modeling. The insight behind the Boltzmann machine is that probability distributions can be modeled by using an energy function according to the Boltzmann distribution. The insight underlying the Born machine is that probability distributions can be modeled by using a quantum state per the Born rule. The two methods are complementary. The Boltzmann machine is the traditional method aimed at supervised learning on classical platforms. The Born machine is a contemporary probabilistic method designed to accommodate unsupervised generative learning on quantum platforms. Conceptually, both methods target the same problem of trying to describe the emergent collective behavior of complex systems with a large number of degrees of freedom by identifying probability distributions in a large possibility space. The aim of both is to find a function that describes input data, generically a function with the Boltzmann machine, and specifically a wavefunction with the Born machine (Table 17.2).

Table 17.2. Boltzmann machine versus Born machine.

| Topic | Boltzmann Machine | Born Machine |
|---|---|---|
| Model characterization | Classical probabilistic model | Modern probabilistic model |
| Machine learning focus | Classical machine learning | Quantum machine learning |
| Learning domain | Supervised learning (discriminative algorithms) | Unsupervised learning (generative algorithms) |
| Approach derivation | Statistical physics | Quantum physics |
| Probability distribution | Energy-based model | Quantum state-based model |
| Probabilistic model | Boltzmann distribution | Born rule |
| Implied implementation | Classical platform: Neural networks, GPU | Quantum platform: Tensor networks, quantum circuits |
| Emblematic reference | Ackley *et al.* (1985) | Cheng *et al.* (2018) |

Originally proposed in 1985 (Ackley *et al.*, 1985), the Boltzmann machine has become the backbone of modern machine learning. Boltzmann machines are named after the Boltzmann distribution in statistical mechanics, which is used in the machine learning algorithm's sampling function, structured as an energy minimizing probability function. The energy-based function incorporates the Boltzmann distribution. The Boltzmann distribution is a probability distribution that gives the probability that a system is in a certain state as a function of the state's energy and the temperature of the system. The formula includes Boltzmann's constant ($k$B) as the proportionality factor that relates the average relative kinetic energy of particles in a gas with the thermodynamic temperature, and has a specific value of $1.380\ 649 \times 10^{-23}$ Joules-Kelvin$^{-1}$ (Tiesinga *et al.*, 2021, p. 025010–3). The Boltzmann distribution can be used to calculate various problems ranging from single atoms to a large container of gas. The distribution indicates that states with lower energy always have a higher probability of being occupied.

## 17.1.2 *Supervised versus unsupervised learning*

The Born machine can be used for wavefunction ansatz and also unsupervised generative learning. Statistical classification (machine learning) consists of two main strategies, the discriminative approach and the generative approach. Whereas discriminative algorithms learn directly from the data, generative algorithms learn the distribution of the data. Generative methods study how the probability of the data is generated, and from this, can generate or produce new samples (Goodfellow *et al.*, 2014). Generative methods can but do not necessarily create new data; the point is that the distribution is understood well enough to be able to generate additional samples.

The discriminative approach performs well in supervised learning, by classifying new data samples based on having learned from a labeled training dataset. However, most real-life data are not cleanly labeled and annotated as datasets conducive to supervised learning. Hence, generative modeling is a tool for characterizing unknown data by modeling probability distributions to elicit features, categories, dimension, and other attributes. Generative modeling may be able to identify natural features in datasets, and can use sampling methods which supervised learning cannot. The generative approach is thus being developed for unsupervised learning (Table 17.3).

In the canonical task of classification, the two approaches compute classifiers with different statistical modeling methods. Discriminative classifiers model the conditional probability distribution, or no distribution, whereas generative classifiers model the joint probability distribution. Discriminative algorithms learn directly from the data and then try to classify new data. Generative algorithms learn the distribution of the data,

Table 17.3. Supervised (discriminative) versus unsupervised (generative) learning.

| Topic | Discriminative | Generative |
|---|---|---|
| Learning domain | Supervised learning | Unsupervised learning |
| Model focus | Learn directly from data | Learn probability distribution of data |
| Probability focus | Model conditional probabilities | Model joint probabilities |
| Status | Established | Emerging and expanding |
| Notable examples | Ongoing results from labeled datasets: Iris, MNIST, ImageNet | Generative adversarial networks, variational autoregressive networks |

and then try to classify new data or produce new data. Discriminative algorithms may outperform on targeted classification and regression tasks, and generative algorithms perform better at characterizing unknown datasets. In general, the two classes of models are complementary views of the same procedure, either modeling the data directly (discriminative approach) or modeling the distribution of the data (generative approach). Generative modeling learns the joint probability distribution of data.

### 17.1.3 *Unsupervised generative learning*

Several quantum machine learning projects use the Born rule to determine the output probabilities, rather than a Boltzmann distribution-based energy function as in classical machine learning (Table 17.4). In quantum machine learning, datasets are often mapped to the basis vectors of a Hilbert space. Then the algorithm proceeds by learning the two-point correlations (joint probabilities in the generative model) between pairs of variables that are located at short or long distance from one another. First, Han *et al.* (2018) deploy a Born machine for unsupervised generative learning using matrix product states (a tensor network formulation) to model the probability distribution of unlabeled data samples. The probabilistic model is structured as a matrix product state, which allows for adaptive learning and direct sampling (which is not possible in classical machine learning). Once the matrix product state wavefunction is identified, learning is achieved by adjusting the parameters of the wavefunction such that the distribution represented by the Born rule is as close as

Table 17.4. Born machine implementation examples.

| No. | Project | Input Data | Platform |
|---|---|---|---|
| 1 | Unsupervised generative learning | Bit string samples from Bars and Stripes, MNIST | Tensor network Born machine |
| 2 | Generative modeling to train shallow quantum circuits (NISQ devices) | Quantum state data | Quantum circuit Born machine |
| 3 | Variational autoregressive networks | Bit string samples of thermal states | Quantum circuit Born machine |

possible to that of the data distribution. The generative modeling method is tested on standard datasets including Bars and Stripes (random binary patterns) and MNIST (handwritten digits). Data are translated to binary strings which are mapped to the basis vectors of a Hilbert space of dimension $2^n$. These are the input data for the matrix product state tensor network to model in terms of joint probability distribution interpreted with the Born rule.

Second, Benedetti *et al.* (2018) propose a hybrid quantum-classical approach for generative modeling on gate-based NISQ devices. The $2^n$ amplitudes of the wavefunction are obtained from an $n$-qubit quantum circuit designed to construct and capture the correlations observed in a dataset, and a Born rule is used to determine the output probabilities. The Born rule is implemented by simulating a quantum circuit executed on NISQ hardware. The method is tested by learning a GHZ state preparation process for an ion trap quantum computer. The method is further tested by training circuits to prepare approximations of thermal states (which demonstrates the power of Born machines to approximate Boltzmann machines when the data have thermal-related features). The method might be implemented to prepare GHZ states and approximations of thermal states on NISQ platforms.

Third, the further reach of the Born machine approach can be seen in Liu *et al.*'s (2019) work in studying thermal quantum states. Born machines are good for the quantum machine learning of classical data, and also for the quantum machine learning of quantum problems involving thermal data that are inaccessible with other models. Liu *et al.*'s (2019) approach extends the variational quantum eigensolver (VQE) to accommodate thermal quantum states. The algorithm uses a variational autoregressive network to generate bit string samples of thermal states as input quantum states for the quantum circuit. The Born machine approach is used to interpret probability distribution results. Thermal observables can be examined such as variational free energy, entropy, and heat. A variational ansatz is obtained for the density matrix. The resulting model allows the ability to perform variational free energy calculations over density matrices efficiently. Applications of the approach are demonstrated for systems with thermal properties and excitations of quantum lattice models.

#### 17.1.3.1 *Born machine implications for quantum computing*

Studying quantum mechanical systems (both baseline ground states and higher energy levels in the form of thermal states) presents a variety of challenges to classical computational approaches. First, classical algorithms generally encounter the difficulties of diagonalizing (effectively representing in a matrix form) exponentially large Hamiltonians. Second, classical algorithms confront the sign problem that originates from the quantum nature of the problem. Third, even if the system can be written on an eigenbasis (factorized basis), there is still an intractable partition function (the configuration integral of all correlation functions in a quantum system) which involves the summation of an exponentially large number of terms.

Quantum computing offers an attractive alternative for solving a number of these problems and modeling the complexities of thermal states in quantum mechanical systems. The most straightforward way to address the difficulties of classical computing is to directly realize the physical Hamiltonian on an analog quantum device and study the system at thermal equilibrium (van Houcke *et al.*, 2012). Such an approach has been demonstrated in the observation of topological phenomena in a programmable lattice of 1,800 qubits (King *et al.*, 2018). However, this entails storing the entire wavefunction, which with $2^n$ complex numbers, is not a scalable method.

A more general approach to quantum computing would be to study thermal properties with a universal gate model quantum computer. To accommodate the ground state, numerous modeling projects have been proposed. However, for more complex thermal systems at higher energy levels and away from equilibrium, additional algorithmic innovations are needed to prepare thermal quantum states on quantum circuits, particularly taking into account their unitary nature. As one example, quantum algorithms have been proposed for preparing thermal Gibbs states on quantum computers (Terhal & DiVincenzo, 2000). Unfortunately, even a straightforward Gibbs state may not be feasible on NISQ devices with limited circuit depth. In a more complicated example, a variational quantum algorithm is proposed for preparing thermofield double states (Wu & Hsieh, 2018), but implementation still requires additional quantum resources such as ancilla qubits, as well as measuring and extrapolating Rényi entropies which are not feasible with NISQ devices. Further, assessing quantum time evolution in dynamical systems requires methods such as performing exponentially difficult tomography (quantum state reconstruction) on a growing number of qubits and the synthesis of multi-qubit unitaries.

To facilitate the modeling of more complex quantum systems such as thermal states, Martyn and Swingle (2019) develop an approach to prepare the thermal density matrix as a classical mixture of quantum pure states in the eigenbasis. The approach is useful for addressing certain situations. However, in this and other related proposals, the classical probabilistic model is either assumed to be factorized or expressed as an energy-based model (Boltzmann machine). The result is that the factorized distribution is only an approximation of the Gibbs distribution in the eigenbasis. Energy-based models thus still face the problem of an intractable partition function which prevents the method from adequately sampling and learning.

Instead, the Born machine as a generative method might offer a solution to the intractable partition function since the goal of generative modeling is to directly represent, learn, and sample from complex high-dimensional probability distributions (Liu *et al.*, 2019). Examples of generative models including autoregressive models, variational autoencoders, and generative adversarial networks have been demonstrated classically. For the quantum context, autoregressive models stand out since they support an unbiased gradient estimator for discrete variables, direct sampling, and tractable likelihood at the same time. The autoregressive models have reached state-of-the-art performance in modeling realistic data and found real-world applications in synthesizing natural speech and images. Variational optimization of the autoregressive network has been used for classical statistical physics problems. Quantum generalization of the autoregressive network has also been employed for ground state analysis of quantum many-body systems (Sharir *et al.*, 2019).

Liu *et al.* (2019) propose and approach that combines quantum circuits and classical autoregressive neural networks. The combined model parametrizes a variational density matrix as a classical mixture of quantum pure states, and the autoregressive network generates bit string samples as input states to the quantum circuit. One result is that the VQE is extended to accommodate thermal quantum states. The Born machine approach is used to interpret probability distribution results. Thermal observables can be examined such as variational free energy, entropy, and heat. A variational ansatz is obtained for the density matrix. The resulting model allows variational free energy calculations to be performed over density matrices efficiently. Applications of the approach are demonstrated for systems with thermal properties and excitations of quantum lattice models.

The quantum circuit acts as a canonical transformation that brings the density matrix to a diagonal representation. Also, since the circuit approximately diagonalizes the density matrix, it can be used for other purposes such as accelerated time evolution (Cirstoiu *et al.*, 2020). One use of the approach could be to study the thermal properties of frustrated quantum systems which are otherwise prevented by the sign problem. It is also possible to employ the qubit efficient VQE scheme developed by Huggins *et al.* (2019) to study the thermal properties of quantum many-body systems on a quantum computer with the number of qubits being smaller than the number of degrees of freedom. In this scenario, the ansatz for the density matrix is a classical mixture of matrix product states. Variational ansatz for the density matrix can also be used in the quantum algorithm for nonequilibrium dynamics and steady states.

## 17.2 Probabilistic Methods: Reduced Density Matrix

The Born machine is one example of the bigger theme of probabilistic quantum models that use quantum-based methods to perform probability-related tasks such as machine learning. There is a thought progression from merely considering the encoding of a binary-valued qubit in a quantum circuit to having in mind a full-blown quantum state. A quantum state is all of the statistical information that describes a quantum system, namely, vectors of potential particle movement in a complex Hilbert space. One of the first steps toward the quantum state mindset is Cheng *et al.*'s (2018) noticing that the quantum mechanical Born rule can be used to determine the output probabilities in a machine learning algorithm. Then Bradley *et al.* (2019) notice that classical probability distributions can be modeled using quantum states. This quickly becomes standard as

Martyn *et al.* (2020) encode classical data into a quantum state as the routine process of embedding data into an exponentially large vector space, in which the vectors are wavefunctions that are tensor products that can be taken up easily by a quantum machine learning platform. What is different compared to earlier quantum machine learning implementations (Farhi & Neven, 2018; Grant *et al.*, 2018) is that whereas the earlier focus was encoding qubits, the later focus is encoding a quantum state. To perform more sophisticated applications with a quantum computer, the input data must be encoded in a quantum state.

### 17.2.1 *Modeling classical data with quantum states*

Bradley *et al.* (2019) propose an algorithm for unsupervised generative learning based on a standard setup for a density matrix renormalization group (DMRG) tensor network model. The same formalism that is used to interpret the wavefunction in quantum mechanics is employed as a framework to treat classical data, and further, take advantage of the quantum entanglement formulation to identify otherwise inaccessible correlations in classical data.

The mathematical problem of interest is determining the probability distribution of a generic set of sequences from a finite set of samples. Obtaining such probability distributions on datasets is a first and obvious analysis function in the characterization of data. A key insight is that classical probability distributions can be modeled using quantum states. The work models classical input data with quantum states (both pure and entangled) and machine learns the probability distributions. Mathematically, the idea is to transition from finite sets to functions on finite sets. Functions on sets have more structure (such as entanglement) than the sets themselves, and the extra structure is meaningful.

The work is part of the ongoing shift from classical computing to quantum computing. The expansion from finite sets to functions on finite sets is relevant to quantum problem formulation because functions on finite sets have a natural Hilbert space structure. The work employs two known probabilistic quantum reformulations: The reduced density matrix as the quantum version of the marginal probability distribution, and the partial trace as the quantum version of marginalization (Table 17.5).

Table 17.5. Comparison: Classical-quantum statistics.

| No. | Classical Statistics | Quantum Statistics |
|---|---|---|
| 1 | Finite sets | Functions on finite sets |
| 2 | Fixed space structure | Hilbert space structure |
| 3 | Probability distribution | Density matrix |
| *Complexity reduction techniques* | | |
| 4 | Marginal probability distribution | Reduced density matrix |
| 5 | Marginalization | Partial trace |

The quantum version of the standard classical statistical probability distribution is the density matrix. The density matrix results from a density operator acting on the Hilbert space of the system, and provides the information describing a quantum state, in a statistical format. Complexity reduction techniques are applied to reduce unwieldy statistical models in both the classical and quantum setting. In classical statistics, a marginal probability distribution is often calculated to approximate the salient attributes of the data as opposed to computing the full probability distribution which may be costly and unfeasible. The quantum version of the marginal probability distribution is the reduced density matrix, which is generated by a reduced density operator. The distinction is that the reduced density matrix holds enough information to reconstruct the entire joint probability distribution whereas the marginal probability distribution does not. The upshot is that the quantum approach is more effective at modeling classical probability distributions than classical methods.

### 17.2.1.1 *Quantum entanglement found in classical data*

The reduced density matrix contains more information than the marginal distribution. Since there is entanglement in quantum states, the reduced density matrix that describes the subsystems in the quantum system includes entanglement (information about relationships between complementary subsystems). This is in contrast to the classical picture in which the marginal probability distribution integrates out any information about complementary subsystems. From a quantum information-theoretic perspective, the reduced density matrix is a less-lossy form of information compression than the marginal probability distribution and may contain both short-range and long-range correlations. The additional information (entanglement) preserved in the reduced density matrix can be used to study the system in greater depth. Classical data would not be thought to have entanglement, but applying the quantum entanglement formalism, indeed correlations in the underlying data may be accessed.

The result is that classical data and classical probability distributions can be modeled with quantum states and exploited with the concept of entanglement. The ability to exploit quantum entanglement allows more system information to be encoded naturally in the model, and this leads to an enhanced ability to analyze the system of interest. The premise is that extra information is included in the quantum encoding structure in the reduced densities (in a richer but more compact format). The innovation is that with probabilistic quantum methods, quantum entanglement can be used to reveal correlations in classical data.

#### 17.2.1.2 *Practical implementation*

In Bradley *et al.*'s (2019) implementation, the data are a generic set of sequences from a finite set of samples in classical data, represented as reduced density matrices, in which entanglement is preserved. The machine learning network and machine learning algorithm are the standard setup also used in the team's other work (Stoudenmire & Schwab 2017; Reyes & Stoudenmire, 2020). The machine learning network is a matrix product state tensor network. The machine learning network is trained with an adaptive algorithm (using alternating least squares) based on the DMRG algorithm.

Entanglement, as the "extra information" available in the quantum method of the reduced density matrix as compared to the classical marginal probability distribution, is useful both for studying the underlying system and the model. In this case, the underlying system is the classical data encoded as quantum states such that entanglement reveals correlations that are not accessible with classical methods. The model is the tensor network, built to incorporate entanglement in the modeling of quantum many-body systems. Entanglement as the renormalized quantity in the quantum states instantiated in the tensor network model reveals other kinds of information about the model. The training algorithm uses entanglement as feedback information contained in the reduced densities that allows the mechanics the algorithm to be refined by tabulating the generalization error of the resulting model. The feedback information (entanglement) is further used to produce an error estimate for the training.

#### 17.2.1.3 *Advantages of probabilistic quantum methods*

Several benefits of quantum machine learning on tensor networks with probabilistic quantum methods are demonstrated. First, probabilistic quantum methods allow the creation of better models that do not integrate out relevant information. This leads to data compression as the second advantage. For quantum data, including a renormalization quantity such as entanglement allows the system to be compressed so that it may be tractably computed. For classical data, entanglement allows the system to be compressed such that it contains a richer level of information about relationships within the system for a greater level of computation about the system. From a practical perspective, probabilistic quantum methods can be used to construct efficient information compression protocols for the transfer of quantum information. Third, an important benefit of using tensor networks as opposed to neural networks for machine learning is their transparency. Tensor networks can be viewed as a sequence of related linear maps, which act together on a high-dimensional space. This allows generates a machine learning model which is particularly expressive, and can be investigated to assess which architectural effects are having the greatest contribution. The probabilistic quantum methods are portable to other machine learning techniques, including because the linear operations of the tensor network can be inspected (unlike the usual "black box" of machine learning methods).

### 17.2.2 *Density matrices and density operators*

The density matrix is the quantum analog to the classical probability distribution. The density matrix is a matrix that describes the statistical state of a quantum system in complete detail. Using density matrices is complicated but unavoidable since even if an overall system might be in a pure state, the various subsystems that comprise it might be in a variety of mixed states (states that are written as a combination of other states). Hence, a density matrix is used to describe the state of the composite system. Since a quantum system cannot be observed directly, the density matrix describes the system state as produced by the density operator. The density operator acts on the system to produce expectation values of system observables to generate the overall system state. The density matrix is the overall state, and the density operator produces the overall state.

The density matrix is a representation of all possible information about a quantum state or system. Since the density matrix is comprehensive and elaborate, a reduced density matrix distilled from the overall system may be better for addressing a particular problem. Dirac proposed the notion of the reduced density matrix in 1930. The reduced density matrix is the partial trace of the density matrix. The reduced density matrix is calculated as the partial trace of the density matrix with fewer complex coefficients. For example, the state vectors in the full system might have over a hundred complex coefficients but the reduced density operator has only four. The reduced density operator describes the properties of the system leaving parts of it unobserved. Just as the density operator is used to produce the density matrix, the reduced density operator is used to produce the reduced density matrix. The reduced density operator describes the state of a composite system by reducing pure states and mixed states with many complex coefficients using a partial trace of the matrix.

The DMRG tensor network structure is designed specifically to accommodate the complexity of quantum mechanical system density matrices. The DMRG is extended to the calculation of reduced density matrices and partial trace matrix operations as the quantum analogs in complexity reduction. In classical probability distribution modeling, the marginal distribution is the probability distribution of a subset of variables without reference to other variables in the system (this contrasts with the conditional distribution which includes the relationships of the subset of variables with the other variables in the system). Marginalization is the technique of marginalizing or discarding the variables that are not needed for a particular analysis as a complexity reduction technique. The corresponding technique to marginalization in the quantum domain is the partial trace in the sense that the reduced density matrix is calculated as the partial trace of the density matrix with fewer complex coefficients.

## 17.3 Tensor Networks: Pixel = Spin (Qubit)

Stoudenmire and Schwab (2017) propose one of the first machine learning implementations using tensor networks. A key insight is that an image pixel equates to a spin value in a quantum system (and hence its later translatability to a qubit in a quantum computing environment). The program includes a quantum-inspired tensor network model for supervised machine learning, using tensor networks to encode pixel data as qubits or spins, and an adaptive loss function for the weight tensor. The work demonstrates how algorithms for optimizing tensor networks can be translated to supervised learning tasks by using matrix product states (or tensor trains) to parametrize models for classifying images. The method is tested on the MNIST dataset (handwritten images) with a classification error of less than one percent.

### 17.3.1 *Decomposition of high-dimensional vectors*

The broad problem space is reducing the high dimensionality of the large vectors that arise in many areas of both quantum mechanical science (for example, chemistry, condensed matter, and materials science) and machine learning. The solution is simplifying more complicated problems into smaller solvable ones. Precisely one such a strategy for manipulating large vectors in quantum mechanics is decomposing them into a tensor network representation. Tensor networks incorporate low-order tensors, which yet still accurately reproduce high-order tensors through a particular geometry of tensor contractions.

Tensor networks are a strategy for truncating the possibility space into salient prospects. The idea behind tensor networks is decomposing a large tensor into contractions of smaller tensors. In a graph-theoretic representation, the tensors are the network nodes and the contractions are the lines (edges) connecting them. Consequently, a large tensor, under a decomposition, becomes a network. The wavefunction is precisely a large and unwieldy tensor in the form of $2^n$ complex numbers. In the tensor network, the wavefunction is decomposed into a $2n \times M$ expression (M is parameters or degrees of freedom), which is solvable. A tensor network approximates the exponentially large set of components of a high-order tensor in terms of a much smaller set of parameters whose number only grows polynomially in the size of the input space. An important variable is the bond dimension (tensor rank) which controls the number of parameters of the model and can be tuned up or down to find the optimal model based on cost, expressibility, and lack of overfitting.

In the quantum mechanical application, tensor networks are good at focusing on a small part of the Hilbert space with relevant local structure, such as determining a ground state Hamiltonian, as captured by the tensor product structure. Tensor network states have been shown to be a tool for modeling many-body quantum states. For example, the matrix product state (one-dimensional tensor network geometry) representation of ground states has been proven to be efficient for one-dimensional gapped local Hamiltonian (Landau *et al.*, 2015). The idea is to apply the same kinds of tensor network techniques to machine learning for feature extraction, dimensionality reduction, and analyzing the expressibility of neural networks. The tensor network machine learning algorithm Stoudenmire and Schwab (2017) propose is outlined in Table 17.6.

#### 17.3.1.1 *Machine learning algorithm: Weighted data features*

A standard structure for a machine learning algorithm is as follows. The method draws from kernel learning methods in which there are large vectors that arise in nonlinear kernel learning, and these input vectors are mapped into a higher dimensional space via a feature map before being classified by a decision function. The aim is to find a function that is in the form of a weighted average of relevant features in input data. The expression is a weight coefficient (a weight vector as a coefficient) multiplied with the input data (which is structured as vectors of features). The learning network manipulates the weights in the weights times the features expression to identify the most relevant features and weights.

Table 17.6. Implementations steps: Tensor network.

| No. | Implementation Steps (weight tensor × feature tensor = probability distribution) |
|---|---|
| 1 | Encode data: Make a wavefunction (tensor product) of the feature map of the input data. The data feature tensor of the overall system (wavefunction) is a tensor product of individual image data feature tensors obtained by applying the local feature map to each input |
| 2 | Network architecture: Set up the regularization and optimization of the weight tensor as a matrix product state tensor network representation |
| 3 | Training the network: Train the matrix product state tensor network with an adaptive algorithm based on the density matrix renormalization group (DMRG), sweeping iteratively back and forth through the network |
| 4 | Testing the network: Use the machine learning tensor network to solve specific problems such as image classification |

Through this structural formulation, the network's optimization algorithms learn (test with small trail-and-error changes) a function that approximates the probability distribution of the underlying data. The challenge is that both the feature vector and the weight vector can be exponentially large or even infinite. The decomposition concept is applied in the tensor network approach to both elements. The process can be considered in two steps, first encoding the feature tensor from the input data, and second optimizing the weight tensor for the learning process. The overall aim is to approximate the probability distribution of the data. For data input, this means making a wavefunction (tensor product) of the feature map. The data feature tensor of the overall system (wavefunction) is a tensor product of individual image data feature tensors obtained by applying the local feature map to each input.

#### 17.3.1.2 *Step 1: Encoding input data into tensor networks*

In quantum mechanics, tensor networks are used to combine independent system elements by taking the tensor product of individual state vectors to obtain the overall system state. Likewise, in applying tensor networks to machine learning, individual feature vectors are combined to obtain the overall feature map of the system. The feature map of the system is written as a tensor product of the individual feature vectors (which are generated as the local feature map applied to each input). Each data input is mapped to a $d$-dimensional vector. The overall feature map can be viewed as a vector in a $d^n$-dimensional space or as an order-$n$ tensor. The feature map has the same structure as a product state or a wavefunction.

A concrete example of the feature map construction can be seen with MNIST data inputs. The data are gray scale images with $n$ pixels, each pixel ranging in value from 0.0 for white to 1.0 for black, and gray scales in between. The MNIST digits (originally $28 \times 28$ pixels) are scaled down to $14 \times 14$ by averaging clusters of four pixels. Each pixel value is mapped to a normalized two-component vector. The feature map for each pixel is the normalized wavefunction of a single qubit in which the spin-up state corresponds to a white pixel, the spin-down state to a black pixel, and a superposition corresponds to a gray pixel. The local feature maps thus map each input component to a $d$-dimensional vector. The full image is represented as a tensor product of the local vectors, and the overall feature map is a tensor product of the individual image feature vectors. In this representation, the input data images are encoded into the tensor network.

#### 17.3.1.3 *Step 2: Selecting network architecture*

The second step is selecting the network architecture, which in this case is approximating the weight tensor with matrix product states. The overall machine learning formulation is the weight tensor multiplied with the feature vector tensor. Although both the feature vector tensor and the weight tensor may be unwieldy, the data encoding has already been specified and so special attention is given to the weight tensor. A way to regularize and optimize the weight tensor efficiently is needed. The tensor network strategy is to represent this high-order weight tensor as a tensor network, meaning as the contracted product of lower-order tensors.

A tensor network approximates the exponentially large set of components of a high-order tensor in terms of a much smaller set of parameters whose number only grows polynomially in the size of the input space. Here, the weight tensor is approximated as a matrix product state (one-dimensional tensor network geometry), which has the advantage that methods for manipulating and optimizing matrix product states are well understood and highly efficient. Hence, a matrix product state decomposition of the weight tensor is defined. The matrix product state representation gives the learning network the ability to efficiently optimize the weights and adaptively change their number by varying a few tensors at a time (in close analogy to the DMRG algorithm used in physics). The matrix product state tensor network operates by taking the tensor products of the weights tensor and the data features tensor (the data feature tensor of the system is the tensor product of the individual data feature tensors).

#### 17.3.1.4 *Step 3: Training the network*

The matrix product state tensor network is trained using an adaptive algorithm based on the DMRG algorithm. The machine learning goal is to find a suitable overall weight vector that gives the probability distribution of the data, structurally by minimizing a cost function corresponding to the model output. The learning algorithm manipulates the weights (in the weights times the features expression) to identify the most relevant features and weights. The weight tensor is optimized with a sweeping algorithm. The sweeping algorithm is based on the DMRG formulation which renormalizes across system dimensions, meaning in the sense of compactifying multiple scales in a system while preserving meaningful correlations.

Here, the sweeping algorithm optimizes the weights by sweeping back and forth along a matrix product state tensor network, iteratively minimizing a cost function that defines the classification task. The strategy for reducing the cost function is to vary two neighboring matrix product state tensors at a time. The pairwise optimization of the tensors highlights the adaptability advantage of tensor networks. The usual machine learning method only varies just one parameter at a time in the loss function. However, the tensor network formulation provides the ability to vary two tensors thus giving a more sophisticated method for adaptively changing the matrix product state bond dimension (tensor rank). Per the singular value decomposition (a known decomposition method), the dimension of the matrix product state bond dimension can be chosen adaptively (based on number of large singular values defined by a threshold chosen in advance). Through the pairwise optimization, the matrix product state form of the weight tensor can be maximally compressed, including by different amounts on each bond, while still ensuring an overall decision function that is optimal.

#### 17.3.1.5 *Step 4: Testing real-life data*

The machine learning tensor network is tested by executing the machine learning process on MNIST data. The MNIST dataset consists of 10,000 handwritten digits that are gray scale images of the digits zero through nine. The sweeping algorithm is used to train the weights, and the algorithm quickly converges in the number of passes, or sweeps over the matrix product state tensor network. In this analysis, typically only two or three sweeps were needed to see good convergence, with test error rates changing only by hundredths of a percent thereafter. Specifically, test error rates decreased rapidly as a function of the maximum matrix product state bond dimension. A bond dimension of 10 resulted in a 5% testing and training error rate, and with a bond dimension of 20, the error dropped to only 2%. The largest bond dimension tried was 120. After three sweeps, the error rates obtained were a test error of 0.97% (97 misclassified images out of the test set of 10,000 images) and a training set error of 0.05% (32 misclassified images).

The bond dimension (tensor rank or Schmidt rank) is the dimension of the bond index connecting one tensor in the chain to the next. In typical physics applications, the matrix product state bond dimension can range from 10 to 10,000 or even more. For the most challenging physics systems, the idea is to allow as large a bond dimension as possible since a larger dimension means more accuracy. However, there is more of a focus on bond dimension optimization in the machine learning context. When using matrix product state in machine learning, the bond dimension controls the number of parameters of the model. Thus, in contrast to physics applications, taking too large a bond dimension in machine learning might not be desirable as it could lead to overfitting. Also, more parameters are more costly. Sample code based on the ITensor library for Stoudenmire and Schwab's machine learning tensor network model is available at https://github.com/emstoudenmire/TNML.

#### 17.3.1.6 *Advantages of tensor networks for machine learning*

The key advantages of a tensor network model for machine learning are dimensionality reduction, adaptivity, and direct sampling. First, the dimensionality advantage of tensor networks is that training the model scales linearly in the size of the training set. The cost for evaluating a data input is independent of the training set size. More specifically, the tensor network method delivers a family of learning models with a cost that is linear in the training set size for optimization, and independent of training set size for evaluation, despite using an expressive feature map (in which the dimension of feature space can be exponential in the size of the input space). Second, tensor networks are adaptive in ways that other machine learning techniques are not. The adaptivity advantage is that the dimensions of tensor indices internal to the network grow and shrink during training to concentrate resources on the particular correlations within the data that are most useful for learning. Third, the tensor network form can be sampled directly unlike other "black box" machine learning methods. The tensor network presents opportunities to extract information hidden within the trained model and accelerate training by using techniques such as optimizing different internal tensors in parallel. This further means that given the sophistication of the tensor network model, certain subprocesses can be optimized directly. Overall, the tensor network machine learning method of mapping data into an extremely high-dimensional Hilbert space is likely to advantageous for producing models sensitive to high-order correlations among features in many contexts, such as analyzing the brain.

## 17.4 Tensor Networks: Wavelet = Spin (Qubit)

Another example of training of a tensor network structure to carry out a machine learning task is presented as follows. Reyes and Stoudenmire (2020) propose an algorithm for supervised learning using tensor networks. The algorithm first conducts a pre-processing step (to reduce the feature space representing the data and therefore the number of parameters of the model) through a series of wavelet transforms approximated by the layers of a MERA tensor network. The algorithm second uses a matrix product state tensor network to act on the coarse-grained data, performing supervised learning on sequential data (DCASE audio files and mean temperature data). The matrix product state tensor network is trained using an adaptive algorithm (using alternating least squares) based on the DMRG method. The matrix product state tensor network is used to represent the top layer of trainable weights.

The machine learning tensor network model presented by Reyes and Stoudenmire (2020) is used to learn sequential data (sound clip and average daily temperature) with a wavelet as the elemental unit or spin value that could be further encoded in a quantum computing environment. The method is extended from the Stoudenmire and Schwab (2017) machine learning tensor network model used to learn image data (MNIST) with the pixel being the elemental spin unit (Table 17.7).

Table 17.7. Supervised tensor networks: Pixel and wavelet.

| | Image: Pixel = Spin (Qubit) | Sound/Time Series: Wavelet = Spin (Qubit) |
|---|---|---|
| Goal | Find function = weight tensor × feature tensor (feature vectors, label) | |
| Architecture | Image pixel/MPS TN | Wavelet transform/MPS TN |
| Spin (qubit) | Pixel = Spin (qubit) | Wavelet = Spin (qubit) |
| Step 1: Data encoding | The data feature tensor of the overall system (wavefunction) is a tensor product of individual image data feature tensors obtained by applying the local feature map to each input | The data feature tensor of the overall system (wavefunction) is a tensor product of wavelet transform amplitudes obtained by data preprocessing through a MERA tensor network |
| Step 2: Network architecture | Matrix product state tensor network | |
| Step 3: Training the network | Network trained with an adaptive algorithm (using alternating least squares) based on the DMRG algorithm | |
| Step 4: Testing real-life datasets | MNIST | DCASE audio files (classification), mean temperature (linear regression) |
| Sequential data | No (images) | Yes (sequence is important) |
| Reference | Stoudenmire and Schwab (2017) | Reyes and Stoudenmire (2020) |

### 17.4.1 *Wavelet transform*

A *wavelet* is a wave-like oscillation with an amplitude that begins at zero, increases, and then decreases back to zero. Wavelets are crafted to have specific properties that make them useful for signal processing (for example, to combine with the known portion of a damaged signal to rebuild the full signal). A *wavelet transform* is a manipulation that transforms a wavelet such that it changes in time extension, but not in overall shape. This is allowed per the uncertainty principle of signal processing which describes the trade-off between time and frequency, much like the trade-off between position and velocity in the Heisenberg uncertainty principle.

For simple stationary signals, a Fourier transform is often applied as a signal processing technique, whereas a wavelet transform is used for nonstationary signals. The Fourier transform is a ubiquitous transformation which can be used to translate an input signal from the time domain to the frequency domain. Nonstationary signals, however, require analysis in both the time and the frequency domains. Wavelet transforms facilitate this type of analysis by transforming a signal into the time-frequency domain in which one or the other axis can be manipulated per the signal processing uncertainty principle.

To execute the wavelet transform, the wavelet is written as a vector and the inner product is taken for a subset of the signal. An integral performs a summation over all the elements within that subset, and there is some degree of overlap with neighboring subsets. Using this method, the wavelet transformations of an input signal can be used to average and rescale the initial signal to one half its size (from size $n$ to size $n/2$), while preserving local information in both the time and frequency domains. The preserved information is that which is associated with the part of the signal that varies most smoothly with the time index. Two standard types of wavelet transforms are the Haar transformation and the Daubechies-4 transformation, respectively, summing over two or four elements of the subset of vector inner products. The benefit is reducing the size of the data by one half with each wavelet transform while preserving relevant information (local time and frequency information). By preserving relevant local information across scales, the wavelet transform is a renormalization method.

#### 17.4.1.1 *Wavelet transform equates to MERA tensor network*

The key point for the tensor network context is that the wavelet transform equates to a MERA (multi-scale entanglement renormalization ansatz) tensor network. The MERA tensor network renormalizes entanglement across scales. The wavelet transform likewise renormalizes time and frequency information across scales. In fact, preserving local time and frequency information across system scales can be seen as constituting a definition of entanglement. Generically, entanglement is conceived as correlations between system elements. Local time and frequency relations amount to correlations. The wavelet transform/MERA implementation is proposed and demonstrated by Evenbly and White (2018). The data are fermionic modes. A wavelet transform of fermionic modes is realized in the form of a quantum circuit which is mapped to a MERA tensor network. The model is used to calculate the ground state of a quantum critical Ising model. The insight is that the wavelet transform is a renormalization process just as MERA instantiates in the tensor network format. Hence, it is possible to realize a wavelet transform with a MERA tensor network.

#### 17.4.1.2 *Step 1: Data encoding: MERA tensor network*

The machine learning algorithm used by Reyes and Stoudenmire (2020) first conducts a pre-processing step (to reduce the feature space representing the data and therefore the number of parameters of the model) through a series of wavelet transforms approximated by the layers of a MERA tensor network. The MERA is a tensor network model whose geometry and structure implements multiple coarse-grainings (renormalization) of input variables (Vidal, 2007). The MERA network consists of alternating tree tensor layers (isometries) and disentangler layers as a family of tensor network factorizations that process information hierarchically. MERA preserves the computational advantages associated with tree-tensor networks, such as efficient marginalization, yet can be more expressive and powerful due to extra disentangler layers which mix branches of the tree.

Introducing tensors which connect subtrees could make computations with the resulting network prohibitively expensive. However, the MERA disentangler tensors are constrained to being unitary. Likewise, the main layers of the network, tree tensors or isometry tensors, are constrained to obeying isometric conditions (one-to-one mappings). Due to these constraints, MERA computations can be carried out with a cost that scales polynomially in the dimensions of the internal indices of the network (i.e. efficiently). A typical operation for the MERA tensor network is to represent a probability distribution and calculate the marginal distribution and correlation functions. A specific application for a MERA tensor network is calculating the ground state of a local Hamiltonian in both gapless and gapped systems. The point is that the MERA architecture is comprised of alternating layers of tree tensors (isometries or one-to-one data mappings) and disentangler tensors (which capture information from other subtrees in the overall network).

In the wavelet analysis, specific isometries and disentanglers are used to parametrize the MERA layers which approximately compute the wavelet coarse-graining transformations of input data. The process includes selecting different ways to approximate the Haar and Daubechies wavelet transforms. Specifically, each input data element is mapped into a rank-1 matrix product state, and then acted on by MERA layers approximating Daubechies-4 wavelet transformation. Each subsequent layer of the MERA is constructed by encoding wavelet transforms into the disentangler and isometry tensors. The work draws on the wavelet transform-MERA relationship established by Evenbly and White (2016). Taking the input data, the MERA tensor network is used to perform a series of discrete wavelet transforms to reduce the overall size of the data while simultaneously preserving local information within it (local relationships formatted as time and frequency relations). The result is that applying the MERA tensor network to the data is a pre-processing step which reduces the overall feature space representing the data and therefore the number of parameters required by the machine learning model.

Both MERA tensor networks and machine learning networks are composed of the same structure of alternating layers. MERA's isometry (one-to-one) mappings followed by disentanglers (renormalizers) are similar to machine learning's pooling layer followed by consolidation (convolution and activation) layer. Quantum machine learning structures can be further generalized to functions of alternating linear and nonlinear transformations (Han & Hartnoll, 2020).

### 17.4.1.3 *Steps 2 and 3: Network architecture and training*

The machine learning algorithm is comprised of two steps, first is the coarse-graining of the input data through some number of discrete wavelet transforms, implemented as MERA tensor network layers. Second, the matrix product state tensor network developed by Stoudenmire and Schwab (2017) is used to represent the top layer of trainable weights. As in the previous work, the matrix product state tensor network is trained using an adaptive algorithm (using alternating least squares) based on the DMRG method. The technique sweeps back and forth between the first tensor and the last to optimize the algorithm (network structure).

The two-phase model is very powerful because it is essentially two tensor networks bolted together. The model's capability derives from the fact that not only is the regular machine learning process adaptive (with trainable weights), but the process of coarse-graining the input data is also adaptive, and the two phases can feed and adapt relative to each other. The insight is that since tensors are multi-linear, controlled transformations of one tensor network into another are possible through established techniques such as matrix factorization and tensor contraction. Thus, this construction takes advantage of the capability of one tensor network to transform into another. The benefit is that the amount of coarse graining can be adjusted during the training phase to adaptively discover the right number of coarse-graining steps needed to obtain the best results. The compound formulation is enabled by MERA's structure as a tensor network composed of multi-linear transformations. The model is trained by the network initially defining a larger number of coarse-graining steps, and then a smaller number of fine-grained steps in favor of the top tensor containing the adjustable model weights to reach the desired architecture.

The result of coarse-graining the input data through the series of wavelet transformations effectively reduces the size of the data by a factor of two after each transformation. Then the MERA tensor network optimization portion of the process works as follows. The form of the wavelet, as a wave-like oscillation with an amplitude that begins at zero, increases, and then decreases back to zero, suggests being written in a wavefunction format with different coefficients corresponding to the different amplitudes. Deploying this format to encode the input data, the wavelet coefficients are decomposed into sequentially applied transformations. The interpretation is that each local feature vector can be considered as a "particle" whose state has coefficients given by the input components. The path the particle takes can be traced through the MERA, assigning appropriate transformations to it as it propagates through the tensors. With this construction, the optimal flow of data particles through the MERA can be derived (working out the result of applying the MERA layer to a patch of four adjacent input tensors at a time).

Thus, this two-phase process is followed to obtain the optimal machine learning function. The first step is the data encoding as wavelet transforms processed with a MERA tensor network and the second step is an MPS tensor network learning the feature weights tensor. The new wrinkle in this method is using MERA layers to approximate wavelet scaling functions as a preprocessing step. Relying on the presence of disentanglers, the MERA network is able to approximate non-trivial families of wavelets with overlapping support such as Daubechies-4 wavelets. The resulting algorithms are tested with real-life datasets.

#### 17.4.1.4 *Step 4: Testing real-life datasets*

The model was tested by performing supervised learning on DCASE audio files data and linear regression tasks on mean temperature data evaluated on the basis of the percentage of correctly labeled samples. For supervised learning, the DCASE set of audio classification data were used. The dataset consists of 15 batches (one batch per label), each containing 234 ten-second audio clips for training. Each audio clip is a vector of 441,000 samples, and was embedded into a vector of $2^{19}$ elements by padding with zeros. The problem was constrained to focus on binary classification, specifically distinguishing between "bus" and "beach" environment audio clips. Each dataset for the selected labels was coarse-grained through Haar transformations before encoding the data into the Daubechies-4 wavelet MERA. The optimization was carried out over five sweeps.

For linear regression, a dataset of four years of daily temperature data ($n$ = 1,462) was used. These data are available in a single data file of the average daily temperatures of the Fisher River (near Dallas, Texas) recorded from January 1, 1988 to December 31, 1991 were used to construct input datasets for regression. Temperature data were labeled singly and in blocks to have a contiguous block of p temperatures as input for the MERA tensor network. The temperature immediately following this $p$ block was assigned as the label for that training example. By shifting the starting index of the $p$ block of temperatures, multiple examples could be constructed. In this way, the regression task was recast as a classification task over a continuous label. The optimization was carried out over forty sweeps.

The overall result is that the methods were tested by performing a classification task on audio data and a regression task on temperature time-series data, studying the dependence of training accuracy on the number of coarse-graining layers and showing how fine-graining through the network may be used to initialize models with access to finer-scale features. The further benefit of the chosen network architecture can be seen as follows. The accuracy of the model depends on the number of wavelet layers, and the input data can exhibit correlations at length scales that can be lost through the wavelet transformations. It is therefore important to tailor the number of wavelets and initial size to the specific dataset being analyzed in order to maintain a desirable accuracy. The tensor network setup gives an affordable and adaptive way to strike a balance between the efficiency and generalization gains obtained by coarse-graining versus model expressivity by trading off one for the other through the fine-graining procedure. One way to select the best number of layers would be to use too many intentionally, and then fine-grain until the gains in model performance begin to saturate.

## References

Ackley, D.H., Hinton, G.E. & Sejnowski, T.J. (1985). A learning algorithm for Boltzmann machines. *Cog. Sci.* 9(1):147–69.

Alcazar, J., Leyton-Ortega, V. & Perdomo-Ortiz, A. (2020). Classical versus quantum models in machine learning: Insights from a finance application. arXiv:1908.10778v2.

Benedetti, M., Garcia-Pintos, D., Perdomo, O. *et al.* (2019). A generative modeling approach for benchmarking and training shallow quantum circuits. *NPJ Quantum Inf.* 5(45):1–9.

Born, M. (1926). Zur quantenmechanik der stoßvorgänge. *Zeitschrift Physik.* 37:863–67.

Bradley, T.-D., Stoudenmire, E.M. & Terilla, J. (2019). Modeling sequences with quantum states: A look under the hood. *Mach. Learn.: Sci. Technol.* 1:035008.

Carleo, G. & Troyer, M. (2017). Solving the quantum many-body problem with artificial neural networks. *Science*. 355(6325):602–26.

Chen, J., Cheng, S., Xie, H. *et al.* (2018). Equivalence of restricted Boltzmann machines and tensor network states. *Phys. Rev. B*. 97(8):085104.

Cheng, S., Chen, J. & Wang L. (2018). Information perspective to probabilistic modeling: Boltzmann machines versus Born machines. *Entropy*. 20(583).

Cirstoiu, C., Holmes, Z., Iosue, J. *et al.* (2020). Variational fast forwarding for quantum simulation beyond the coherence time. arXiv:1910.04292v2.

Evenbly, G. & White, S.R. (2016). Entanglement renormalization and wavelets. *Phys. Rev. Lett.* 116(14):140403.

Farhi, E. & Neven, H. (2018). Classification with quantum neural networks on near term processors. arXiv:1802.06002. MIT-CTP/4985.

Glasser, I., Sweke, R., Pancotti, N. *et al.* (2019). Expressive power of tensor-network factorizations for probabilistic modeling. *Adv. Neural Info. Proc. Sys*. 32:1498–1510.

Goodfellow, I.J., Pouget-Abadie, J., Mirza, M. *et al.* (2014). Generative adversarial nets. *Adv. Neural Info. Proc. Sys*. 27:2672–80.

Grant, E., Benedetti, M., Cao, S. *et al.* (2018). Hierarchical quantum classifiers. *NPJ Quantum Info*. 4(65):1–16.

Han, X. & Hartnoll, S.A. (2020). Deep quantum geometry of matrices. arXiv:1906.08781v2.

Han, Z.-Y., Wang, J., Fan, H. *et al.* (2018). Unsupervised generative modeling using matrix product states. arXiv:1709.01662v3.

Huggins, W., Patel, P., Whaley, K.B. & Stoudenmire, E.M. (2019). Towards quantum machine learning with tensor networks. *Quantum Sci. Technol.* 4(2):024001.

King, A.D., Carrasquilla, J., Raymond, J. *et al.* (2018). Observation of topological phenomena in a programmable lattice of 1,800 qubits. *Nature.* 560:456–60.

Landau, Z., Vazirani, U. & Vidick, T. (2015). A polynomial time algorithm for the ground state of 1D gapped local Hamiltonians. *Nat. Phys*. 11(7):566–9.

Liu, J.-G., Mao, L., Zhang, P. & Wang, L. (2019). Solving quantum statistical mechanics with variational autoregressive networks and quantum circuits. arXiv:1912.11381v1.

Liu, J.-G. & Wang. L. (2018). Differentiable learning of quantum circuit Born machine. *Phys. Rev. A*. 98(6):062324.

Martyn, J. & Swingle, B. (2019). Product spectrum ansatz and the simplicity of thermal states. *Phys. Rev. A*. 100(3):032107.

Reyes, J. & Stoudenmire, E.M. (2020). A multi-scale tensor network architecture for classification and regression. arXiv:2001.08286v1.

Sharir, O., Levine, Y., Wies, N. *et al.* (2019). Deep autoregressive models for the efficient variational simulation of many-body quantum systems. arXiv: 1902.04057.

Stoudenmire, E.M. & Schwab, D.J. (2017). Supervised learning with quantum inspired tensor networks. *Adv. Neural Info. Proc. Sys*. 29:4799.

Terhal, B.M. & DiVincenzo, D.P. (2000). Problem of equilibration and the computation of correlation functions on a quantum computer. *Phys. Rev. A*. 61(2):022301.

Tiesinga, E., Mohr, P.J., Newell, D.B. & Taylor, B.N. (2021). CODATA recommended values of the fundamental physical constants: 2018. *Rev. Mod. Phys*. 93(2):025010.

van Houcke, K., Werner, F., Kozik, E. *et al.* (2012). Feynman diagrams versus Fermi-gas Feynman emulator. *Nat. Phys*. 8:366–70.

Vidal, G. (2007). Entanglement renormalization. *Phys. Rev. Lett*. 99(22):220405.

Wu, J. & Hsieh, T.H. (2018). Variational thermal quantum simulation via thermofield double states. *Phys. Rev. Lett*. 123(22):220502.

# Chapter 18

# Quantum Kernel Learning and Entanglement Design

*Just like quantum computing, kernel methods perform implicit computations in a possibly intractably large Hilbert space through the efficient manipulation of data inputs*

— Schuld and Killoran (2019, p. 1)


### Abstract

This chapter discusses how quantum methods are used to improve machine learning techniques (Q/ML). The main approaches to machine learning are neural networks, tensor networks, and kernel learning, each of which has a quantum counterpart. Quantum kernel learning methods obeying the RKHS (reproducing kernel Hilbert space) formalism can be used to compute kernel functions at other scale dimensions of the system and have applications in quantum finance. The point is to have an analytical model that grows more slowly than the underlying system. Modeling classical data with wavefunctions finds hidden correlations, namely, how the system is entangled, which can be used as quantum system design principles.

# 18.1 Quantum Kernel Methods

## 18.1.1 *Machine learning approaches*

There are three main approaches to machine learning: Neural networks, tensor networks, and kernel methods. Kernel methods is the technique of embedding data into a higher-dimensional feature space for simplified analysis. Functions in the higher-dimensional feature space are not computed directly on data coordinates, but rather on a relevant *kernel* of the data supplied by kernel functions (distance measures between data points in the feature space). Kernel methods were deployed earlier in the history of machine learning (most successfully in the 1990s (Schuld & Killoran, 2019, p. 1)), but were surpassed by neural networks in the "big data" and cloud computing era. However, the advent of quantum machine learning demands a wider range of approaches that include neural networks, and also emphasize tensor networks (to model quantum many-body problems) and kernel methods (to address high dimensionality).

Of the three machine learning approaches, neural networks are the least ready for quantum platforms and must be adapted. Tensor networks are "already-quantum" in the sense of having been derived to approximate wavefunctions, accommodate entanglement and renormalization, and solve other quantum mechanical problems. As such, tensor networks have a more straightforward path to implementation on quantum hardware than neural networks. Kernel methods are also "already-quantum" in that they share many parallels with quantum computing and can be readily constructed as quantum circuits. Both quantum computing (generally) and kernel methods (specifically) target the challenge of performing computations efficiently in an intractably large Hilbert space. Kernel methods have the additional benefit of being straightforward to implement using quantum optical computing (favored for its more expansive qudits) with squeezed light states and optical coherent states (Table 18.1).

## 18.1.2 *Kernel methods*

Kernel methods are a class of machine learning algorithms used for pattern analysis. In pattern analysis, the task is to find relations in datasets such as clusters, rankings, principal components, and correlations. Kernel

Table 18.1. Machine learning approaches and quantum status.

| Approach | Quantum Readiness Status | Quantum Platform |
|---|---|---|
| Neural networks | Must be quantum-adapted | NISQ simulation (Farhi and Neven, 2018) |
| Tensor networks | Already-quantum: Solve quantum many-body problems | IBM Q demo (Grant *et al.*, 2018) |
| Kernel methods | Already-quantum: Compute problems in an intractably large Hilbert space | NISQ & Optical (Schuld and Killoran, 2019) |

methods are named for their use of kernel functions. Kernel functions operate in an implicit high-dimensional feature space. They do not compute the coordinates of the underlying data in the space, but rather calculate the inner products between all the pairs of data in the feature space. The *kernel*, or salient description of the data, emerges as a similarity function over the inner products of the pairs of data points. The idea is that the kernel function operation is computationally cheaper than the explicit computation of the coordinates, but nevertheless yields relevant results. Kernel methods is an indirect technique and the approach of implicitly mapping data inputs into high-dimensional feature spaces for simplified calculation is sometimes called the *kernel trick*. These kinds of kernel functions are used to analyze many kinds of data including images, text, graphs, and sequential data. One of the best-known examples of kernel methods is support vector machines (SVMs).

SVMs are a supervised learning method applied to binary classification problems. Given a set of training examples, each marked as belonging to one of two categories, the SVM training algorithm builds a model to assign new examples to one category or the other. The SVM model represents the data as points in space, mapped so that the examples of the separate categories are divided by a clear gap. New examples are then mapped into that same space and predicted to belong to a category based on the side of the gap on which they fall.

The challenge is that when executed in a classical computing environment, both SVMs and kernel methods more generally do not scale well with the size of the feature space both in terms of data points and dimensionality. One of the most significant limitations of classical algorithms using nonlinear kernels is that the kernel function has to be evaluated for all pairs of input feature vectors which themselves may be of substantially high dimension. This can lead to computationally excessive times during training and during the prediction process for a new data point. Hence, the ability to access quantum formulations provides an opportunity to resolve some of the scaling limits of kernel methods as deployed on classical platforms.

#### 18.1.2.1 *Kernel methods reduce dimensionality*

Conceptually, kernel methods are a dimensionality reduction technique. The surprising discovery is that data become easier to analyze once they are mapped into a higher-dimensional feature space (Scholkopf & Smola, 2002). In a high-dimensional space, it is easier to classify data as lines can be drawn (literally) to separate different classes of data into different spaces. The high dimensional environment makes it easier to identify relevant features by which to classify the data. The kernel methods consist of formally embedding data into a higher-dimensional feature space and then using simple (linear) models to describe the data.

In the standard kernel method of SVMs, algorithms draw a decision boundary between two classes of data points by mapping the data into a feature space where they become linearly separable into categories. The dimensionality-management technique is that the algorithm does not explicitly perform computations with vectors in the feature space, but uses a kernel function that is defined on the domain of the original input data. The kernel function measures the distance between data points in the standard method by taking the pairwise inner products of two data inputs that have been mapped into the feature space. Many iterations of the kernel functions are performed for the classification algorithm to learn the best possibly function for the pattern recognition task at hand. A structural benefit of the kernel learning setup is that in the learning process, the machine learning algorithm can switch between kernels (data representation models) to test different model permutations. The practical benefit of kernel methods is having an iterative testing structure for a machine learning algorithm to learn by quickly cycling between many different possibilities. The theoretical benefit of kernel methods is being able to define a lower-dimensional model that operates in a higher-dimensional space.

#### 18.1.2.2 *Dimensionality reduction and squeezed light states*

The aim of many quantum algorithms is to perform efficient computations in a Hilbert space that grows rapidly with the size of the quantum system. "Efficient" typically means that the number of operations applied to the system will grow at most polynomially with the system size. A standard quantum algorithm is the quantum Fourier transform (which is part of Shor's factoring algorithm). The quantum Fourier transform uses polynomial operations to perform a discrete Fourier transform on $2^n$ amplitudes. Other kinds of quantum algorithms are used in quantum optical computing, for example, in global fiberoptic networks to produce squeezed states of light. Squeezed states are oscillatory waves whose phase or amplitude is squeezed (resulting in a reduced shape wave form) in order to reduce quantum noise (fluctuations and interference). Squeezed light states are used in communications networks as they have less quantum uncertainty (noise) than other kinds of quantum states. The quantum algorithm for light state squeezing is a single operation applied to a light mode which formally manipulates the quantum state in an infinite-dimensional Hilbert space.

#### 18.1.2.3 *Quantum algorithm design*

The consistent theme of the quantum algorithms in the quantum Fourier transform and light state squeezing examples is operating in a lower-dimensional space than that of the quantum system being analyzed (the same premise as kernel methods). A quantum system that is growing exponentially needs to be matched with a corresponding algorithm that grows only linearly or polynomially if the problem is to remain tractable.

It would not be possible to compute quantum systems without techniques for managing dimensionality growth. Hence, there are two related requirements for quantum algorithm design. First is the idea of calculating quantum systems on the basis of a lower-dimensional operation being performed in a higher-dimensional space. Second is incorporating growth dynamics in that the lower-dimensional model needs to accommodate exponential growth in the underlying quantum system while itself scaling only linearly or polynomially. The result is that the elements in the quantum system are not being calculated exactly, only approximately or on average. Quantum algorithms and quantum computing in general can be seen as a technique that performs implicit (indirect) computations in an intractably large Hilbert space by efficiently manipulating the underlying quantum system. The three dimensionality reduction methods of the quantum Fourier transform, squeezed states, and kernel methods all instantiate the similar structure of performing indirect computations in an intractably large-dimensional space by efficiently manipulating data inputs (Table 18.2).

### 18.1.3 *Quantum kernel methods*

Schuld and Killoran (2019) formulate kernel methods for quantum machine learning. They develop a quantum machine learning algorithm that encodes inputs in a quantum state as a nonlinear feature map that then maps the data to a quantum Hilbert space. The quantum state data are generated by squeezed states of light. Quantum algorithms are run to analyze the input data in the high-dimensional feature space. Two approaches are developed, a hybrid classical-quantum method and a fully quantum method. In the hybrid approach, a classically intractable kernel is computed by using a quantum device to estimate the inner products of the quantum states in the feature space. The kernel can then be fed into any

Table 18.2. Dimensionality reduction techniques.

| No. | Technique | Lower-Dimensional Computational System | Higher-Dimensional Quantum System |
|---|---|---|---|
| 1 | Fourier transform | $n$-qubit system | $2^n$-amplitude Hilbert space |
| 2 | Squeezed states | Single operation (squeezing) | Infinite-dimensional Hilbert space |
| 3 | Kernel methods | Kernels as inner products of the distance between two data points | Higher-dimensional feature space |

classical kernel method downstream such as SVMs. In the quantum approach, a variational quantum circuit operates directly as an explicit classifier in the feature space to learn the decision boundary of the kernel function. The two approaches are tested with quantum simulators operating on standard two-dimensional datasets (circles, moons, and blobs). For example, with the fully quantum circuit model, the derived Fock space (multi-particle Hilbert space) classifier worked well on a "moons" dataset with 32 parameters, having a loss converging on zero after about 200 iterations of a stochastic gradient descent algorithm. The method can be deployed on currently available NISQ devices.

The steps for implementing the quantum kernel method appear in Table 18.3. First, input data are encoded into feature maps. Then the feature maps are mapped into vectors (distance measures) in a Hilbert space. The inner products of the feature vectors (distance measures) are taken to write the kernel function. Each feature map has a separate kernel function (meaning that each different data encoding leads to a different feature map which leads to a different kernel function).

#### 18.1.3.1 *Quantum kernel methods: Feature map approach*

A key point is that Schuld and Killoran's (2019) method is not just a usual quantum kernel methods approach to machine learning algorithms that learn the best kernel functions to approximate data. Instead, the method

Table 18.3. Implementation steps: Quantum kernel methods.

| | |
|---|---|
| 1 | Encode data (classical or quantum) and obtain feature map of data |
| 2 | Map feature map to Hilbert space = "feature Hilbert space" |
| 3 | Take inner products of the vectors in the feature Hilbert space |
| 4 | Obtain kernel function (measure of distance between data points) |
| 5 | Vary data encodings to obtain different kernel functions (kernel trick) |
| 6 | Find the best kernel function that describes the data |
| | (a) Classical: Quantum device evaluates classically intractable kernel function and passes results to support vector machine or other classical interpretation method |
| | (b) Quantum: Quantum device operates as a variational quantum circuit to learn the decision boundary of the kernel function directly in the Hilbert feature space |

uses the intermediary step of the feature map as a potentially generic theoretical structure for quantum kernel methods. In the team's adaptation of kernel methods for quantum machine learning, the core idea remains the same, namely, encoding data into a higher-dimensional feature space in which it is easier to analyze. The quantum kernel method encodes data inputs (classical or quantum) into a quantum state that is interpreted as a feature map, which is mapped to a potentially vastly higher-dimensional feature space. The data feature map on the Hilbert space can be called generically the "Hilbert feature space".

The quantum kernel method derives kernels that are given by the inner product of quantum states in the Hilbert feature space. The same structural benefit of classical kernel methods persists in running the kernel trick. The machine learning algorithm cycles through different kernel function permutations to learn the best model for the problem at hand (which in the quantum version means testing various data encodings among other aspects of the model). Also, as in classical kernel methods, the same argument holds in that even simple classifiers such as linear models may have enormous power in the Hilbert feature space. A further benefit of the feature map approach is that nonlinear transformations on the data are outsourced to the procedure of encoding inputs into a quantum state. The quantum circuit implements linear transformations and other formalisms for the task of performing nonlinear translations on the data, which in other quantum setups, usually involve costly workarounds such as post-selection and repeat-until-success circuits.

### 18.1.4 *Embedded data Hilbert spaces*

A key innovation is the broader implication of the Hilbert feature space (data encoded as a Hilbert space feature map). The general idea is embedding data into a quantum Hilbert space. Such embedded-data Hilbert spaces could become a standard feature in quantum machine learning. A generic pattern recognition capability could be built into quantum devices. Quantum devices could be machine learning-enabled from the beginning as a standard feature. Such a capability would further underline machine learning as a core infrastructural technology.

The idea of embedding data into Hilbert spaces as a generic computational method, for machine learning or otherwise, highlights the even more fundamental concept of embedding. Embedding in quantum systems is not only useful for potentially enabling quantum circuits with a generic pattern recognition (machine learning) capability, but also for working with entanglement. Many exploitable features in quantum computing depend on the ability to embed or entangle data in systems. A standard technology feature of embedded-data Hilbert spaces could likewise standardize entanglement management in the ability to harness short-range (UV) and long-range (IR) correlations in quantum systems. A list of generic features for quantum system design, many based on information-theoretic formulations, appears in Table 18.4.

## 18.1.5 *Quantum finance*

### 18.1.5.1 *Reproducing kernel Hilbert space formalism*

The intent is to write a kernel function in the structure of a known formalism called a reproducing kernel Hilbert space (RKHS). An RKHS is a Hilbert space generated by a kernel function that reproduces every possible function in the space. The RKHS is a bit like a short-cut or renormalization tool for moving between system scales. The benefit of the RKHS

Table 18.4. Generic feature set for quantum computing.

| No. | Feature | Description |
|---|---|---|
| 1 | Machine learning | Pattern recognition, probability distribution function-finding |
| 2 | Entanglement manipulation | Exploit short-range (UV) and long-range (IR) correlations |
| 3 | Renormalization | View system at multiple scales per attribute compression |
| 4 | Quantum error correction | Use ancilla (ancillary) qubits to correct and secure data |
| 5 | Information compression protocols | Transfer quantum states between locations |

formalism is being able to identify a kernel function at any scale tier of the underlying system without having to compute it directly. The underlying system can be discrete or continuous, and involve nonlinear kernel functions.

The key idea is that with the RKHS formalism, kernel functions at even higher dimensions in the system can be readily obtained. The RKHS method avoids having to map the data feature vectors to higher-dimensional spaces and compute individual inner product pairwise similarity functions directly, effectively rederiving the kernel function for the system for each new set of dimensions. Instead, the laborious process of inner product calculations of vectors can be streamlined. Having found the initial kernel function for the system in the form of an RKHS formalism means that the time-saving measure can be applied to extend the analysis to other higher-dimensional characterizations of the system, according to the RKHS property that kernels are additive.

#### 18.1.5.2 *Time series analysis and AdS/RKHS*

A specific example of an RKHS formalism for kernel function derivation is in the quantum finance application of quantum SVMs proposed by Chatterjee and Yu (2017). The work uses optical coherent states (which have an inherent RKHS property) for the rapid calculation of radial kernels (a nonlinear kernel function which is classically intractable). The inner products of the coherent states are used to write a Gaussian (radial) kernel function which can be used in the machine learning of patterns in large datasets, such as those generated in financial markets. The research is partially supported by the Chicago Mercantile Exchange (CME) foundation. The quantum finance use case is deploying quantum kernel methods to find salient relationships in very large datasets extremely quickly, much faster than classical methods.

The quantum SVMs approach shows that coherent states reproduce the same kinds of radial kernels seen in classical SVMs, but substantially reduce the computational times of such kernels, especially in the high dimensional feature spaces of very large datasets. Further, an AdS/RKHS application may be possible. The use of reproducing kernels (RKHS) is not usually possible in classical algorithms due to their complexity.

However, algorithms such as those from anti-de Sitter space coherent states and Bessel function kernels from Poschl-Teller coherent states are now conceivable using coherent state-driven quantum kernel method approaches (Gazeau, 2009). The next step in this research trajectory is to understand more about the relationship between coherent states and the RKHS formalism.

In another quantum finance application, Alcazar *et al.* (2020) test quantum circuit Born machines on ion-trap quantum computers, outperforming classical methods (restricted Boltzmann machines) in a well-known portfolio optimization problem in finance using time-series pricing data from asset subsets of the S&P500 stock market index. The work is also partially supported by the banking and finance industry.

### 18.1.6 *Squeezed states of light*

The quantum kernel method feature map approach developed by Schuld and Killoran (2019) uses squeezed states of light as a quantum data source. Squeezed states of light are interpreted as a feature map from the one-dimensional real input space of the squeezed states to the Hilbert space of Fock states (the Fock space, a multi-particle Hilbert space). The squeezing parameter can be changed to vary the machine learning model. An increased squeezing parameter (more highly squeezed input data) may improve model performance, up to some threshold. The resulting squeezing-based quantum machine learning classifier can be implemented by optical quantum computers.

#### 18.1.6.1 *Squeezed states: Quantum noise reduction technique*

Squeezed states are a manipulation applied to any kind of quantum wave or oscillatory state, by squeezing the phase or amplitude in order to have less quantum uncertainty than "regular" coherent (oscillating) states. The aim is to reduce the quantum uncertainty associated with measurement and noise. Squeezed states are particularly relevant in applications related to optics. Squeezed states of light were proposed in 1983 (Walls, 1983) and demonstrated in 1985–1986 (Slusher, *et al.*, 1985; Wu, 1986).

Squeezed states are a practical means of reducing and coping with quantum uncertainty. The problem is that quantum uncertainty becomes obvious when *identical* measurements of the same quantity (observable) on *identical* objects (such as modes of light) give *different* results (computed as eigenvalues). In order to obtain the full picture, measurement statistics need to be recorded at many different phases. Squeezed states (wave forms with either phase or amplitude squeezed into a reduced shape) provide a more manageable solution to working with quantum uncertainty (which cannot be fully eliminated).

#### 18.1.6.2 *Global telecommunications networks*

Squeezed states of light are the way that light is produced and managed in the global fiberoptic communication industry, and have also become workhorse techniques used in scientific applications such as gravitational wave analysis (Schnabel, 2017). The observables in squeezed light experiments correspond exactly to those used in optical communication. Amplitude modulation and frequency modulation are the usual means of imprinting information on a carrier field. The measurement object is the *mode* that is characterized by the statistics of the eigenvalues in the phase measurement calculation. This particular measurement object is the modulation mode that is carried by the light beam. Signal reconstitution can be performed from the continuous spectrum of many modulation modes carried by the same light beam in standard communications network equipment. The observables also correspond to the measurement quantities in laser interferometers, such as Sagnac interferometers which measure rotation changes and Michelson interferometers which are used in observing gravitational waves. Squeezed states of light thus have many applications in optical communication and measurement. Squeezed light states can be produced with off-the-shelf nonlinear optical equipment.

#### 18.1.6.3 *Continuous basis quantum systems*

Quantum systems with a continuous basis are complicated to analyze. Many Hilbert space formulations produce the Dirac delta equation as a potential system kernel, but the expression is not square integrable, which means that it cannot be an RKHS. Instead, it is necessary to incorporate the generalized coherent states formulation (for example, as elaborated by Klauder and Skagerstam (1985)). Coherent states are oscillatory quantum states, the quantum state of the quantum harmonic oscillator (a state with dynamics closely resembling the oscillatory behavior of a classical harmonic oscillator). Whereas all quantum states are presumed to be in the form of a wavefunction, not all quantum states obey a regular oscillating form. Generalized coherent states is a formulation that offers a representation of the Hilbert space with the reproducing property which is necessary to define an RKHS in which the kernel is not the Dirac delta function. The best-known type of coherent states are optical coherent states which are the eigenstates of the non-Hermitian bosonic creation operator, with the associated kernel whose square is a radial basis function or Gaussian kernel as discussed by (Chatterjee & Yu, 2017) and expanded by Schuld and Killoran's (2019) feature map method.

### 18.1.7 *RHKS and machine learning*

In the machine learning context, a RKHS is a Hilbert space of continuous linear functions. Such RKHSs have wide application in machine learning, quantum mechanics, complex systems, and harmonic analysis. This is because they reduce infinite-dimensional problems to finitely calculable problems. RKHSs are practically useful as a means of simplifying a loss minimization problem from an infinite-dimensional to a finite-dimensional optimization problem. Instead of explicitly optimizing over an infinite-dimensional RKHS, a machine learning setup can start with an implicit ansatz (guess) and solve a convex optimization problem based on certain parameters (Schuld & Killoran, 2019, p. 3).

The machine learning deployment is that RKHSs are used to construct ReLU-like nonlinear functions. ReLU (rectified linear unit) functions are commonly used activation functions in machine learning. The rectangular shape activates more quickly than slower acting s-curve shaped functions. The RKHS construction of ReLU functions implies the representation power of neural networks that use ReLU activations in the Hilbert space of continuous functions. Per the representer theorem, every function in a RKHS that minimizes a risk function can be written as a linear combination of the kernel function evaluated at the training points (Scholkopf *et al.*, 2001). RKHSs can be represented as bounded continuous functions and as feature maps.

## 18.2 Entanglement as a Design Principle

This section considers entanglement as a design tool. Four deployment methods are discussed including entanglement in tensor network design, entanglement in modeling classical data with quantum states, entanglement entropy as a quantum information measure, and entanglement for sequential data analysis (via wavelet transform). These are listed in Table 18.5 as, first, Martyn *et al.* (2020) explore entanglement properties

Table 18.5. Entanglement design for quantum systems.

| No. | Method | Entanglement Use | Findings |
|---|---|---|---|
| *Entanglement as a tensor network design tool* | | | |
| 1 | Supervised learning on block product state TN | Measure range and extent of tensor network entanglement | IR correlations not needed for classification |
| *Entanglement in modeling classical data with quantum states* | | | |
| 2 | Generative learning: DMRG-based MPS TN | Write classical data as quantum states & reduced density matrix | Entanglement preserves classical correlations |
| *Entanglement entropy as a quantum information measure* | | | |
| 3 | 8-qubit quantum circuit TTN and MERA TN | Use entanglement entropy to identify the best model class | Obtain best quantum circuit |
| 4 | Unitary tensor network: Hierarchical tree structure | Use entanglement entropy to calculate gain of whole given part | Useful for image pre-processing and fidelity |
| *Entanglement for sequential data analysis (via wavelet transform)* | | | |
| 5 | Wavelet transform MERA & DMRG-based MPS TN | Renormalize entanglement as time and frequency correlations | Entanglement is key to adaptive learning |

as the amount and range of entanglement within a system with a supervised learning tensor network using block product states.

Second, Bradley *et al.* (2019) model classical data as quantum states, applying the quantum probabilistic method of the reduced density matrix instead of the classical marginal probability distribution, which retains salient system information across scales eliminating it via integration. The "extra information" or entanglement can be used as a design principle to study both the underlying system (classical data) and the tensor network model being used to analyze the data. The same formalism used to interpret the wavefunction is used as a framework to treat classical data, and further, take advantage of the quantum entanglement formulation to identify correlations in the classical data.

Then, two projects incorporate entanglement as a quantum information measure in the design of their models. Grant *et al.* (2018) use entanglement entropy as a core property of synthetic quantum states and model testing to identify the best models. Liu *et al.* (2019) calculate the entanglement entropy of the underlying images as a pre-processing step before the classifier assesses fidelity. Finally, Reyes and Stoudenmire (2020) use wavelet transforms to effectively renormalize entanglement (in the form of local time and frequency correlations in sequential data).

### 18.2.1 *Entanglement and tensor networks*

Entanglement is an important property for characterizing a quantum system. Having a method for quantifying entanglement (identify the correlations between the parts of a system) is crucial. Some of the most relevant entanglement properties are the amount and range of entanglement within the system. This information can be used to obtain an UV–IR correlation profile of the interrelatedness of the subsystems. One team investigates quantum system entanglement properties with a supervised learning tensor network model applied to MNIST data (Martyn *et al.*, 2020). The work proposes a block product state (as opposed to a matrix product state) as a more restricted form of tensor network model for identifying the entanglement properties of the quantum system. In this research, the finding is that long-range correlations in the quantum system may not be important for image classification. The practical implication is that quantum machine learning systems may not need to include long-range correlations, which reduces cost. Also, the work reminds one of information compression algorithms in video streaming that also use mostly short-range correlations. These emerging universal principles and methods are a structural problem akin to that of the brain which also optimizes long-range correlations maintained by the white matter.

The work begins with the pioneering effort of Stoudenmire and Schwab (2017) which has become a standardized basis for many machine learning tensor network models. Stoudenmire and Schwab's model uses tensor networks for supervised image classification tested on the MNIST data set of handwritten digits. The more fundamental theoretical question raised by the model is exactly what quantum state the tensor network might be learning during the training. To identify this quantum state, Martyn *et al.* (2020) propose a plausible candidate state (constructed as a superposition of product states corresponding to the images in the training set) and investigate its entanglement properties. The resulting candidate quantum state is so robustly entangled that it cannot be approximated by the tensor network used by Stoudenmire and Schwab that incorporates matrix product states, and an alternative is needed.

To obtain a better understanding of the entanglement properties of a quantum-type system modeled with tensor networks, the team proposes a block product state structure instead of using the more familiar matrix product state structure. This method effectively treats the system as smaller blocks rather than as a whole. The block product structure restricts the entanglement to being within small blocks of $n \times n$ pixels (qubits). Different forms of block product states are examined, including nearest neighbor block product states and snake block product states, to assess the amount and range of entanglement in the machine learning system. The snake block product state performs best (snaking through the blocks in an s-curve fashion). The result is that block states in this model are extremely expressive (achieving a training accuracy of 99.97% with only $n = 2$). The interpretation is that long-range entanglement (correlations) may not be essential for image classification. The downside is that the current model overfits, and test accuracies are not competitive with other contemporary machine learning approaches. The model's value is as a theoretical investigatory tool for uncovering general principles regarding entanglement in quantum machine learning tensor networks.

#### 18.2.1.1 *Blocks as a renormalization method*

Blocks are a known renormalization method. Martyn *et al.* (2020) use a block product state tensor network as opposed to the more familiar MERA (multi-scale entanglement renormalization ansatz) tensor network. The aim of both is to renormalize entanglement across multiple scale levels within a system. There is a long history of blocks as a renormalization method. Renormalization refers to the renormalization group which is a mathematical apparatus that allows for the systematic investigation of the changes of a physical system as viewed at different scales. Particularly to address the $2^n$ problem of quantum mechanical systems, the idea is to calculate smaller subsets or blocks of the system instead of the system as a whole. The $2^n$ problem in quantum mechanics is that the Hilbert space grows exponentially with size (a spin-1/2 chain of length $n$ has $2^n$ degrees of freedom). The "blocking idea" of block spin (considering blocks of spins) was proposed by Kadanoff (1966) to define the components of a system at large distances as aggregates of components at shorter distances. Wilson (1971) provided the numerical formulation to formally calculate systems with the block idea. One modern tensor network version of renormalization is the density matrix renormalization group (DMRG) method which further develops the concept of blocks in a completely new way as self-resizing smart entities.

#### 18.2.1.2 *Density matrix renormalization group*

The DMRG is a numerical variational technique (sampling method) used in quantum mechanical problem solving such as finding the lowest energy wavefunction of a Hamiltonian. The technique was proposed by White (1992) and is one of the most efficient methods for calculating one-dimensional systems.

The method deploys blocks in an ingenious manner. The central idea is smart decomposition units that resize iteratively. The overall quantum system is decomposed into superblocks consisting of a sandwich of two blocks plus a middle. The insight is to expand each block iteratively (staying within the system and retaining renormalization attributes). This improves on the previous method of appending an exogenous test block to a system block (resulting in failure as the external test block does not have access to information within the system). The problem is framed as having a complex multi-dimensional system and needing a means of expanding and testing permutations of sub-blocks within the system to determine its properties, and using some kind of smart decomposition structure to do so. The self-resizing block is a smart renormalization structure.

The DMRG method operates as follows. After a warm-up cycle, the method splits the system into two subsystems (blocks), which do not need to have equal size, and two sites in between. A set of *representative states* (for the ground state) has been chosen for the block during the warm-up. The set of the left block plus two sites in the middle plus the right block is known as the superblock. Now a candidate for the ground state of the superblock, which is a reduced version of the full system, may be found. The accuracy may not be good, but the method is iterative and improves as the process cycles.

The candidate ground state that has been found is projected into the Hilbert subspace for each block using a density matrix (juggernaut apparatus of all information about a quantum state), hence the name DMRG method. The *relevant states* for each block are updated. One of the blocks grows at the expense of the other and the procedure is repeated. When the growing block reaches maximum size, the other starts to grow in its place. Each time the process returns to the original situation of blocks of equal size, a sweep is said to have been completed. In practice, only a few sweeps may be needed, for example, to obtain the precision formulation of a one-dimensional lattice.

The success of the DMRG method is due to overcoming the problems of previous renormalization group methods by connecting two blocks with the two sites in the middle rather than adding a single site to a block at each step, and by using the density matrix to identify the most important states to keep at the end of each step.

### 18.2.2 *Classical data and quantum states*

A key insight in quantum computing is that classical data can be modeled with quantum states, and that this provides surprising visibility into otherwise inaccessible correlations in the underlying data. One example is modeling classical probability distributions with quantum states (Bradley *et al.*, 2019). The implication is that the same formalism used to interpret the wavefunction in quantum mechanics can be used as a framework for treating classical data, and take advantage of quantum entanglement formulations to identify correlations in the classical data. Classical statistics are represented with a probability distribution, and further, to reduce complexity, a marginal probability distribution. The quantum mechanical statistical equivalents are the density matrix and the reduced density matrix. The density matrix encapsulates all information about a quantum state in a statistical format.

The point is that the reduced density matrix contains more information than the marginal distribution. The reduced density matrices hold efficient information to reconstruct the entire joint probability distribution whereas marginal probability distributions do not. The quantum method is therefore a more effective means of modeling classical probability distributions. Since there is entanglement in quantum states, the reduced density matrix that describes the subsystems in the quantum system includes entanglement, which carries along information about complementary subsystems. This is in contrast to the classical picture in which the marginal probability distribution integrates out information about complementary subsystems.

A training algorithm based on the DMRG procedure uses the extra information (entanglement) contained in the reduced density matrices and instantiates it into a tensor network model. The extra information (entanglement) is used to find previously unseen correlations in the underlying system (classical data) and is also used to study the model, by producing an error estimate for the training such that the model can be improved as well.

Entanglement, as the additional system information available in the quantum method of the reduced density matrix as compared to the classical marginal probability distribution is a design principle that can be deployed both for studying the underlying system and the model used to study it. Entanglement is the first and primary design principle as a quantity that is present in quantum systems, increasingly accessible with quantum probabilistic methods, and routinely renormalized in quantitative models such as tensor networks.

### 18.2.3 *Entanglement entropy*

Two projects use entanglement as a quantum information measure in the design of their models. Grant *et al.* (2018) develop an 8-qubit quantum circuit to classify both classical data (Iris and MNIST) and entangled quantum data (self-generated) with tensor network models (TTN and MERA), and test the circuit with Iris data on a currently available quantum computer (IBM QX4). Synthetic quantum states are created as an entangled data source with which to test and develop the quantum circuit. A key advance is the algorithm that is able to classify highly entangled quantum states, for which there is no known efficient classical method.

Ten different versions of the 8-qubit quantum circuit are produced and tested with the quantum data. A dataset of 5,000 quantum states is generated for each circuit. A quantum state is generated by randomizing all the single-qubit gates, and then executing the circuit on the initial state. The process is repeated many times to produce the quantum dataset for each circuit. The benefit of having quantum states data is that they can be fed directly into the quantum computer without additional processing. The quantum computer executes a machine learning classification algorithm with the task of identifying which of two circuit layouts generated a particular quantum state. The aim is to correctly classify the states most of the time and reduce the error in doing so.

Entanglement entropy is calculated to assess the results of the synthetic classification task based on the bipartite entanglement measure proposed by Bennett and DiVincenzo (2000). For each state (each of the 5,000 states of data for each circuit), the maximum bipartite entanglement entropy is computed over all possible partitions A and B of the 8 qubits. The maximum bipartite entanglement entropy is the degree to which the maximum entropy in partition A is equal to the maximum entropy in partition B. The assumption is that a circuit is implied to be well-formed if the entropy between its parts are equal. The more equally the entanglement entropy is balanced within the system, the better the circuit. Entanglement entropy is calculated to identify the best circuits. The range of entanglement entropy distributions is examined with the aim of finding an optimal threshold that classifies states correctly most of the time. Such a result indicates that the classification task is meaningful and reflected in the circuits.

Liu *et al.* (2019) also use entanglement entropy as a machine learning tensor network design tool. Here, the entanglement entropy is computed for each individual instance, not as quantum states, but as the underlying data (MNIST images). A four-way bipartite entanglement (up/down and left/right) measure is employed to assess the images before loading them into the classifier. Entanglement entropy is further used as a quantum information measure to distinguish the amount of information in one subsystem that can be gained by measuring an entangled subsystem. Entanglement entropy is used to calculate the information gain from the whole given a part. The implied correspondence is between seeing a partial image and measuring the subsystem of the quantum state. The implication is that given a partial image, entanglement entropy quantifies the additional information that can be obtained from the whole image.

## References

Alcazar, J., Leyton-Ortega, V. & Perdomo-Ortiz, A. (2020). Classical versus quantum models in machine learning: Insights from a finance application. arXiv:1908.10778v2.

Bennett, C.H. & DiVincenzo, D.P. (2000). Quantum information and computation. *Nature*. 404:247–55.

Bradley, T.-D., Stoudenmire, E.M. & Terilla, J. (2019). Modeling sequences with quantum states: A look under the hood. *Mach. Learn.: Sci. Technol.* 1:035008.

Chatterjee, R. & Yu, T. (2017). Generalized coherent states, reproducing kernels, and quantum support vector machines. *Quantum Inf. Commun.* 17(15-16): 1292–1306.

Farhi, E. & Neven, H. (2018). Classification with quantum neural networks on near term processors. arXiv:1802.06002. MIT-CTP/4985.

Gazeau, J.-P. (2009). *Coherent States in Quantum Physics*. New York: Wiley.

Grant, E., Benedetti, M., Cao, S., *et al.* (2018). Hierarchical quantum classifiers. *NPJ Quantum Inf.* 4(65):1–8.

Kadanoff, L.P. (1966). Scaling laws for Ising models near $T_c$. *Physics Physique Fizika*. 2:263–72.

Klauder, J.R. & Skagerstam, B.-S. (1985). *Coherent States: Applications in Physics and Mathematical Physics*. London: World Scientific.

Liu, D., Ran, S.-J., Wittek, P. *et al.* (2019). Machine learning by unitary tensor network of hierarchical tree structure. arXiv:1710.04833v4.

Martyn, J., Vidal, G., Roberts, C. & Leichenauer, S. (2020). Entanglement and tensor networks for supervised image classification. arXiv:2007.06082v1.

Reyes, J. & Stoudenmire, E.M. (2020). A multi-scale tensor network architecture for classification and regression. arXiv:2001.08286v1.

Schnabel, R. (2017). Squeezed states of light and their applications in laser interferometers. *Phys. Rep.* 684:1–51.

Scholkopf, B., Herbrich, R. & Smola, A. (2001). *Computational Learning Theory.* London: Springer, pp. 416–26.

Scholkopf, B. & Smola, A.J. (2002). *Learning with Kernels: Support Vector Machines, Regularization, Optimization, and Beyond.* Cambridge: MIT Press.

Schuld, M. & Killoran, N. (2019). Quantum machine learning in feature Hilbert spaces. *Phys. Rev. Lett.* 122(4):040504.

Slusher, R.E. *et al.* (1985). Observation of squeezed states generated by four wave mixing in an optical cavity. *Phys. Rev. Lett.* 55(22):2409.

Stoudenmire, E.M. & Schwab, D.J. (2017). Supervised learning with quantum inspired tensor networks. *Advances in Neural Information Processing Systems*. 29:4799.

Vidal, G. (2007). Entanglement renormalization. *Phys. Rev. Lett.* 99(22):220405.

Walls, D.F. (1983). Squeezed states of light. *Nature*. 306(5939):141–6.

White, S.R. (1992). Density matrix formulation for quantum renormalization groups. *Phys. Rev. Lett.* 69(19):2863–6.

Wilson, K.G. (1971). Renormalization group and critical phenomena. I. Renormalization group and the Kadanoff scaling picture. *Phys. Rev. B.* 4:3174–83.

Wu, L.-A. (1986). Generation of squeezed states by parametric down conversion. *Phys. Rev. Lett.* 57(20):2520–3.

# Chapter 19

# Brain Modeling and Machine Learning

*[T]he human brain, the ultimate machine*

— Paul Allen (2011, p. 304)

**Abstract**

This chapter discusses brain modeling approaches including compartmental neuroscience simulation, classical machine learning, and spiking neural networks in neuromorphic architectures. It is clear that quantum methods and platforms could extend these efforts. Of particular interest is the need to model the effects of nonlinear calcium signaling in synaptic integration which requires the diffusion-reaction mathematics of partial differential equations (PDEs). Spiking neural network methods propose useful alternatives to classical machine learning's backpropagation as real-life temporal models cannot go backward to iteratively update network weights as permutations of the model cycle.

## 19.1 Brain Modeling

The brain, and particularly neural signaling, has long been the target of various modeling strategies. A fundamental advance was Hodgkin and Huxley's (1952) proposal for how ion channels give rise to the action potential. The work resulted in the 1963 Nobel Prize in Physiology or Medicine for describing the propagation of electric signals in squid axons.

Contemporary neural signaling is often analyzed by starting with the Hodgkin–Huxley model as the basis for articulating the conduction of electrical impulses through the axon. What is new in neuroscience is the contemporary era of "big data" connectomics and imaging technologies and computational tools such as machine learning and quantum computing becoming standardized approaches. At present, there are three approaches to neuroscience modeling and the study of neural signaling — classical computational neuroscience, classical machine learning, and neuromorphic architectures and spiking neural networks (Table 19.1).

An open challenge is the situation that most computational platforms do not yet include full functionality for synaptic integration, one of the biggest problems in the domain. Synaptic integration (or dendritic integration) is the neuron's information processing capability of aggregating thousands of incoming synaptic inputs from other neurons. Although many neuroscience modeling platforms support dendritic trees, most do not include full synaptic integration (Poirazi & Papoutsi, 2020). The problem is that the main method for modeling the effects of nonlinear calcium signaling in dendritic spiking activity requires the diffusion-reaction mathematics of partial differential equations (PDEs) which are difficult to include in neuroscience modeling applications. In classical computational neuroscience, some multicompartmental models (having separate compartments for axon-soma and dendritic activity) attempt to include a basic level of spatial synaptic integration functionality. Classical machine learning is primarily focused on neuron reconstruction and synapse detection in connectome projects, and hence synaptic integration is not yet a concern. Neuromorphic architectures and spiking neural networks generally do not offer synaptic integration functionality. As the challenge is complex, three-dimensional, and involves diffusion equations, it might be

Table 19.1. Neuroscience modeling approaches.

| No. | Modeling Category | Platforms |
|---|---|---|
| 1 | Computational neuroscience | NEURON, GENESIS, BRIAN, NEST |
| 2 | Classical machine learning | Connectomics: TeraVR, *DeepNeuron* |
| 3 | Neuromorphic architectures and spiking neural networks | Neurogrid, SpiNNaker, BrainScaleS, DYNAP-SE, Pohoiki Beach, True North |

appropriate for quantum computing. Synaptic integration could be a key opportunity for quantum computing for the brain applications, including the possible emergence of a subfield devoted to quantum machine learning for synaptic integration.

### 19.1.1 *Compartmental neuroscience models*

Tikidji-Hamburyan *et al.* (2017) conduct a review of contemporary computational neuroscience simulation platforms. The simulators are software programs that accommodate a range of single-neuron and brain network modeling (Table 19.2). Four simulators are selected as the three most popular (determined by the number of models using them in the ModelDB database), NEURON, GENESIS, and BRIAN, plus NEST as the leading simulator of the Human Brain Project. The standard platform is NEURON, which focuses on the intricacies of single-neuron modeling, and at the other end of the spectrum is NEST, which is used for network modeling and most easily maps to high-performance computing environments. BRIAN might be the most "quantum-ready" as it is a simulator for spiking neural networks (Goodman & Brette, 2008), and already incorporates machine learning, which is an add-on to the other simulators. Brette *et al.* (2007) also survey the market.

Although the brain processes to be modeled have simple intuitive explanations (for example, diffusion or voltage propagation in dendrites), the mathematical and computational implementation is not straightforward and requires knowledge of PDEs and numerical methods.

Table 19.2. Computational neuroscience simulators.

| Range | Single-Neuron | | Whole-Brain | |
|---|---|---|---|---|
| Simulator | NEURON | GENESIS | BRIAN | NEST |
| Notable features | Detailed interaction models, education | Diffusion-reactions, nonlinear reconstruction | Most structured computational language | Large-scale networks, human connectome projects |
| Citations | 1 (most) | 2 | 3 | 4 (least) |

Neuroscientists and computer scientists typically work together to outline the problems and workflows, and implement the simulators. Ultimately, the simulators compile the most computationally intensive procedures into binary code, with the aim of maximizing computational performance. A detailed example of single-neuron modeling is described by Mainen and Sejnowski (1996), and brain networks in the Blue Brain and Human Brain Projects (Markram, 2012). Simulators can be categorized along the single-neuron to brain networks continuum (as in the table), by dynamics (with dynamics that are absent, discontinuous, or continuous), or by model class (single-compartment, two-compartment, or multicompartment). The four simulators support all of the versions of neural dynamics and model classes, though in different ways and with a varying intensity of custom programming required. In the simulators, models of discontinuous dynamics include minimal complexity, and although continuous dynamics models include some more complex features (the general dynamics of membrane potential as well as different types of neuron excitability), the biophysical nature of temporal integration is still extremely simplified.

#### 19.1.1.1 *Compartment model classes*

In terms of model classes, the single-compartment model focuses on the axon and soma relation, and attempts to accurately model the biophysical processes of membrane potential dynamics. This includes factors such as cross-membrane currents and membrane capacitance, but not their spatial integration (the distribution of ion channels along dendrite trees). These are conductance-based models in which each cross-membrane current is represented as a nonlinear conductance that is connected to a battery with voltage equal to Nernst's reversal potential. The conductance is a complex dynamic model with one or more dynamic variables. The classical example of a single-compartment conductance-based model is the Hodgkin–Huxley model (Hodgkin & Huxley, 1952).

Two-compartment models are the start toward a fuller spatial reconstruction of neural signaling, and feature a basic representation of the axon and soma of a neuron in one compartment and the dendrites in the other. The strength of electrical coupling between the compartments and their size is used to imitate different neuron morphologies. Ion channels are typically described by two voltage-dependent gating variables and one calcium-dependent variable with Boltzmann rate functions. A typical example is an implementation of the McCormick two-compartment model of a cortical pyramidal cell. This consists of a minimum of ten ion channels with sixteen activation-inactivation variables, each of which has two rate functions, plus calcium and sodium dynamics, and synaptic dynamics.

A multicompartment model is used for the full spatial reconstruction of neuron morphology including both axon-soma and dendrite activity. The difference between the two-compartment model and the full spatial reconstruction is a more detailed dendritic process in the form of the distribution of ion channels along dendrite trees. Multiple compartments are used to model different aspects of the signaling process, particularly the complex diffusion-reaction system of calcium signaling. Whereas the simpler axon-soma and dendrite processes can be modeled with ordinary differential equations (ODEs), a PDE formulation is required for the diffusion-reaction of dendrites (Dayan & Abbott, 2001, p. 806) (Table 19.3).

The treatment of cross-membrane potential is at the heart of simulation models. A cross-membrane electrical current depends on both inner and outer ion concentrations. The usual example of such a dependency is a calcium-dependent potassium current, in which conductance is a function of the intracellular calcium concentration. In simple models, calcium kinetics is usually defined as a first-order ODE, which is easy to embed into a single-compartment or two-compartment model. However, the dynamics of calcium concentration is much more complex than a

Table 19.3. Computational neuroscience model classes.

| Parameter | Single-Compartment | Two-Compartment | Multicompartment |
|---|---|---|---|
| Model topic | Axon-soma | Axon-soma and dendrite (basic) | Axon-soma and dendrite (advanced) |
| Signaling functionality | Electric signaling | Electric signaling | Electric and calcium signaling |
| Model focus | Membrane dynamics | Ion channels | Diffusion-reaction system |
| Mathematics | ODE | ODE | PDE |

first-order ODE in a real neuron. Calcium may be buffered by calmodulin and many other molecules pumped into or released from mitochondria and endoplasmic reticula. Calcium ions can diffuse inside a neuron both radially and along dendrites (longitudinal diffusion). A dendrite model is essentially a nonlinear diffusion-reaction system and hence the simulator must support diffusion-reaction systems and their modeling method, PDEs.

The four simulators generally support the different model classes and dynamics. NEURON and GENESIS are more modular and BRIAN and NEST are more attuned to large-scale network models with simple individual neurons. NEURON and GENESIS can fully support the complex intracellular diffusion-reaction system, while in NEST, individual neurons are considered mostly as point processes without geometrical representation. NEURON has a graphical user interface and allows various single-compartment and multicompartment models that do not require any coding and is therefore more accessible and widely used for educational purposes. A further consideration is neuron-to-neuron communication, in which synapses (modeled as gap junctions) may require updating at each simulation step.

#### 19.1.1.2 *Synaptic integration*

Synaptic integration is the neuron's information processing capability of aggregating thousands of incoming synaptic inputs from other neurons. A problem that arises in modeling synaptic integration with computational neuroscience platforms is that real-life synaptic currents from other neurons have complex nonlinear dynamics. However, in models, input currents are often treated as a direct current that is static, which results in linear current inputs, and overall an incomplete spatiotemporal progression in computational neuroscience models even when using multicompartmental models.

An overlay method is proposed as one solution to the too-basic linear dynamics of incoming signaling currents problem (Li *et al.*, 2019). The work proposes an overlay to the existing point neuron model (in NEURON), in the form of a synaptic integration current that can capture a greater range of dendritic effects. The overlay consists of parametrizing the interaction between each pair of synaptic inputs on the dendrites with a single coefficient. The result is a fast algorithm for neuronal simulation that includes the more realistic dynamics of a neuron with detailed dendritic morphology within the standard computational framework. The enhanced point neuron model incorporates an additional synaptic integration current arising from the nonlinear interaction between synaptic currents across spatial dendrites. The model captures the somatic voltage response of a neuron with complex dendrites and is capable of performing rich dendritic computations. This leads to an improved analysis of the decomposition of excitatory and inhibitory synaptic inputs, and the finding that the impact of spike inhibition may have been underestimated in previous studies. The model includes the known dendritic filtering effect (that far-off signals are attenuated).

An unrelated team also presents a more robust model of nonlinear synaptic integration (Li *et al.*, 2020). The finding is that excitatory synaptic currents (both fast and slow) have a much more complex dynamics (via oscillatory fluctuations) than expected, and that normal activity has a greater impact on integration than noise. Another consideration of nonlinear synaptic integration models the postsynaptic density and dendritic shape as elliptical spheroids (Cugno *et al.*, 2019). The research indicates that the curvature of dendritic geometry gives rise to pseudo-harmonic functions that can be used to predict the locations of minimal and maximal dendrite concentrations along the spine head and how this might be related to the processing of incoming signals.

In terms of testing models on neuromorphic processors (that imitate spiking neural networks by firing per a thresholding effect), synaptic integration is not always part of on-board chip functionality. Two neuromorphic computing projects may begin to incorporate greater support for dendritic trees in *BrainScaleS* (Schemmel *et al.*, 2017) and for shared dendritic encoding in *Neurogrid* (Boahen *et al.*, 2020). There is at least one existing neuromorphic processor, DYNAP-SE (Dynamic Neuromorphic Asynchronous Processor) from aiCTX, which offers neuron and synapse functionality (Moradi *et al.*, 2018). The DYNAP-SE is a reconfigurable, general-purpose, mixed-signal Spiking Neural Network processor with analog circuits that can be used to emulate the biophysics of neurons and synapses in real-time. Nilsson *et al.* (2020) make use of the DYNAP-SE neuromorphic chip, together with an excitatory-inhibitory pair combination method for synaptic integration. The method solves a problem in being less computationally and energetically costly than other multi-compartmental and neuromorphic circuit methods, but is also a little less flexible.

For possible encoding on the *BrainScaleS* neuromorphic platform, Stockel and Eliasmith (2020) extend an existing neural engineering framework (Eliasmith & Anderson, 2003) with nonlinear conductance-based synapses. This addresses the problem that postsynaptic currents are usually treated as a linear superposition of filtered presynaptic events. Instead, the work develops biophysical phenomena as computational primitives, namely, synaptic filtering, and the nonlinear relationship between somatic input currents and neural response. The proposal reinforces the argument that biological computational models are much more powerful than is currently being exploited.

#### 19.1.1.3 *The future of compartmental models*

The longer-term future of neuroscience modeling could feature a wider range of models including those that are compartmental among others. On the one hand, there are critiques of the insufficiencies of the compartmental model (Almog & Korngreen, 2016). The work argues that the compartmental method's focus on single neurons is ad hoc and unrealistic. Given the interconnected behavior of the brain, an "immense expansion" in computer power might allow the instantiation of more realistic multineuron models. Likewise, others argue that the intricacies of dendritic phenomena such as the integration of spatially distributed synaptic inputs are beyond the scope of the existing point neuron models (Herz *et al.*, 2006; Gerstner & Naud, 2009).

On the other hand, advances also continue to be made with the compartmental model, including in multineuron interaction. Mel (2016) uses a detailed compartmental model setup in NEURON in an ongoing body of work that investigates the dense network of connections through which pyramidal neurons exchange information. The compartmental model is applied to study the symmetry or asymmetry between a proximal and distal location on one dendrite. Individually, input signals behave differently, but the problem of interest is characterizing the symmetry or asymmetry of the interaction between the two inputs when they are applied together. Various patterns arise, in particular a two-dimensional asymmetric sigmoidal function (a left-shifting in the sigmoid) and eventually a linearization of the input–output curve. The effect of a distal modulator on a proximal input is not an increase in the excursion size but a left-shifting of the sigmoid. A two-dimensional asymmetric sigmoidal function is produced that is a two-dimensional nonlinearity. The implication is the brain has the ability to steer inputs proximally and distally and by doing so these modulatory effects can be tailored to nonlinear asymmetric multi-dimensional sigmoidal interaction functions (Jin *et al.*, 2018).

### 19.1.2 *Theoretical neuroscience*

The broader theoretical neuroscience concern is the right kinds of modeling approaches to address the complex reality of the brain. In the contemporary era of greater real-life data capture and computational modeling capacity, stalwart models are being examined and possibly superseded by new models. A key theme is extending the single neuron view to also consider the brain as an interconnected network of multiple neurons. Historical views have directed modeling activity. These include the "neuron doctrine" proposing that the elementary biological unit in the brain is the active cell of the neuron (Ramon y Cajal, 1894), and Hebbian plasticity which suggests modeling the brain as a single primitive at the single neuron level (Hebb, 1949). In one extension to Hebbian plasticity, Valiant (2018) proposes that cortical activity is built on a small collection of base primitives at the intermediate systems level. The four primitives are based on resource constraints on neuron numbers, connection numbers, and synaptic strengths, and include association, memorization, inductive learning, and hierarchical memory assignment.

#### 19.1.2.1 *Network neuroscience modeling*

In ongoing work, Bassett *et al.* (2018) develop a brain networks view, instantiating neuroscience modeling with the graph-theoretic approach of network science. An attractive aspect of the work is the systematic approach in attempting to elicit the bulk properties of the brain (Table 19.4). The method proposes theoretical model development in four phase-based transitions.

The first phase is the transition from data representation to first-principles theories. Concretely in the graph-theoretic approach, the data representation might be stored as a simple, temporal, multilayer, or annotated graph. To reach a theory-based model, operations are performed on the data, for example, by combining the graph with a differential equation to specify the dynamics, evolution, and function of the network nodes and edges. The second phase is the transition from structure to function, a key aim in connectome projects. For example, a synthesis of extensive prior work in the macaque suggests that the pattern of 305 structural connections among 32 visual areas is consistent with a distributed hierarchy of information processing. The third phase is the transition from elementary descriptions to coarse-grained approximations, which might involve various renormalization methods. Where, in quantum mechanical physics, individual quarks are a basic description that gives way to small masses, likewise in the brain, the firing of individual neurons is studied in larger-scale models of neural behavior such as mean-field theories and neural mass models. The fourth phase is the transition from simplicity to complexity as partial brain models are now giving way to an insistence on three-dimensional, whole-brain, full-volume descriptions.

Table 19.4. Network neuroscience phase transitions.

| No. | Model Phase Transition | Transition Example |
|---|---|---|
| 1 | From data representation to first-principles theory | Simple graph representation -> differential equation specifying dynamics |
| 2 | From structure to function (connectome projects) | 305 macaque connectome structural connections -> 32 visual areas distributed hierarchy of information processing |
| 3 | From elementary descriptions to coarse-grained approximations | Quarks -> small mass; individual neuron firing -> mean-field or neural mass model |
| 4 | From simple to complex | Partial brain -> whole-brain |

### 19.1.2.2 *Empirical context: Brain–computer interfaces*

Accurate neuroscience modeling is crucial to the operation of real-life brain–computer interfaces (BCIs). BCIs or brain–machine interfaces (BMIs) are a direct communications pathway between a wired brain and an external device. They seek to establish real-time bidirectional links between living brains and artificial actuators (in prosthetics, for example). Various BCI applications exist for the neural control of robotic and virtual actuator movement to direct upper and lower limb functions (Lebedev & Nicolelis, 2017). In the other direction, BCIs also deliver sensory feedback generated by external actuators to the brain. Studies find that BCIs, though artificial tools, are assimilated into the neurophysiological schema of the body (in primates).

A contemporary research topic in BCIs is more efficient algorithms for signal decoding and real-time control. Some of the approaches to control algorithms include machine learning, manifold geometry, and spiking neural networks. Machine learning methods are frequently used in the algorithmic decoders of brain signals in BCIs (Lebedev & Nicolelis, 2017, p. 792). New machine learning techniques are proposed based on the application of the least-squares complex-valued filter to analyze real-time EEG data related to BCIs (Smetanin *et al.*, 2020). Such algorithms are relevant for the real-time control of BCIs for applications in which participants learn to modulate their own brain activity, previously prohibitive due to feedback delays. Other research from Petrosuan *et al.* (2020) proposes the use of convolutional neural networks to decode BCI signals in a compact spatiotemporal format. What is new is the ability to tune both toward the decoding of target signals and away from interference, in both the spatial and the frequency domains. Such data might be conducive to wavelet transforms and implementation in the MERA-based quantum machine learning tensor networks proposed by (Reyes & Stoudenmire, 2020).

Another team, Trautmann *et al.* (2019), propose a more scalable geometric approach to estimate neural population dynamics that does not involve the traditional technique of spike sorting. Spike sorting is the attribution of action potentials to individual neurons. However, the method is not scalable as future generations of BCIs might have increasing numbers of electrodes, instead of hundreds, maybe thousands or even millions (Stevenson & Kording, 2011). The geometric approach uses the theory of random projections which suggests the possibility of accurately estimating the geometry of low-dimensional manifolds from a small number of linear projections of the data. Multi-unit threshold crossings are used in place of sorted neurons. The threshold crossings method applies to population-level analyses but is not applicable to situations involving only single neurons. Finally, the deployment of spiking mechanisms has been suggested as a more natural activation of spike processing in BCIs (Serb *et al.*, 2020).

## 19.2 Classical Machine Learning and Neuroscience

### 19.2.1 *Machine learning and biomedicine*

> *To mathematical biophysics, the [all-or-none threshold firing] theory contributes a tool for rigorous symbolic treatment of known nets and an easy method of constructing hypothetical nets*
>
> — McCulloch and Pitts (1943, p. 132)

McCulloch and Pitts propose one of the first models of artificial neural networks, suggesting that the "all-or-none" threshold firing character of neurons can be treated with propositional logic (1943, p. 115). Machine learning has ensued as a highly successful area of computer science for image, speech, and text recognition. Classical machine learning methods have also gained attention in the biomedical context, primarily in the use of imaging applications for pathology diagnosis. Several studies have indicated achieving expert-level performance in medical image interpretation tasks with machine learning algorithms.

One of the first projects was the demonstration of dermatologist-level classification of skin cancer with deep neural networks (Esteva *et al.*, 2017). A deep convolutional neural network is trained using a dataset of 129,450 clinical images consisting of 2,032 different diseases. The neural network's performance is tested against 21 board-certified dermatologists examining biopsy-proven clinical images. The neural network achieves performance on par with tested experts. The implication is that neural networks might be able to help with diagnostic preprocessing and extend the reach of dermatologists. The human-level performance of medical professionals has been similarly demonstrated in other medical imaging tasks such as lymph node metastases detection in breast cancer (Bejnordi *et al.*, 2017) and diabetic retinopathy detection (Gulshan *et al.*, 2016).

In a more complicated diagnostic situation, Rajpurkar *et al.* (2018) demonstrate human-level performance in the evaluation of chest X-rays. A deep learning algorithm is used to classify clinically important abnormalities in chest radiographs at a performance level comparable to that of practicing board-certified radiologists. Chest radiography is the most common type of worldwide imaging examination, with over two billion procedures performed each year. A convolutional neural network (CheXNeXt) is developed to concurrently detect the presence of fourteen different pathologies, including pneumonia, pleural effusion, pulmonary masses, and nodules in frontal-view chest radiographs. The network was trained and validated with a set of 420 images held out of the training data, containing at least 50 cases of each of the original pathology labels.

### 19.2.2 *Machine learning and neuroscience*

#### 19.2.2.1 *Machine learning and brain tumors*

Accurate pathological diagnosis is crucial for the optimal management of cancer patients. However, for the 100 known central nervous system tumor entities, standardization of the diagnostic process has been particularly challenging. There is a high degree of variability in the histopathological diagnosis of many tumor types. To address this problem, Capper *et al.* (2018) present a machine learning approach to DNA methylation-based central nervous system tumor classification across all tumor types and age groups. The machine learning method consists of an unsupervised clustering analysis of reference cohort samples ($n$ = 2,801) including using a dimensionality reduction technique. Individual samples are coded into respective pathology classes ($n$ = 91). The algorithm then classifies new tissue methylation data based on these labels. The result suggests a prospective change in diagnosis in 12% of cases examined.

The work is notable as central nervous system tumors are highly diverse clinically and biologically. Tumors encompass a wide spectrum from benign neoplasms that may be cured by surgery alone (such as pilocytic astrocytoma) to highly malignant tumors that respond poorly to any therapy (such as glioblastoma). The research incorporates the full range of over 100 brain tumor types defined by the WHO classification of central nervous system tumors, including glioblastoma, ependymomas, glioneuronal tumors, and choroid plexus tumors (Louis *et al.*, 2016).

#### 19.2.2.2 *Machine learning and neuropathologies of aging*

In one practical application of machine learning and neuroscience, an automated machine learning technique for the EEG-based classification of Parkinson's disease patients is proposed (Koch *et al.*, 2019). The method consists of extracting 794 features from each of the 21 EEG channels, which results in a massive feature space that is classified with a Bayesian method. The approach is compared to the features commonly used during the clinical evaluation of EEG data, with the result that the automated model achieves a significantly higher accuracy (84.0%). Having a set of data-driven biomarkers for Parkinson's disease could be helpful in decision-making about whether the invasive implantation of Deep Brain Stimulation devices would help patients.

In another practical application of machine learning and neuroscience, convolutional neural networks are used to analyze the aging of the human brain. Cole *et al.* (2016) perform machine learning analysis on fMRI neuroimaging data ($n = 2{,}001$) to accurately predict the chronological age of healthy people and deviations from healthy brain aging that have been associated with cognitive impairment and disease. The age predictions are generated using raw imaging data. The convolutional neural network brain-predicted age appears to represent an accurate, highly reliable, and genetically valid phenotype that has potential to be used as a biomarker of brain aging. The benefit of a baseline standard is substantially reducing the computation time for novel data, which speeds up the possibility of providing real-time information on brain health in clinical settings.

In similar research, Levakova *et al.* (2019) present a deep learning framework for the prediction of chronological age from structural MRI scans ($n = 10{,}176$). The analysis examines the biomarkers of neurological disorders and brain aging in more detail. Using a convolutional neural network to analyze raw imaging data allows the identification of the brain regions that have the biggest contribution to brain aging, and an analysis of the underlying processes. The finding is that cavities containing cerebral spinal fluid, previously identified as general markers of atrophy, have the highest contribution to predicting brain age, and may be an early warning signal of pathology. These kinds of information about human brain aging health and pathology might be further combined with synapse lifespan data (Cizeron *et al.*, 2020) to further indicate early-onset neuropathologies.

### 19.2.3 *Machine learning and connectomics*

One of the fastest-growing applications in machine learning neuroscience is connectomics. Connectome imaging is producing more data than most other biomedical fields (Motta *et al.*, 2019). With the widespread use of high-throughput recording techniques for data acquisition, data analysis is now the current bottleneck, particularly neuron reconstruction and synapse detection. Other data analysis imaging challenges include tracking cells in high-resolution videography, analyzing spike data from large-scale electrode arrays, and detecting action potentials from calcium-based fluorescence transients, all of which might be facilitated with machine learning-related methods for image classification.

#### 19.2.3.1 *Neuron reconstruction: TeraVR and DeepNeuron*

One of the primary focal areas in high-throughput connectomics and neuroinformatics is neuron reconstruction. Such reconstruction entails converting high-resolution micro-imaging data to a usable description of morphology, distinguishing between neurons and glia, and including the three-dimensional spatial locations of a cell's parts and its topological connections. The task involves single-neuron tracing (identification) and connectivity (synapse) detection. Neuron reconstruction is the first data annotation step toward being able to understand cell type, function, connectivity, and development.

The Allen Institute continues to develop various brain atlases, annotation tools, and methods. Toward the task of whole-brain single-neuron reconstruction, an open-source virtual reality annotation system is proposed, TeraVR (Wang *et al.*, 2019). TeraVR is a virtual reality neuron reconstruction platform designed to manage terabyte-scale (whole-brain) imaging data. TeraVR integrates immersive and collaborative three-dimensional visualization, interaction, and hierarchical streaming of tera-voxel-scale images. The benefit of TeraVR is being able to annotate the precise full morphology of long-projecting neurons in whole mouse brains. TeraVR is based in intelligent tracing algorithms which can be bundled with deep learning neural networks such as *DeepNeuron* for accelerated neuron reconstruction. *DeepNeuron* is an open-source toolbox using deep learning networks for neuron reconstruction, in particular, detecting neuron signals, connecting neuronal signals into a tree, pruning and refining the tree morphology, and classifying dendrites and axons in real time (Zhou *et al.*, 2018). *DeepNeuron* has been implemented as an Open-Source plugin in Vaa3D.

#### 19.2.3.2 *Neural connectivity: Synapse detection*

In neuron reconstruction, after tracing a single neuron, the next step is identifying neural connectivity by detecting synapses. Unfortunately synapse detection may be equally as complex as neuron reconstruction and hence machine learning methods could likewise be indispensable (Dorkenwald *et al.*, 2017). Steady improvements in automated electron microscopy segmentation suggest that the detection of synaptic connectivity could become the next focal point for innovation in the overall neuron reconstruction process (Staffler *et al.*, 2017). In other work, Parag *et al.* (2018) present a method for automated synapse detection. The approach proposes a general-purpose synaptic connectivity detector that attributes the location and direction of a synapse simultaneously. In the algorithm, first, one deep fully convolutional neural network generates candidate synaptic connections from three-dimensional voxel data proximity predictions. Then a second three-dimensional convolutional neural network prunes the set of candidates to produce the final detection of cleft and connectivity orientation. Experimental results indicate that the algorithm outperforms the existing methods for determining synapses in both rodent and fruit fly brain projects.

#### 19.2.3.3 *Brain atlas annotation and deep learning network*

Machine learning is also used in connectomics to check and backstop other methods, for example, in improving the quality of neuroscience tools such as brain atlases (Iqbal *et al.*, 2019). The aim of a brain atlas is to serve as a standard reference guide to anatomical regions of interest in the brain. However, there can be considerable variability in acquired data due to brain size and form differences across individuals. Thus, machine learning techniques are applied to identify potential holes and inconsistencies in the registration to render atlas data more coherent. The work proceeds from a project implementing a solution for neuron detection at multiple scales of analysis. A high-performance deep neural network detects neurons labeled with different genetic markers in a range of imaging planes and imaging modalities. The work introduces a fully automated artificial intelligence-based method for whole-brain image processing to detect neurons in different brain regions during development (*DeNeRD*). The benefit is facilitating the task of mapping the structure of the mammalian brain at cellular resolution that requires capturing key anatomical features at the appropriate level of analysis.

#### 19.2.3.4 *Generative machine learning for unlabeled data*

Since volumetric brain data is high-dimensional, machine learning connectomics can move more quickly to generative machine learning methods that use unsupervised learning to classify unlabeled data. The higher dimensionality allows generative algorithms the ability to learn the distribution of the data, as compared to discriminative algorithms that are restricted to learning directly from already-labeled data in supervised learning (Goodfellow *et al.*, 2014). The upshot for connectomics is that large datasets can be labeled using only a small fraction of raw image data for training (Motta *et al.*, 2019).

The functional imaging data of intracellular calcium transients is a good example. The source of calcium transients is action potentials in the soma occurring at certain time points. The transformation of an action potential to the somatic calcium influx, calcium binding to the sensor proteins and its decay dynamics, as well as the sources of imaging noise, are all relatively well understood. Therefore, the generative model describing action potential-to-calcium data transformation is well constrained. This means that by optimizing the action potential time points to generate data that best resembles the measured data, it is possible to obtain the action potential time points as a result, which helps to create a temporal profile of activity.

However, significant advance may be required for the fully automated connectomic machine learning of unsupervised data. One estimate is that methods would need an improvement in classifier accuracy of about two orders of magnitude to reconstruct one neuron, and another seven orders of magnitude for the automated reconstruction of an entire mouse brain (Helmstaedter, 2015, p. 27). This can be compared to the automation improvements in classifying handwritten digits in the MNIST dataset which took fifteen years to gain one order of magnitude in machine learning error rate improvement.

### 19.2.4 *Rapprochement*

Given that machine learning was originally inspired by real-life models of the brain (Hopfield, 1982), an ongoing question is the right relationship between the fields of neuroscience and machine learning. Although there is some intuition that the disciplines are aligned, how to further enact this collaboration is unclear. For example, Arbib's text book of brain theory and neural networks (2003) cites the two central questions, namely, "How does the brain work?" and "How can we build intelligent machines?" but does not discuss how the two might come together.

#### 19.2.4.1 *Machine learning applied to neuroscience*

There are more proposals made by computer scientists for how neuroscience might benefit from machine learning than the converse. In one example, a group of machine learning industry practitioners presents a deep learning framework for neuroscience (Richards *et al.*, 2019).

The three central components of such a deep learning framework are the learning goal (expressed as an objective function (loss function) to be maximized or minimized), a set of learning rules (expressed as synaptic weight updates), and the network architecture (the pathways and connections for information flow in the brain). Earlier work from the Google DeepMind team (Marblestone *et al.*, 2016) highlights the cost function as a central principle in the operation of both the brain and artificial neural networks. In machine learning, cost functions and training procedures have become more complex and varied across layers and over time, complexities which could likewise inform the study of the brain.

### 19.2.4.2 *Machine learning and neuroscience at odds*

Chance *et al.* (2020) note that structural differences between neuroscience and machine learning may prevent a closer collaboration. They argue that differing priorities and perspectives exist between the two fields, largely motivated by end goals. On the one hand, neuroscience is directed by funding sources toward identifying disease pathologies for potential therapeutic targets. This translates into a culture that emphasizes defining and describing specific system components. As a result, neuroscience is primarily focused on an understanding of form, the components of biological neural circuits, and mechanism, how neural circuits work. On the other hand, machine learning focuses on a much higher level of abstraction, in generating functions that describe data. Machine learning seeks to increase performance (with respect to an objective function), and requires demonstrated improvements on the performance of a specific task. Machine learning is primarily aimed at understanding how a system produces a solution at an algorithmic-level, rather than understanding the underlying mechanisms or the biological neural architectures. In contrast to neuroscience, machine learning is not interested in the underlying form. Therefore, it is not necessarily immediately clear how neuroscience can help in improving machine learning algorithms, or how machine learning can contribute to the understanding of form and mechanism in neuroscience. However, the two fields continue to influence each other and there could be a broader exploration of potential synergies.

#### 19.2.4.3 *Next-generation machine learning*

A further problem surfaces regarding the potential limits of machine learning in general, suggesting that new approaches, biologically inspired and otherwise, are needed for further advance. Sejnowski, one of the scientists who introduced the Boltzmann machine (Ackley *et al.*, 1985) acknowledges the progress of deep learning, but thinks that "major breakthroughs" will be needed to achieve greater insight into the operation of the brain (Sejnowski, 2020). Similarly, an earlier opinion from Google DeepMind argued that machine learning methods had reached a plateau, and called for a return to neuroscience-inspired artificial intelligence (Hassabis *et al.*, 2017). The work posits that a better understanding of biological brains could play a vital role in building the intelligent machines of the future, and suggests resynchronizing the fields of machine learning and neuroscience.

On the other hand, quantum machine learning, as one of the biggest advances in machine learning, is not biologically inspired. Neither are other recent advances such as generative neural networks (Goodfellow *et al.*, 2014) and transformer neural networks (Vaswani *et al.*, 2017). The longer-term future of machine learning could also draw from the physics-based approach of random tensors (for dimensionality of three and greater), making use of color theory (the minimum number of colors to fill in a graph) and additional symmetries in the advance of finding the $1/N$ expansion (a perturbative expansion of quantum field theories) (Gurau, 2016, 2011). Other approaches to machine learning and brain modeling such as neuromorphic computing and spiking neural networks are a return to a closer linkage with biological underpinnings.

## 19.3 Neuromorphics and Spiking Neural Networks

### 19.3.1 *Neuromorphic computing*

Neuromorphic computing refers to computing systems that mimic the neuro-biological architectures of the human nervous system (Monroe, 2014). They are proposed as a next-generation computing platform that could extend beyond the limits of classical von Neumann architectures and operate on classical, quantum, and quantum optical platforms.

The idea behind neuromorphic computing is to closely imitate natural neural structures, including by building time and dynamics into functioning. Instead of transmitting information constantly or at each propagation cycle as in classical computing systems, neuromorphic computing mechanisms (like the neurons in the brain) transmit information only via thresholding, when a membrane potential (an intrinsic quality of the neuron related to its membrane electrical charge) reaches a specific value. Neuromorphic engineering aims to build machines that better interact with natural environments by applying the principles of neuronal computation, including robust analog signaling, real-time dynamics, distributed complexity, and learning. These kinds of cognitive computing platforms suggest advantages in efficiency, fault tolerance, and adaptability over von Neumann architectures. Tasks for neuromorphic architectures involve pattern analysis, decision making, optimization, and real-time system control.

#### 19.3.1.1 *Neuromorphic computing chips and projects*

There are various large-scale neuromorphic chips and hardware projects. One of the first neuromorphic chips was introduced by Intel in 2017, Loihi, composed of 130,000 neurons. The chip uses an asynchronous spiking neural network to implement adaptive self-learning and event-driven behavior (Davies *et al.*, 2018). Meanwhile, other similar projects were announced, IBM's TrueNorth brain-inspired computer chip with 1 million neurons and 256 million synapses (Merolla *et al.*, 2014), and Brainchip's Akida neuromorphic system-on-chip with 1.2 million neurons and 10 billion synapses (Pele, 2019). In July 2019, Intel announced an 8 million neuron neuromorphic system (Pohoiki Beach) comprised of 64 Loihi chips. Other efforts involved with the EC Human Brain Project include Spikey (Pfeil *et al.*, 2013), SpiNNaker (Furber *et al.*, 2014) and BrainScaleS (Schemmel *et al.*, 2017) (Table 19.5).

Neurogrid is an example of neuromorphic hardware architecture. There is a circuit board with 16 custom-designed chips (NeuroCores). Each core's analog circuitry emulates 65,536 neurons. The neurons are connected using digital circuitry designed to maximize spiking throughput and minimize energy consumption. The group filed for a patent in

Table 19.5. Large-scale neuromorphic computing projects.

| No. | Name | Location/Sponsor | Research Program |
|---|---|---|---|
| 1 | Neurogrid | Stanford University | Brains in Silicon program |
| 2 | True North | IBM | SyNAPSE program (DARPA) |
| 3 | Spikey | University of Heidelberg | FACETS/EC human brain project |
| 4 | SpiNNaker | University of Manchester | EC human brain project |
| 5 | BrainScaleS | Kirchhoff Inst. for Physics | EBRAINS/Human brain project |

2020 (Boahen *et al.*, 2020) based on previous work (Boahen, 2014, 2017). A spiking neural network computing infrastructure is envisioned based on multi-layer kernel architecture, shared dendritic encoding, and the thresholding of accumulated spiking signals.

### 19.3.2 *Spiking neural networks*

One of the main applications of neuromorphic computing is spiking neural networks, which are the spiking-activation version of traditional artificial neural networks. Although artificial neural networks were initially inspired by the brain's architecture, there are fundamental differences in their structure, neural computations, and learning rules as compared to the brain (Tavanaei *et al.*, 2019). Spiking neural networks incorporate more of the rich features that are able to imitate real-life brain processing.

Spiking neural networks are a more recently developed technology than traditional artificial neural networks. One of the earliest feedforward hierarchical convolutional networks of spiking neurons was proposed by Masquelier and Thorpe (2007), notably for unsupervised learning. Work has ensued with over forty projects demonstrating a variety of spiking neural networks in deep, convolutional, and recurrent spiking neural networks (Tavanaei *et al.*, 2019, p. 5). Although at present spiking neural networks sometimes lag behind traditional artificial neural networks in terms of performance, the gap is shrinking. Spiking neural networks also have advantages in requiring less programming and being more hardware friendly and energy-efficient than the alternative.

#### 19.3.2.1 *Spike-based activation*

One aspect that distinguishes neuromorphic computing from traditional computing is a threshold-based spike activation method. This is in contrast to nonspike activated artificial neural networks, in which neurons are typically characterized by a single, static, continuous-valued activation (despite the fact that activation is an evolving research frontier in artificial neural networks). Biological neurons, however, use discrete spikes to compute and transmit information, and the spike time and rate convey additional information (Gerstner *et al.*, 2014). Theoretically imitating the brain, in neuromorphic computing, a spike primitive orchestrates inputs from multiple sources by temporally integrating their weighted sum and fires a single spike when this value crosses a threshold.

Spikes are discrete events that occur at analog times, and thus the spiking encoding scheme represents a hybrid between traditional analog and digital approaches that is capable of both expressiveness and robustness to noise. The information representation scheme influences computational efficiency. Spike encoding as a cortical encoding strategy for neuronal computation algorithms is a sparse coding scheme with justification in coding theory (Borst & Theunissen, 1999). The spiking activation integrates a small set of basic operations (delay, weighting, spatial summation, temporal integration, and thresholding) into a single device, which is capable of performing a variety of computations depending on how its parameters are configured. Such a distributed, asynchronous model processes information using both space and time, and is amenable to algorithms for unsupervised learning (Maass, 1997).

#### 19.3.2.2 *Backpropagation and the learning problem*

A known challenge with spiking neural networks is the learning problem. Spiking neural networks are not able to learn with backpropagation as traditional artificial neural networks do. Backpropagation propagates error signals backward through time to update network weights, and allows neurons to participate in a network computation several times iteratively. Such a method is not possible in biological networks which are necessarily subject to the forward-arrow of time, only "running time once".

Traditional artificial neural networks "learn" by varying the weights of individual nodes in a trial-and-error process by which the computational performance of the network improves. Gradient descent is calculated for a loss function that measures errors in the current network performance and gradients of the loss function are propagated backward through all network layers to each node. The backpropagation of errors method is a standard technique that has made a substantial contribution to the progress of artificial neural networks in optimizing the loss function, calculating the error contribution of each neuron after a batch of data is processed (Rumelhart *et al.*, 1986). Backpropagation allows a significant reduction in combinatorial complexity as the highest-yield neurons can be upweighted retrospectively. In spiking neural networks, however, the potential use of backpropagation runs into the challenge that biology is subject to the forward-arrow of time. Also, from a technical perspective in algorithm implementation, the transfer function in spiking neural networks is usually nondifferentiable, which prevents the use of backpropagation.

#### 19.3.2.3 *Eligibility propagation synaptic plasticity*

Ongoing work proposes e-prop (eligibility propagation) as the equivalent of backpropagation to enable learning in spiking recurrent neural networks (Bellec *et al.*, 2020). The presence of slowly changing hidden variables offers a solution to the problem of how a spiking neural network can learn without error signals that propagate backward in time. In the experimental setup, the hidden variables of neurons are changed slowly, generating eligibility traces that propagate forward over longer time spans, which coincide with instantaneous error signals arising later in the system. The e-prop method cannot make backward use of time, but does incorporate the future use of time, coordinating two separate temporal trajectories.

E-prop thus provides a synaptic plasticity rule that performs a function similar to backpropagation, by indicating which neurons are contributing more to the solution and should be up-weighted, but without having to go back in time (Gerstner *et al.*, 2018). Drawing from neuroscience research, e-prop is based on a compound measure of two location-based features that have been discovered in the brain: Local eligibility traces and targeted top-down learning signals. The first mechanism, local eligibility traces, is a finding that neurons in the brain maintain traces of preceding activity on the molecular-level (for example, in the form of calcium ions or activated CaMKII enzymes).

The second mechanism, targeted top-down learning signals, refers to an abundance of top-down neurotransmitter signaling involving dopamine, acetylcholine, and neural firing (Sajad *et al.*, 2019). Such targeted top-down signaling is related to a feedback loop called error-related negativity in which effective behavior requires evaluating the outcomes of actions and adapting performance to optimize consequences. Dopamine signals in particular have been found to be differentially directed to target populations of neurons, rather than being global (Engelhard *et al.*, 2019). The effect of the two locality measures (local eligibility traces and targeted top-down learning signals) functioning together is that the brain maintains a fading memory of events in which the presynaptic neuron fired before the postsynaptic neuron, which induces synaptic plasticity if followed by a top-down learning signal.

The e-prop method is implemented as a learning algorithm for a spiking recurrent neural network. The result is that e-prop learns more slowly than backpropagation, but approximates the same performance. The e-prop algorithm is tested with a classical benchmark task (Mnih *et al.*, 2016) for learning intelligent behavior with a reward structure, winning Atari video games provided by the Arcade Learning Environment (Bellemare *et al.*, 2013). To win the games, the agent must learn to extract salient information from the pixels of the game screen, and to infer the value of specific actions, even if rewards are obtained in the future. At the well-known Atari game of Pong, the e-prop method produced a competitive score. In the more complicated Fishing Derby game requiring a memory-type function, the e-prop method exhibited two different learned behaviors, evading the shark and collecting fish. The salient skill demonstrated was that the agent had to learn how to switch between the two behaviors as required by the situation.

The implication is that it is not possible to solve the problem of synaptic plasticity in the brain without solving the problem of time, in coordinating earlier time events that persist and later time events that influence them (local eligibility traces and targeted top-down learning signals).

This suggests the possibility of modeling synaptic plasticity with quantum information scrambling, such as with a thermofield double state (Brown *et al.*, 2019) or a time superfluid (Lin *et al.*, 2019) for coordinating the early and late-time arrival of signals. This could include testing it on existing quantum simulation platforms such as Rydberg atoms.

#### 19.3.2.4 *Wider application of spiking neural networks*

Spiking neural networks is an active area of research. The main focus is solving the learning problem by finding alternatives to backpropagation, but the research also extends to other brain-inspired machine learning structures (using brain architectures to inspire new machine learning designs), and using spiking neural networks and machine learning to study the brain (Table 19.6). As there is ML/Q and Q/ML, there is ML/SNN and SNN/ML. The potential benefit is not just an effective spiking neural network structure for artificial intelligence computing, but understanding more about how the brain may actually function.

Bellec *et al.* (2020) propose e-prop as an alternative to backpropagation that is a compound measure of local firing eligibility traces (calcium activations) and targeted top-down learning signals (dopamine signals). Another solution to the learning problem is bundling two networks together, a traditional neural network using backpropagation to produce analysis and inputs, that are then mapped to a spiking neural network (Kim *et al.*, 2019). The method involves training a continuous-variable

Table 19.6. Spiking neural networks research applications.

| No. | Problem Target | Description | Network |
|---|---|---|---|
| 1 | Backpropagation | Eligibility propagation not backpropagation | RNN |
| 2 | | Run two RNNs, transfer ANN input to SNN | RNN |
| 3 | | Approximate gradient backpropagation | CNN |
| 4 | Brain-inspired machine learning | Dendrites as threshold-based linear units | CNN |
| 5 | | Multicompartmental neurons in deep learning | CNN |
| 6 | Neuroscience | Synaptic integration in fingertip response | CNN |
| 7 | | Sequential analysis of audio in the brain | RNN |

rate recurrent neural network with biophysical constraints and transferring the learned dynamics and constraints to a spiking recurrent neural network. In another approach, Kaiser *et al.* (2020) employ learning algorithms that approximate backpropagation, using only local error functions, that can be implemented in spiking neural networks. The key to the problem is realizing that learning dynamics in artificial neural networks and synaptic plasticity in spiking neural networks are similar. The method is tested on MNIST data.

Other research focuses on converting convolutional neural networks to spiking neural networks. Lee *et al.* (2020) propose an alternative machine learning algorithm to backpropagation that uses pseudo-derivatives to produce the leaky integrate-and-fire spiking temporality of spiking neural networks, thereby effectively training a deep convolutional spiking neural network. On the one hand, spiking neural networks are a powerful computing paradigm, but only have shallow architectures. It is difficult to train deep spiking neural networks due to the discontinuous, nondifferentiable nature of the spike generation function. On the other hand, previous attempts to convert convolutional neural networks to spiking neural networks were unable to produce the threshold-based spiking threshold-spiking temporal dynamics of spiking neural networks. Instead, the work uses a pseudo-derivative method that accounts for the leaky effect in the membrane potential of neurons. The algorithm approximately estimates the leaky effect by comparing total membrane potential value and obtains the ratio between leaky and nonleaky neurons. During the backpropagating phase, the pseudo-derivative of leaky neuronal function is estimated by combining the straight-through estimation and the leak correctional term. The deep spiking neural networks obtained superior classification accuracies in MNIST, SVHN, and CIFAR-10 datasets in comparison to the other networks trained with the spike-based algorithm.

Aside from focusing on alternatives to backpropagation in artificial neural networks, drawing from the computational power of brain architectures to inspire new machine learning designs is another research theme. Jones and Kording (2020) develop a simple model of SNN/ML implementing the dendrite as a sequence of threshold-based linear units as a special case of a sparse network. The resulting sparse ANN with binary dendritic tree constraints made up of nonlinear nodes was tested on

MNIST and CIFAR-10 datasets. The implication is that traditional neural network models may be severely underestimating the computational power of biological neurons, and that could be incorporated in machine learning networks. Guerguiev *et al.* (2017) likewise use spiking neural networks as brain architecture to inspire machine learning, here deploying multicompartmental neurons in the framework of a deep learning network. Like neocortical pyramidal neurons, neurons in the model receive sensory information and higher-order feedback in (electronically) segregated compartments. Due to the segregated feedback, neurons in different layers of the network are able to coordinate synaptic weight updates. As a result, the network learns to categorize images better than a single layer network. The result is that the algorithm takes advantage of multilayer architectures to identify useful higher-order representations which are the hallmark of deep learning.

Hay and Pruszynski (2019) use machine learning to model and explain the brain in regard to fingertip tactile response, proposing a synaptic integration method with convolutional machine learning. The work focuses on a description of how the human tactile processing pathway innervates the fingertips of the hand and rapidly processes the orientation of edges moving across the fingertip. The synaptic integration is as follows. First, the work derives spiking models of human first-order tactile neurons that fit and predict responses to moving edges with high accuracy. Second, the model neurons are used in simulating the peripheral neuronal population that innervates a fingertip. Third, machine learning is applied to train classifiers to perform synaptic integration across the neuronal population activity. The result is that the synaptic integration across first-order neurons processes edge orientations with high acuity and speed. The machine learning model includes both fast-decaying and slow-decaying excitatory and inhibitory synapses in the classifiers. The models suggest that the integration of fast-decaying (AMPA-like) synaptic inputs within short timescales is critical for discriminating fine orientations, whereas integration of slow-decaying (NMDA-like) synaptic inputs refines discrimination and maintains robustness over longer timescales.

Also applying machine learning to studying the brain, for sequential analysis, Nicola and Clopath (2017) deploy a model of supervised learning in spiking neural networks in sequential data models of songbird singing and storing and replaying a movie sequence.

## 19.4 Optical Spiking Neural Networks

The spiking neural network is developed for the optical platform (Tait *et al.*, 2014). Just as spiking neural networks complement and extend the artificial neural networks, the optical spiking neural network is the similar complement to the optical neural network. Neuromorphic photonics is an emerging field incorporating photonics and neural network processing models, combining the advantages of both optics and electronics to build systems with high efficiency, high interconnectivity, and extremely high bandwidth (Shastri *et al.*, 2018). Neuromorphic silicon photonics have the potential to integrate processing functions that might eventually vastly exceed the capabilities of electronics (Tait *et al.*, 2017). Artificial neural networks began with Hopfield (1982) and were extended to spiking neural networks by Masquelier and Thorpe (2007). Optical neural networks were demonstrated by Woods and Naughton (2012), and extended to optical spiking neural networks by Tait *et al.* (2014) (Table 19.7).

In the optical setup, amplifiers manage the thresholding for the spike activation in optical spiking neural networks and the nonlinear activation in optical neural networks (Pierangeli *et al.*, 2018). Feldmann *et al.* (2019) propose an all-optical spiking neurosynaptic network for supervised and unsupervised learning. The technique exploits wavelength division

Table 19.7. Optical spiking neural networks.

| No. | Network | Description | Year |
|---|---|---|---|
| 1 | Artificial neural network | Computing system inspired by biological neural networks | 1982 |
| 2 | Spiking neural network | Threshold activated neural network (more biologically realistic, adaptive) | 2007 |
| 3 | Optical neural network | Neural network implementation using optical components | 2012 |
| 4 | Optical spiking neural network | On-chip optical architecture for high-performance spiking laser neurons | 2014 |

multiplexing techniques to implement scalable circuit architecture for photonic neural networks.

Ultrafast laser neurons are one of the latest concepts (Nahmias *et al.* 2020). A laser neuron is a nonlinear optoelectronic device that uses excitable laser dynamics to achieve biologically inspired spiking behavior. The functionality is demonstrated with simultaneous excitation, inhibition, and summation across multiple wavelengths. Ultrafast laser neurons could contribute to the implementation of linear operations such as matrix multiplications using photonic integrated circuit technology. The laser neuron is able to perform nonlinear operations in the photonic domain, including with a wavelength multiplexing protocol for large-scale system integration. Laser neurons represent an emerging class of optoelectronic nonlinear processors that can be used to harness the bandwidth density and energy efficiency of photonic computing.

## References

Ackley, D.H., Hinton, G.E. & Sejnowski, T.J. (1985). A learning algorithm for Boltzmann machines. *Cog. Sci.* 9(1):147–69.

Allen, P. (2011). *Idea Man: A Memoir by the Cofounder of Microsoft*. New York: Penguin.

Almog, M. & Korngreen, A. (2016). Is realistic neuronal modeling realistic? *J. Neurophysiol.* 116:2180–209.

Arbib, M.N. Ed. (2003). *The Handbook of Brain Theory and Neural Networks*. 2nd Edition. Cambridge: The MIT Press.

Bassett, D.S., Zurn, P. & Gold, J.I. (2018). On the nature and use of models in network neuroscience. *Nat. Rev. Neurosci.* 19(9):566–78.

Bejnordi, B.E., Veta, M., Johannes van Diest, P. *et al.* (2017). Diagnostic assessment of deep learning algorithms for detection of lymph node metastases in women with breast cancer. *J. Am. Med. Assn.* 12:318(22):2199–210.

Bellec, G., Scherr, F., Subramoney, A. *et al.* (2020). A solution to the learning dilemma for recurrent networks of spiking neurons. *Nat. Commun.* 11:3625.

Bellemare, M.G., Naddaf, Y., Veness, J. & Bowling, M. (2013). The arcade learning environment: An evaluation platform for general agents. *J. AI Res.* 47:253–79.

Boahen, K. (2014). Neurogrid: A mixed-analog-digital multichip system for large-scale neural simulations. *Proc. IEEE.* 102(5):699–716.

Boahen, K. (2017). A neuromorph's prospectus. *Comput Sci Eng*. 19(2):14–28.

Boahen, K.A., Fok, S.B., Neckar, A.S. *et al.* (2020). Methods and apparatus for spiking neural network computing based on threshold accumulation. U.S. Pat Appl. #20200019839.

Borst A. & Theunissen, F.E. (1999). Information theory and neural coding. *Nat. Neurosci.* 2:947–57.

Brette, R., Rudolph, M., Carnevale, T. *et al.* (2007). Simulation of networks of spiking neurons: A review of tools and strategies. *J. Comput. Neurosci.* 23(3):349–98.

Brown, A.R., Gharibyan, H., Leichenauer, S. *et al.* (2019). Quantum gravity in the lab: Teleportation by size and traversable wormholes. aXiv:1911.06314v1.

Capper, D., Jones, D.T.W., Sill, M. *et al.* (2018). DNA methylation-based classification of central nervous system tumors. *Nature.* 555:469–74.

Chance, F.S., Aimone, J.B., Musuvathy, S.S. *et al.* (2020). Crossing the cleft: Communication challenges between neuroscience and artificial intelligence. *Front Comput. Neurosci.* 14(39):1–9.

Cizeron, M., Qiu, Z., Koniaris, B. *et al.* (2020). A brainwide atlas of synapses across the mouse life span. *Science*. 369:270–5.

Cole, J.H., Poudel, R.P.K., Tsagkrasoulis, D. *et al.* (2016). Predicting brain age with deep learning from raw imaging data results in a reliable and heritable biomarker. *Neuroimage*. 163:115–24.

Cugno, A., Bartol, T.M., Sejnowski, T.J. *et al.* (2019). Geometric principles of second messenger dynamics in dendritic spines. *Sci. Rep.* 9(1):11676.

Davies, M. Srinivasa, N., Lin T.-H. *et al.* (2018). Loihi: A neuromorphic many-core processor with on-chip learning. *IEEE Micro*. (38):82–99.

Dayan, P. & Abbott, L.F. (2001). *Theoretical Neuroscience*. Cambridge: MIT Press.

Dorkenwald, S., Schubert, P.J., Killinger, M.F. *et al.* (2017). Automated synaptic connectivity inference for volume electron microscopy. *Nat. Meth.* 14(4): 435–42.

Eliasmith, C. & Anderson, C.H. (2003). *Neural Engineering: Computation, Representation, and Dynamics in Neurobiological Systems*. Cambridge: MIT Press.

Engelhard, B., Finkelstein, J., Cox, J. *et al.* (2019). Specialized coding of sensory, motor and cognitive variables in VTA dopamine neurons. *Nature*. 570: 509–13.

Esteva, A., Kuprel, B., Novoa, R.A. *et al.* (2017). Dermatologist-level classification of skin cancer with deep neural networks. *Nature.* 542:115–8.

Feldmann, J., Youngblood, N., Wright, C.D. *et al.* (2019). All-optical spiking neurosynaptic networks with self-learning capabilities. *Nature*. 569(7755): 208–14.

Furber, S.B., Galluppi, F., Temple, S. & Plana, L.A. (2014). The SpiNNaker project. *Proc IEEE.* 102:652–65.

Gerstner, W., Kistler, W.M., Naud, R. & Paninski, L. (2014). *Neuronal Dynamics: From Single Neurons to Networks and Models of Cognition*. Cambridge: Cambridge University Press.

Gerstner, W., Lehmann, M., Liakoni, V. *et al.* (2018). Eligibility traces and plasticity on behavioral time scales: Experimental support of neohebbian three-factor learning rules. *Front Neural Circuits.* 12:53.

Gerstner, W. & Naud, R. (2009). How good are neuron models? *Science.* 326:379–80.

Goodfellow, I.J., Pouget-Abadie, J., Mirza, M. *et al.* (2014). Generative adversarial nets. *Adv. Neural Inf. Process Syst.* 27:2672–80.

Goodman, D. & Brette, R. (2008). Brian: A simulator for spiking neural networks in python. *Front Neuroinform*. 2:5.

Guerguiev, J., Lillicrap, T.P. & Richards, B.A. (2017). Towards deep learning with segregated dendrites. *eLife*. 6:e22901.

Gulshan, V., Peng, L., Coram, M., *et al.* (2016). Development and validation of a deep learning algorithm for detection of diabetic retinopathy in retinal fundus photographs. *J. Am. Med. Assn.* 316(22):2402–10.

Gurau, R. (2011). The 1/N expansion of colored tensor models. *Annales Henri Poincare*. 12:829–47.

Gurau, R.G. (2016). *Random Tensors*. Oxford UK: Oxford University Press.

Hassabis, D., Kumaran, D., Summerfield, C. & Botvinick, M. (2017). Neuroscience-inspired artificial intelligence. *Neuron.* 95:245–58.

Hay, E. & Pruszynski, J.A. (2019). Orientation processing by synaptic integration across first-order tactile neurons. bioRxiv: 396705.

Hebb, D.O. (1949). *The Organization of Behavior: A Neuropsychological Theory*. New York: Wiley and Sons.

Helmstaedter, M. (2015). The mutual inspirations of machine learning and neuroscience. *Neuron*. 86:25–28.

Herz, A.V.M., Gollisch, T., Machens, C.K. & Jaeger, D. (2006). Modeling single-neuron dynamics and computations. *Science.* 314:80–85.

Hodgkin, A.L. & and Huxley, A.F. (1952). A quantitative description of membrane current and its application to conduction and excitation in nerve. *J. Physiol*. 116:449–72.

Hopfield, J.J. (1982). Neural networks and physical systems with emergent collective computational abilities. *Proc. Natl. Acad. Sci.* 79:2554–8.

Iqbal, A., Sheikh, A. Karayannis, T. (2019). DeNeRD: High-throughput detection of neurons for brain-wide analysis with deep learning. *Sci. Rep.* 9(1):13828.

Jin, L., Behabadi, B.F., Jadi, M.P. *et al.* (2018). Classical-contextual interactions in V1 may rely on dendritic computations. bioRxiv: 436956.

Jones, I.S. & Kording, K. (2020). Can single neurons solve MNIST? The computational power of biological dendritic trees. arXiv:2009.01269v1.

Kaiser, J., Mostafa, H. & Neftci, E. (2020). Synaptic plasticity dynamics for Deep Continuous Local Learning (DECOLLE). *Front Neurosci.* 14(424):1–11.

Kim, R., Li, Y., Sejnowski, T.J. (2019). Simple framework for constructing functional spiking recurrent neural networks. *Proc. Natl. Acad. Sci.* 116(45): 22811–20.

Koch, M., Geraedts, V., Wang, H. *et al.* (2019). Automated machine learning for EEG-based classification of Parkinson's disease patients. *2019 IEEE International Conference on Big Data (Big Data)*, Los Angeles, CA, 2019, pp. 4845–52.

Lebedev, M.A. & Nicolelis, M.A. (2017). Brain-machine interfaces: From basic science to neuroprostheses and neurorehabilitation. *Physiol. Rev.* 97: 767–837.

Lee, C., Sarwar, S.S., Panda, P. *et al.* (2020) Enabling spike-based backpropagation for training deep neural network architectures. arXiv:1903.06379v4.

Levakova, G., Rosenthal, G., Shelef, I. *et al.* (2019). From a deep learning model back to the brain. bioRxiv: 803742.

Li, S., Liu, N., Zhang, X. *et al.* (2019). Dendritic computations captured by an effective point neuron model. *Proc. Natl. Acad. Sci.* 116(30):15244–52.

Li, X., Luo, S. & Xue, F. (2020). Effects of synaptic integration on the dynamics and computational performance of spiking neural network. *Cogn. Neurodynamics.* 14:347–57.

Lin, H.W., Maldacena, J. & Zhao, Y. (2019). Symmetries near the horizon. *J. High Energ. Phys.* 1908:049.

Louis, D.N., Perry, A., Reifenberger, G. *et al.* (2016). The 2016 world health organization classification of tumors of the central nervous system: a summary. *Acta Neuropathol.* 131(6):803–20.

Maass, W. (1997). Networks of spiking neurons: The third generation of neural network models. *Neural Netw.* 10:1659–71.

Mainen, Z.F. & Sejnowski, T.J. (1996). Influence of dendritic structure on firing pattern in model neocortical neurons. *Nature.* 382:363–66.

Marblestone, A.H., Wayne, G. & Kording, K.P. (2016). Towards an integration of deep learning and neuroscience. *Front Comput. Neurosci.* 10:94.
Markram, H. (2012). The human brain project. *Sci. Am.* 306:50–55.
Masquelier, T. & Thorpe, S.J. (2007). Unsupervised learning of visual features through spike timing dependent plasticity. *PLoS Comput. Biol.* 3(2):e31.
McCulloch W.S. & Pitts, W.H. (1943). A logical calculus of the ideas immanent in nervous activity. *Bull. Math. Biophys.* 5:115–33.
Mel, B.W. (2016). Towards a simplified model of an active dendritic tree. In *Dendrites*. Eds. Stuart, G., Spruston, N. & Hausser, M. Oxford: Oxford University Press, pp. 465–86.
Merolla, P.A., Arthur, J.V., Alvarez-Icaza, R. *et al.* (2014). A million spiking-neuron integrated circuit with a scalable communication network and interface. *Science.* 345:668–73.
Mnih, V., Badia, A.P., Mirza, M. *et al.* (2016). Asynchronous methods for deep reinforcement learning. In *ICML, Proceedings of the 33rd International Conference on Machine Learning*, New York, NY, USA, June 19–24, 2016, pp. 928–37.
Monroe, D. (2014). Neuromorphic computing gets ready for the (really) big time. *Commun. ACM.* 57(6):13–15.
Moradi, S., Qiao, N., Stefanini, F. & Indiveri, G. (2018). A scalable multicore architecture with heterogeneous memory structures for dynamic neuromorphic asynchronous processors (DYNAPS). *IEEE Trans. Biomed. Circuits and Syst.* 12(1):106–22.
Motta, A., Schurr, M., Staffler, B. & Helmstaedter, M. (2019). Big data in nanoscale connectomics, and the greed for training labels. *Curr. Opin. Neurobiol.* 55:180–87.
Nahmias, M.A., Peng, H.-T., de Lima, T.F. *et al.* (2020). A laser spiking neuron in a photonic integrated circuit. arXiv: 2012.08516.
Nicola, W. & Clopath, C. (2017). Supervised learning in spiking neural networks with FORCE training. *Nat. Comm.* 8(1):2208.
Nilsson, M., Liwicki, F. & Sandin, F. (2020). Spatiotemporal features with a dynamic neuromorphic processor. arXiv:2002.04924v1.
Parag, T., Berger, D., Kamentsky, L. *et al.* (2018). Detecting synapse location and connectivity by signed proximity estimation and pruning with deep nets. arXiv:1807.02739v2.
Pele, A.-F., (2019). Neuromorphic promises better AI. *EE Times*. https://www.eetimes.com/neuromorphic-promises-better-ai/.
Petrosuan, A., Lebedev, M. & Ossadtchi, A. (2020). Decoding neural signals with a compact and interpretable convolutional neural network. Biorxiv: 129114v1.

Pfeil, T., Grubl, A., Jeltsch, S. *et al.* (2013). Six networks on a universal neuromorphic computing substrate. *Front Neurosci.* 7:11.

Pierangeli, D., Marcucci, G., Moriconi, C. *et al.* (2018). Deep optical neural network by living tumor brain cells. arXiv:1812.09311.

Poirazi, P. & Papoutsi, A. (2020). Illuminating dendritic function with computational models. *Nat. Rev. Neurosci.* 21:303–21.

Rajpurkar, P., Irvin, J., Ball, R.L. *et al.* (2018). Deep learning for chest radiograph diagnosis: A retrospective comparison of the CheXNeXt algorithm to practicing radiologists. *PLoS Med.* 15(11):e1002686.

Ramon y Cajal, S. (1995, 1894). *Texture of the Nervous System of Man and the Vertebrates*: Volume I. Trans. Swanson, N. & Swanson, L.W. Oxford: Oxford University Press.

Reyes, J. & Stoudenmire, E.M. (2020). A multi-scale tensor network architecture for classification and regression. arXiv:2001.08286.

Richards, B.A., Lillicrap, T.P., Beaudoin, P. *et al.* (2019). A deep learning framework for neuroscience. *Nat. Neurosci.* 22(11):1761–70.

Rumelhart, D.E., Hinton, G.E. & Williams, R.J. (1986). Learning representation by back-propagating errors. *Nature.* 323:533–36.

Sajad, A., Godlove, D.C. & Schall, J.D. (2019). Cortical microcircuitry of performance monitoring. *Nat. Neurosci.* 22:265–74.

Schemmel, J., Kriener, L., Muller, P. & Meier, K. (2017). An accelerated analog neuromorphic hardware system emulating NMDA- and calcium-based nonlinear dendrites. arXiv:1703.07286v1.

Sejnowski, T.J. (2020). The unreasonable effectiveness of deep learning in artificial intelligence. *Proc. Natl. Acad. Sci.* 117(48):30033–38.

Serb, A., Corna, A., George, R. *et al.* (2020). Memristive synapses connect brain and silicon spiking neurons. *Sci. Rep.* 10:2590.

Shastri, B.J., Tait, A.N., Nahmias, M.A. & Prucnal, P.R. (2014). Photonic spike processing: Ultrafast laser neurons and an integrated photonic network. arXiv:1407.2917v1.

Smetanin, N., Belinskaya, A., Lebedev, M.A. & Ossadtchi, A. (2020). Digital filters for low-latency quantification of brain rhythms in real-time. *J. Neural. Eng.* 17(4):046022.

Staffler, B., Berning, M., Boergens, K.M. *et al.* (2017). SynEM, automated synapse detection for connectomics. *eLife.* 6:e26414.

Stevenson, I.H. & Kording, K.P. (2011). How advances in neural recording affect data analysis. *Nat. Neurosci.* 14:139–42.

Stockel, A. & Eliasmith, C. (2020). Passive nonlinear dendritic interactions as a computational resource in spiking neural networks. arXiv:1904.11713v2.

Tait, A.N., Nahmias, M.A., Shastri, B.J. & Prucnal, P.R. (2014). Broadcast and weight: An integrated network for scalable photonic spike processing. *J. Light. Technol.* 32:3427.

Tait, A.N., Zhou, E., de Lima, T.F. *et al.* (2017). Neuromorphic silicon photonic networks. arXiv:1611.02272v3.

Tavanaei, A., Ghodrati, M., Kheradpisheh, S.R. *et al.* (2019). Deep learning in spiking neural networks. *Neural Netw.* 111:47–63.

Tikidji-Hamburyan, R.A., Narayana, V., Bozkus, Z. *et al.* (2017). Software for brain network simulations: A comparative study. *Front Neuroinform.* 11(46):1–16.

Trautmann, E.M., Stavisky, S.D., Lahiri, S. D.J. *et al.* (2019). Accurate estimation of neural population dynamics without spike sorting. *Neuron.* 103:1–17.

Valiant, L.G. (2018). Toward identifying the systems-level primitives of cortex by in-circuit testing. *Front Neural Circuits.* 12:104.

Vaswani, A., Shazeer, N., Parmar, N. *et al.* (2017). Attention is all you need. In *NIPS'17: Proceedings of the 31st International Conference on Neural Information Processing Systems (NIPS 2017)*, Long Beach, CA, USA, December 4–9, 2017, pp. 6000–10.

Wang, Y., Li, Q., Liu, L. *et al.* (2019). TeraVR empowers precise reconstruction of complete 3-D neuronal morphology in the whole brain. *Nat. Commun.* 10(3474):1–9.

Woods, D. & Naughton, T.J. (2012). Optical computing: Photonic neural networks. *Nature Phys.* 8:257–59.

Zhou, Z., Kuo, H.-C., Peng, H. & Long, F. (2018). DeepNeuron: An open deep learning toolbox for neuron tracing. *Brain Inf.* 5(3):1–9.

# Chapter 20

# Conclusion: AdS/Brain Theory and Quantum Neuroscience

*Creations appear outmoded when viewed from within the future they helped to create*

— Jahren (2017, p. 186)

**Abstract**

This chapter argues that quantum neuroscience applications are needed not only given the complexity of the domain but also to obtain a causal understanding of disease. The AdS/Brain theory is introduced as the first multi-tier renormalized interpretation of the AdS/CFT correspondence, for implementation with bMERA (brain) random tensor networks with Floquet periodicity dynamics. Bulk-boundary pairs are outlined in the multi-tier composite neural signaling model that includes the scales of network, neuron, synapse, and molecule. Standard neuroscience quantum circuits are proposed in a list of Millennium Prize-type challenges, and risks and limitations are discussed.

## 20.1 Quantum Computing for the Brain

The overall finding of this book is that a wide range of foundational physics advances are being applied to neuroscience, and that many aspects of the computational neuroscience research program might migrate in a straightforward though nontrivial manner to quantum computational platforms. Such efforts might greatly extend the kinds of research and explanatory findings that are possible in the context of studying the brain, neural signaling, and neuropathologies. When seen in the light of future standards for neurological study, current approaches might appear primitive. However, these kinds of future-class advances could take years to develop.

## 20.2 AdS/Brain Theory

### 20.2.1 *Quantum neural signaling*

New models for neural signaling are required as quantum computing is implicated as a computational platform and neural signaling is understood as a quantum domain. The "big data" explosion in neuroscience imaging output from connectomics and other projects has made it clear that supercomputers and other existing methods of computation cannot match the need for neural data modeling and interpretation. Simultaneously, quantum computing is emerging as a vastly more scalable platform including with three-dimensional modeling capabilities appropriate to the representation of real-life phenomena such as neural signaling. Also, increasingly in the last decade, neural signaling has come to be appreciated as a far more complicated process than electrical action potential firing alone suggests. A full picture of signaling requires synaptic integration (the neuron's information processing activities aggregating thousands of incoming signals). Synaptic integration involves an understanding of astrocyte calcium signaling, protein cascades in dendritic arbors, and the proton and ion-based transfer of molecules, all of which take place on the quantum (atomic and subatomic) level. The implication is modeling neural signaling processes with quantum-conducive computing systems.

#### 20.2.1.1 *AdS/Brain theory of neural signaling*

Neuroscience and physics are related in the proposal of AdS/Brain as a composite theory of neural signaling at the quantum level. AdS/Brain is an interpretation of the AdS/CFT correspondence as a neural signaling model. An ongoing challenge in both physics and neuroscience is relating the microscale and the macroscale, articulating how collective microscale behavior produces averaged group effects at the macroscale. The AdS/CFT correspondence continues to be one of the best tools for addressing within-system microscale-macroscale interrelation and short-range and long-range correlations. The AdS/Brain theory can be proposed on this basis as a comprehensive theory of neural signaling.

What is new in the AdS/Brain theory is the multi-level correspondence. The bulk-boundary setup of the correspondence is an attractive feature for interrogating one scale level from another, conceptually as nested tiers of Escher *Circle Limit III* (Figure 20.1). The AdS/Brain theory is a composite model of neural signaling in the form of a mathematical framework that incorporates the activity of neurons, glia, synapses, neurotransmitters, and synaptic integration. The four scale tiers of brain network, neuron, synapse, and molecular levels are all involved in the successful orchestration of signal transmission. Each pair of scale tiers has a bulk-boundary relationship, with the implication that the complicated activity occurring in each "bulk" volume can be written in a "boundary" field theory in one less dimension (Table 20.1).

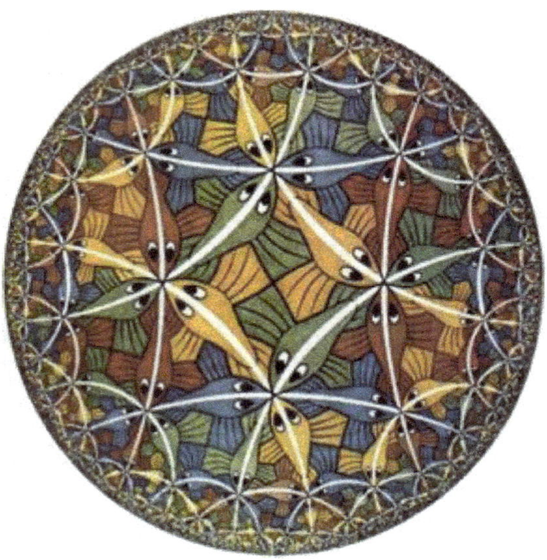

Figure 20.1. M.C. Escher's "Circle Limit III".

*Source*:  www.mcescher.com.

Table 20.1. AdS/Brain: Bulk-boundary scale tiers.

| No. | Tier | Scale | Signal | AdS/Brain | | |
|---|---|---|---|---|---|---|
| 1 | Network | $10^{-2}$ | Local field potential | Boundary | — | — |
| 2 | Neuron | $10^{-4}$ | Action potential | Bulk | Boundary | — |
| 3 | Synapse | $10^{-6}$ | Dendritic spike | — | Bulk | Boundary |
| 4 | Molecule | $10^{-10}$ | Ion charge | — | — | Bulk |

The central requirement of the AdS/Brain theory is to provide a model for the consolidation of various spatial and temporal scales, each having a distinct dynamical regime, into one renormalized theoretical framework. The holographic correspondence is an apparatus that renormalizes the system across scale tiers. The result is that AdS/Brain emerges as a theory of comprehensive neural signaling at various renormalized spatial and temporal scales, each having its own dynamics, in a multi-tier interpretation of the AdS/CFT correspondence. The AdS/Brain theory is a composite, renormalization-based multiscalar model of neural signaling.

The AdS/Brain theory treats multiple scale tiers, and is a matrix quantum mechanics interpretation of the AdS/CFT correspondence. Matrix mechanics is a mathematically consistent formulation of quantum mechanics that is equivalent to the Schrödinger wave formulation. The physical properties of particles are interpreted as matrices that evolve over time, in an algebraic method that produces the spectra of energy operators with ladder operators. The matrix quantum mechanics formulation addresses the fact that quantum systems have multiple dimensions, and need to be solved with multiple matrices (Han *et al.*, 2020). With the matrix quantum mechanics format (algebraic operators), the AdS/Brain theory is further poised for implementation with quantum platforms.

### 20.2.1.2 *Information-theoretic black hole-like physics*

Beyond the theoretical renormalization and microscale-macroscale justifications for the AdS/Brain theory, there is also a practical information-theoretic argument that informs the theory's potential implementation. This argument is that the brain, like many complex systems, exhibits aspects of black hole-like physics, and as such, can be studied with black hole models, the marquis example being the AdS/CFT correspondence. Enumerating the brain with black hole-like physics includes concepts such as UV–IR correlations, entropy, thermal states, fluctuations, superconducting phase transitions, quantum error correcting code spaces, and qudits. From a practical perspective, the term "black hole-like" means quantum information-theoretic formulations such as using entropy to measure short-range and long-range correlations in the system (i.e. how interrelated subsystems are within the system). Just as black hole-like physics is producing results studying quantum gravity in the laboratory, so too these methods might be used to study the brain.

#### 20.2.1.3 *Implementation of the AdS/Brain theory*

A key advance in tackling the complexity of quantum mechanical systems is a shift from the analytical methods of traditional quantum mechanics to quantum field theory (Srednicki, 2007). Calculating particle-many systems in a full-fledged quantum field theory enables a progression in methods from cumbersome canonical quantization to path integrals which sum over particle activity. Inherent in the AdS/Brain theory is that the brain too should be seen not only as a quantum mechanical regime as its behavioral size dictates but also as a quantum field theory domain. This is warranted as the particle-many (neuron-many) activity of large-scale (whole-brain) neural signaling has been established in neural field theories expressed with path integral methods (Amari, 1977; Ohira & Cowan, 1993; Buice & Cowan, 2009; Bressloff, 2015; Chow & Buice, 2015).

Path integrals are suggested for the mathematical implementation of the AdS/Brain theory and a model for the tiered structure also needs to be selected. MERA tensor networks are an obvious choice given their renormalization and entanglement management capabilities, easily consolidating short-range and long-range correlations in very-large quantum systems. A bMERA (brain MERA) version is proposed to attend to the specific needs of a neural field theory. This is in parallel with other domain-specific suggested implementations of MERA such as cMERA (continuous spacetime MERA (Nozaki *et al.*, 2012)) and dMERA (deep MERA fast layer contraction on NISQ devices (Kim & Swingle, 2017)).

In the renormalization picture, the neural system correlations and fluctuations (that produce neural signaling behavior) are formatted as entanglement or entanglement entropy (in the AdS/CFT correspondence frame). The renormalization structure allows short-range and long-range correlations to be analyzed for their role in neural signaling. Most relevant to the AdS/Brain theory are UV–IR correlations in time and space. In space, this means local and long-distance connections, and proximal and distal relationships. In time, this means fast and slow time, the relationship between local fast signals and distant slow signals, and fast network processing at the edge and the slower processing at the core.

The bMERA tensor network with the structure for investigating UV–IR correlations can be implemented with the random tensor network format of Hayden *et al.* (2016). This model extends the reach of the AdS/CFT correspondence to more generic setups in time and space, while recapitulating the Ryu–Takayanagi entropy entanglement formula and other known aspects of the holographic correspondence. However, the random tensor network formalism is not generalized to include dynamics. Thus, dynamics would need to be incorporated from correspondence-based formulations for the quantum domain (Engelhardt & Wall, 2019). This could also include Floquet periodicity (Else *et al.*, 2016) and space-time superfluids (Lin *et al.*, 2019), further interpreted into neural dynamics based on bifurcation and oscillating graphs.

The AdS/Brain theory applies to various scale tiers and processes comprising a complicated particle-many bulk volume of activity that results in a clear event-driven action (a neural signal) on the boundary. Several bulk-boundary examples for AdS/Brain study are outlined in Table 20.2.

Overall, the AdS/Brain theory is articulated as a composite, renormalization-based multiscalar model of neural signaling, for implementation with random tensor networks in a bMERA format. In the same research trajectory, the AdS/Brain correspondence has been suggested as an AdS/BCI control theory for BCI neuronanorobot networks managed with quantum platforms (Swan, 2022). This is in the context of proposals for neuronanorobot fleets for on-board connectome mapping and disease-fighting in human brain-cloud interfaces (Martins *et al.*, 2016, 2019). Other related work develops smart network field theories for quantum platforms (Swan *et al.*, 2020).

Table 20.2. Bulk-boundary: AdS/neural signaling.

| No. | Bulk | Boundary |
|---|---|---|
| 1 | Sending neuron axon | Electric action potential |
| 2 | Presynaptic terminal | Glutamate release from active zone |
| 3 | Synaptic cleft | Neurotransmitter transmission |
| 4 | Synaptic cleft | Astrocyte calcium signaling |
| 5 | Postsynaptic density | Ionotropic protein cascade (glutamate, GABA) |
| 6 | Postsynaptic density | Metabotropic protein cascade (dopamine) |
| 7 | Dendritic arbor | Excitatory/inhibitory spike |
| 8 | Dendrite to soma | Outgoing action potential |

### 20.2.2 *Risks and limitations*

There are several potential risks and limitations concerning quantum neuroscience applications and the specific suggestion of the AdS/Brain theory for neural signaling. The first issue is that perhaps it is simply too early for quantum computing as a nascent and untested platform as to whether it will develop into the qubit or qudit sized machines needed to model a system like the brain with 86 billion neurons and 242 trillion synapses. However, it is clear that these kinds of computing platforms may arise and it is in fact precisely the complexity of the brain that could help to define the requirements for the domain. Quantum computing is central to funding objectives and national competitive initiatives for many countries. The second major critique could be that the AdS/CFT correspondence does not have such a liberal application as to extend all the way to holographic neuroscience for the study of neural signaling, and to a multi-tier interpretation. However, the mathematical models that constitute the AdS/CFT correspondence have been proven to elicit new information about many other physical systems such as condensed matter materials that might have seemed improbable at the outset, and thus neuroscience-related applications are not unwarranted. There may be additional subtleties to AdS/Biology applications that the AdS/Brain theory might help to inform. Also, there is nothing to prevent a stratified series of bulk-boundary relationships in a multi-tier system.

A third complaint could be that the brain's space and time constraints, scale range, and diverse dynamical regimes render the overall domain too specific to be contemplated with any external lens, even a versatile model such as the AdS/CFT correspondence. However, this does not preclude the examination of the brain with such a model, and much may be learned in the process as has been found in the application of other physics-intensive formulations to neural signaling both theoretically and empirically. Finally, these proposals could be defeated on the grounds that obtaining the requisite data for testing, particularly for subatomic synaptic integration processes, is unlikely in the near or even intermediate term, and thus the theories are fated to remain untestable conjectures. Here, though, strides in microscopy innovation for single-molecule resolution and sampling techniques in human pyramidal neurons, for example, suggest that data acquisition may be possible to test setups of these theories at least to further direct their formulation. Overall, the potential risks and limitations are outweighed by the much greater possibilities of quantum neuroscience.

## 20.3 Millennium Prize-Type Challenges

### 20.3.1 *NISQ device neuroscience applications*

The bigger picture of grand challenges for quantum computing for the brain is to implement neural signaling theories (particularly related to synaptic integration) on the more capacious quantum computing platform with the large variety of available quantum methods. These include tensor networks, Born machines, reduced density matrices, wavelet transforms, quantum kernel learning, Rydberg atom arrays, ion traps, boson sampling graph-theoretic models, quantum optics, and spiking neural networks.

#### 20.3.1.1 *Physics-based time technologies*

A central problem is studying UV–IR correlations in the brain, short-range and long-range relations in microscale subsystems that produce macroscale behavior. Such UV–IR processes proceed in time and space, possibly with each scale level having its own dynamics. A number of "time technologies" have emerged in foundational physics research that can be used to study nonlinear dynamical systems. These include out-of-time-order correlation functions, information scrambling periods with ballistic and chaotic growth and saturation, Floquet periodicity, Hopf bifurcation, and continuous-time quantum walks. These quantum methods could increase the reserve of tools available for neural behavior investigation.

#### 20.3.1.2 *Standard neuroscience quantum circuits*

Standard quantum circuits could be developed for a variety of known brain modeling problems. One is instantiating the effects of nonlinear calcium signaling in dendritic spiking activity with partial differential equations and diffusion-reaction functions. Another is a quantum circuit for dendritic filtering that instantiates the attenuation properties of the dendritic membrane between the synapse and the soma (including variance in both charge and voltage) and UV–IR correlations, for example, in a bMERA (brain MERA) tensor network setup. A standard framework for integrating the effects of excitatory and inhibitory postsynaptic potentials (EPSPs and IPSPs) is needed. Other standard circuits could instantiate the geometric configuration of dendritic spine heads, metabotropic-ionotropic neurotransmitter protein signaling cascades, and synaptotagmin protein trafficking in the presynaptic terminal. There could be quantum circuits and variational methods as tools for approximating the four main wavefunctions involved in neural signaling: action potentials, neurotransmitter diffusions, astrocyte calcium signaling waves, and dendritic spikes.

Specific research questions could be posed in the structure of Millennium Prize-type challenges as follows:

1. *AdS/Brain*: Develop an AdS/CFT quantum circuit for a four-tier AdS/Brain model (Harlow, 2017; Harlow & Shaghoulian, 2020)
2. *AdS/Brain*: Simulate neural signaling SYK and scrambling Hamiltonians with Rydberg atoms (Belyansky *et al.*, 2020)
3. *AdS/Brain*: Implement an attention-based transformer neural network for neural signaling (Carrasquilla *et al.*, 2019)

4. *Quantum information theory*: Investigate the brain as a fast-scrambler with Lyapunov exponent-based chaotic/ballistic dynamics (Kobrin *et al.*, 2020; Swingle *et al.*, 2016)
5. *Quantum walks for the brain*: Design a continuous-time quantum walk with a Hadamard coin-flip operator for single-neuron tracing in a DeepNeuron network (Flamini *et al.*, 2018; Wang *et al.*, 2019)
6. *Quantum information theory*: Create a Born machine implementation of neural signaling (Cheng *et al.*, 2018)
7. *Quantum information theory*: Implement a bMERA random tensor network with an efficient neural signaling alpha-bit (Hayden *et al.*, 2016; Haydon & Penington, 2019)
8. *Quantum photonics*: Construct a high-dimensional entangled qudit neural signaling model with photonic encoding in a quantum optical neural network (Erhard *et al.*, 2020; Steinbrecher *et al.*, 2019)
9. *Quantum photonics*: Develop holographic teleportation protocols with operator size winding and entanglement heralding to transmit a neural signaling state (Brown *et al.*, 2019; Dahlberg *et al.*, 2019)
10. *Gaussian boson sampling*: Design a neural firing model with graph-theoretic boson sampling (Zhong *et al.*, 2020; Schuld *et al.*, 2019)
11. *Superconducting*: Implement Hopf bifurcation in a superconducting spacetime crystal Floquet model with Glass networks (Lin *et al.*, 2019; Else *et al.*, 2016; Coombes *et al.*, 2018)
12. *Neural field theory*: Instantiate Cowan's neural statistical field theory in a bMERA tensor network (Buice & Cowan, 2009)
13. *Neuronal gauge theory*: Write a neuronal gauge theory with global symmetry rebalancing using gauge fields and a non-energy-based gauge invariant property (Sengupta *et al.*, 2016)

Given that synaptic integration is a central problem in the modeling of neural signaling, a separate list of circuits for these quantum projects is provided as follows:

14. *Synaptic integration*: Write a quantum circuit to model the active nonlinear behavior of EPSP transmission that includes the filtering properties of the dendritic membrane between synapse and soma

integrating both far-off (distal) and near-by (proximate) signals for upstream transmission (Spruston *et al.*, 2016; Williams & Atkinson, 2008)

15. *Synaptic integration*: Develop a quantum algorithm for synaptic integration that includes the effects of both EPSPs and IPSPs, calcium signaling, and ionotropic and metabotropic protein cascades (Sheng & Kim, 2011; Suzuki *et al.*, 2018)
16. *Synaptic integration*: Establish a standard quantum framework for human pyramidal neurons with proximal-distal asymmetric sigmoidal function activation (Mel, 2016; Jin *et al.*, 2018)
17. *Synaptic integration*: Compose a quantum circuit for the wavefunction of graded calcium-mediated dendritic action potentials (Gidon *et al.*, 2020)
18. *Synaptic integration*: Implement a harmonic oscillator quantum circuit to model the elliptical geometry of dendritic spine heads (Cugno *et al.*, 2019)
19. *Spiking neural networks*: Model short and long spiking timescales with out-of-time-order correlation functions to develop a synaptic plasticity rule based on the spatiotemporal aspects of local eligibility traces and targeted top-down learning signals (Bellec *et al.*, 2020; Boahen *et al.*, 2020)
20. *Presynaptic terminal*: Employ a renormalization group method to describe the mathematics of synaptotagmins, calcium ions, and proton gradient transport of neurotransmitters into vesicles (Sudhof, 2013)
21. *Glial behavior*: Test a quantum circuit of calcium signaling and neuron-glia-vasculature temporal integration (Allen & Eroglu, 2017; Jolivet *et al.*, 2015)
22. *Glia and Neuropathology*: Develop a "quantum disease circuit" to study Alzheimer's disease cells in false apoptosis expressing the *Mertk* receptor that triggers microglia and astrocyte phagocytosis (Damisah *et al.*, 2020)
23. *Glia and Neuropathology*: Design a quantum circuit model of astrocyte and oligodendrocyte repair and toxicity in stroke and neurological diseases such as autism and anxiety disorders (Scimemi, 2018; van Veenendaal *et al.*, 2018)

## 20.4 The Future of Quantum Neuroscience

Three factors could indicate tipping points for the quantum computing industry: Chips, routers, and applications. The first is "the Intel of quantum computing chips", the potential advent of universal quantum processing units (QPUs), ostensibly either superconducting chips or quantum optical processing chips, mass-produced in the semiconductor supply chain template. The second is "the Cisco of quantum networks", equipment manufacturers providing all-optical or optical-electrical interconnects with cloud-connected quantum entanglement repeaters, routers, and switches to enable the "quantum internet", global quantum networks for computing and communication. The third is "the GeoCities, MySpace, and Twitter of quantum computing", making easy-to-use application software that end users can readily engage. The mainstream adoption of quantum computation could proceed quickly due to the convenience of cloud services (IDC estimates that in 2023, ~20 percent of organizations will be allocating ~20 percent of their annual IT budgets to quantum computing (West, 2021)). Although it may be possible to probe phenomena such black holes and quantum gravity in the laboratory (as discussed in chapter 4), being able to utilize these experimental domains via cloud services greatly extends their range of accessibility and obviates the need for on-site hardware setups.

Quantum finance (analyzing financial data with wavefunctions and other quantum formalisms) could be one of the first mainstream fields to develop in quantum computing as the industry is typically an early adopter of new technologies. The four main quantum finance application areas are option pricing, trading strategies, risk management, and portfolio optimization. A progression from classical to digital (blockchains) to quantum finance is underway. Applications of interest include quantum amplitude estimation for option pricing (Stamatopoulos *et al.*, 2020), quantum circuit Born machines for portfolio optimization (Alcazar *et al.*, 2020), and quantum photonic support vector machines for risk analysis (Chatterjee & Yu, 2017).

What might hamper the quantum computing industry is the thinking mentality that restricts the platform to a few niche applications such as finance and cryptography. On the one hand, the current idea is not necessarily that individuals would walk around with quantum smartphones (with Ytterbium-171 isotopes at 1 Kelvin (−458°F)) in their pockets, but would use cloud-based applications that could be transparent to end users. On the other hand, the constant advances in miniaturization and materials cannot be discounted. Technology that is increasingly carried alongside or onboard the human (both invasively and noninvasively) is a trend that is likely to continue, and opens greenfield possibilities for the scalability and information security properties of quantum neuroscience applications. A quantum BCI is not out of the question when considering the next several decades of potential technological advance.

There is a wide-spread awareness of quantum computing as a platform, but not of its capabilities. This is not a surprise as any new technology is at first "a better horse" and only later, in the fuller roll-out and advent of novel applications, does its greater realization as "a car" come to be understood. While acknowledging the inherent unknown difficulties in the evolution path of new technologies, it is nevertheless possible to articulate application classes that could be available based on the scalable three-dimensional capability of quantum computing. Entertainment, prototyping, and manufacturing have transitioned to three-dimensional environments more in line with the experience of everyday life (Corke, 2019), but for the most part computing is still flat translations of the physical world. Quantum computing offers the possibility of seamless movement between the domains.

Quantum computing has been known for some time, perhaps initially in the D-Wave Systems (2007) demonstration of quantum computation by adiabatic evolution. Google's announcement of achieving quantum advantage in October 2019 drew further attention to the industry (Arute *et al.*, 2019). The risk, though, is that the thinking is a lot like that at the beginning of the personal computer revolution in the sense of grossly underestimating the possibilities of the platform. For example, Bill Gates and Steve Allen (cofounders of Microsoft) initially tried to refer IBM's PC project (for a 16-bit operating system) to another vendor (Digital Research), and only accepted the work later (Allen, 2011, p. 133). The result was MS-DOS (Microsoft disk operating system) and ultimately a worldwide installed base of a billion copies of Windows in 2010 (*Ibid.*,

p. 181). Steve Wozniak (cofounder of Apple) presented the concept for the Apple II to his employer Hewlett-Packard, but they were not interested (Schlender & Tetzeli, 2015, p. 47). Thomas J. Watson, CEO of IBM likewise famously observed in 1943 that "I think there is a world market for maybe five computers" (Strohmeyer, 2008).

The pervasive industry thinking at the time was that personal computers were a niche market for hobbyists, but the category exploded into the ubiquity of personal computers, smartphones, and tablets, possibly now on the way to on-board quantum-controlled devices. The same could be true for quantum computing. It is known to exist, but not what its capabilities might be in terms of a potentially transformative impact on all industries. The bigger possibility is that quantum computing could bring about a reconceptualization of computation, facilitated by quantum neuroscience circuits with real-time three-dimensional highly secure biological data processing.

Computation at the level of quantum mechanics is required for the brain, not only as dictated by its complexity, but also to address the causal factors of disease. A substantial advance would be that of progressing to a systemic understanding of pathology that extends beyond what is still in many cases treating symptoms instead of underlying causes. Current methods for the study of the brain could be leapfrogged and complemented by the conceptually different approaches offered by quantum neuroscience. Future-class applications could include personalized connectomics, molecular-scale intervention, and local brain area networks with real-time biological data processing and neuronanorobot monitoring. Service delivery could be via quantum BCIs, CRISPR technologies, nanoparticles, and cellular therapeutics, possibly printed with home-based molecular assemblers. Success could be measured by improved quality of life (healthspan) metrics and reduced clinical instances of pathologies due to preventive approaches.

Although quantum computing is a nascent platform in need of error correction for requisite scalability, the present opportunity is to deploy the quantum mindset (thinking in terms of quantum mathematical and algorithmic formulations) to define a new era of neuroscience investigation. A central focus is explaining the electrical and chemical signaling operations of the brain through spatiotemporal nonlinear dynamical models. This work proposes the multi-tier AdS/Brain correspondence model of successive bulk-boundary tiers of network, neuron, synapse, and molecule. Ultimately, quantum neuroscience might enable robust multiscalar models that capture the nuance of the brain's activities, and contribute to the tireless quest for an improved understanding of the sophisticated 1.5-kg organ, in virtue of possibly expanding its capabilities and protecting it from disease and decline.

## References


Alcazar, J., Leyton-Ortega, V. & Perdomo-Ortiz, A. (2020). Classical versus quantum models in machine learning: Insights from a finance application. *Machine Learning: Sci. Tech.* 1(3):035003.

Allen, P. (2011). *Idea Man: A Memoir by the Cofounder of Microsoft*. New York: Penguin.

Allen, N.J. & Eroglu, C. (2017). Cell biology of astrocyte-synapse interactions. *Neuron*. 96:697–708.

Amari, S. (1977). Dynamics of pattern formation in lateral-inhibition type neural fields. *Biol. Cybern*. 27:77–87.

Arute, F., Arya, K., Babbush, R. *et al.* (2019). Quantum supremacy using a programmable superconducting processor. *Nature*. 574:505–11.

Bellec, G., Scherr, F., Subramoney, A. *et al.* (2020). A solution to the learning dilemma for recurrent networks of spiking neurons. *Nat. Commun.* 11: 3625.

Belyansky, R., Bienias, P., Kharko, Y.A. *et al.* (2020). A minimal model for fast scrambling. arXiv:2005.05362v2.

Boahen, K.A., Fok, S.B., Neckar, A.S. *et al.* (2020). Methods and apparatus for spiking neural network computing based on threshold accumulation. U.S. Pat Appl. #20200019839. https://www.freepatentsonline.com/y2020/0019839.html.

Bressloff, P.C. (2015). Path-integral methods for analyzing the effects of fluctuations in stochastic hybrid neural networks. *J. Math. Neurosci.* 5(4):1-33.

Brown, A.R., Gharibyan, H., Leichenauer, S. *et al.* (2019). Quantum gravity in the lab: Teleportation by size and traversable wormholes. aXiv:1911.06314v1.

Buice, M.A. & Cowan, J.D. (2009). Statistical mechanics of the neocortex. *Prog. Biophys. Mol. Biol.* 99:53–86.

Carrasquilla, J., Torlai, G., Melko, R.G. & Aolita, L. (2019). Reconstructing quantum states with generative models. *Nat. Mach. Intel.* 1:155–61.

Chatterjee, R. & Yu, T. (2017). Generalized coherent states, reproducing kernels, and quantum support vector machines. *Quantum Inf. Commun.* 17(15–16): 1292–1306.

Cheng, S., Chen, J. & Wang L. (2018). Information perspective to probabilistic modeling: Boltzmann machines versus Born machines. *Entropy*. 20(8):583.

Chow, C.C. & Buice, M.A. (2015). Path integral methods for stochastic differential equations. *J. Math. Neurosci.* 5(8):1–35.

Coombes, S., Lai, Y.M., Sayli, M. & Thul, R. (2018). Networks of piecewise linear neural mass models. *Eur. J. Appl. Math.* 29(5):869–90.

Corke, G. (2019). Unity for manufacturing. *Develop 3D*. https://develop3d.com/features/unity-visualisation-vr-manufacturing-industrial-design-game-on-simulation/.

Cugno, A., Bartol, T.M., Sejnowski, T.J. *et al.* (2019). Geometric principles of second messenger dynamics in dendritic spines. *Sci. Rep.* 9(1):11676.

Dahlberg, A., Skrzypczyk, M., Coopmans, T. et al. (2019). A link layer protocol for quantum networks. In *SIGCOMM '19. Proceedings of the 2019 Conference of the ACM Special Interest Group on Data Communication*, Beijing, China, August 19–23, 2019, pp. 1159–73.

Damisah, E.C., Hill, R.A., Rai, A. *et al.* (2020). Astrocytes and microglia play orchestrated roles and respect phagocytic territories during neuronal corpse removal in vivo. *Sci. Adv.* 6(26):eaba3239.

D-Wave Systems. (2007). Quantum computing demo announcement. Press Release. http://dwave.wordpress.com/2007/01/19/quantum-computing-demo-announcement. Accessed March 15, 2021.

Else, D.V., Bauer, B. & Nayak, C. (2016). Floquet time crystals. *Phys. Rev. Lett.* 117(9):090402.

Engelhardt, N. & Wall, A.C. (2019). Coarse-graining holographic black holes. *J. High Energ. Phys.* 1905:160.

Erhard, M., Krenn, M. & Zeilinger, A. (2020). Advances in high dimensional quantum entanglement. *Nat. Rev. Phys.* 2:365–81.

Flamini, F., Spagnolo, N. & Sciarrino, F. (2018). Photonic quantum information processing: A review. *Rep. Prog. Phys.* 82(1):016001.

Gidon, A., Zolnik, T.A., Fidzinski, P. *et al.* (2020). Dendritic action potentials and computation in human layer 2/3 cortical neurons. *Science*. 367(6743): 83–87.

Han, X., Hartnoll, S.A. & Kruthoff, J. (2020). Bootstrapping matrix quantum mechanics. *Phys. Rev. Lett.* 125(4):041601.

Harlow, D. (2017). TASI lectures on the emergence of bulk physics in AdS/CFT. In *Proceedings of Theoretical Advanced Study Institute Summer School 2017, "Physics at the Fundamental Frontier"*, Boulder, Colorado, USA, June 4–July 1, 2017. arXiv:1802.01040, PoS(TASI2017)002.

Harlow, D. & Shaghoulian, E. (2020). Global symmetry, Euclidean gravity, and the black hole information problem. arXiv:2010.10539v1. MIT-CTP 5249.

Hayden, P., Nezami, S., Qi, X.L. *et al.* (2016). Holographic duality from random tensor networks. *J. High Energ. Phy.* 11(9):1–57.

Hayden, P. & Penington, G. (2019). Learning the Alpha-bits of black holes. *J. High Energ. Phys.* 1912:007.

Jahren, H. (2017). *Lab Girl.* New York: Alfred A. Knopf.

Jin, L., Behabadi, B.F., Jadi, M.P. *et al.* (2018). Classical-contextual interactions in V1 may rely on dendritic computations. bioRxiv:436956.

Jolivet, R., Coggan, J.S., Allaman, I. & Magistretti, P.J. (2015). Multi-timescale modeling of activity-dependent metabolic coupling in the neuron-glia-vasculature ensemble. *PLoS Comput Biol.* 11(2):e1004036.

Kim, I.H. & Swingle, B. (2017). Robust entanglement renormalization on a noisy quantum computer. arXiv:1711.07500.

Kobrin, B., Yang, Z., Kahanamoku-Meyer, G.D. *et al.* (2020). Many-body chaos in the Sachdev-Ye-Kitaev model. *Phys. Rev. Lett.* 126(3):030602.

Lin, H.W., Maldacena, J. & Zhao, Y. (2019). Symmetries near the horizon. *J. High Energ. Phys.* 1908:049.

Martins, N.R.B., Angelica, A., Chakravarthy, K. *et al.* (2019). Human brain/cloud interface. *Front Neurosci.* 13(112):1–23.

Martins, N.R.B., Erlhagen, W. & Freitas, R.A. Jr. (2016). Human connectome mapping and monitoring using neuronanorobots. *J. Evol. Technol.* (26): 1–25.

Mel, B.W. (2016). Towards a simplified model of an active dendritic tree. In *Dendrites*. Eds. Stuart, G., Spruston, N. & Hausser, M. Oxford: Oxford University Press, pp. 465–86.

Nozaki, M., Ryu, S. & Takayanagi, T. (2012). Holographic geometry of entanglement renormalization in quantum field theories. *J. High Energ. Phys.* 193: 1–43.

Ohira, T. & Cowan, J.D. (1993). Master-equation approach to stochastic neurodynamics. *Phys. Rev. E.* 48:2259–66.

Schlender, B. & Tetzeli, R. (2015). *Becoming Steve Jobs*. New York: Crown Publishing Group.

Schuld, M., Bradler, K., Israel, R. *et al.* (2019). A quantum hardware-induced graph kernel based on Gaussian boson sampling. arXiv:1905.12646.

Scimemi, A. (2018). Astrocytes and the warning signs of intracerebral hemorrhagic stroke. *Neural Plasticity*. 2018(7301623):1–11.

Sengupta, B., Tozzi, A., Cooray, G.K. *et al.* (2016). Towards a neuronal gauge theory. *PLoS Biol.* 14(3):e1002400.

Sheng, M. & Kim, E. (2011). The postsynaptic organization of synapses. *Cold Spring Harb. Perspect. Biol.* 3(a005678):1–20.

Spruston, N., Stuart, G. & Hausser, M. (2016). *Dendrites*. 3rd Edition. Chapter 12: Principles of dendritic integration. Oxford: Oxford University Press, pp. 1–78.

Srednicki, M. (2007). *Quantum Field Theory*. Cambridge: Cambridge University Press.

Stamatopoulos, N., Egger, D.J., Sun, Y. *et al.* (2020). Option pricing using quantum computers. *Quantum*. 4:291.

Steinbrecher, G.R., Olson, J.P., Englund, D. & Carolan, J. (2019). Quantum optical neural networks. *NPJ Quantum Inf.* 5(60):1–9.

Strohmeyer, R. (2008). The 7 Worst Tech Predictions of All Time. *PCWorld*. https://www.pcworld.com/article/532605/worst_tech_predictions.html.

Sudhof, T.C. (2013). Neurotransmitter release: The last millisecond in the life of a synaptic vesicle. *Neuron*. 80:675–90.

Suzuki, T., Kametani, K., Gui, W. & Li, W. (2018). Protein components of postsynaptic density lattice, a backbone structure for type I excitatory synapses. *J. Neurochem.* 144:390–407.

Swan, M. (2022). B/CI: Quantum computing, holographic control theory, and blockchain IPLD for the brain. In *Nanomedical Brain/Cloud Interface: Explorations and Implications*. Ed. Boehm, F. Boca Raton, FL: CRC Press.

Swan, M., dos Santos, R.P. & Witte, F. (2020). *Quantum Computing: Physics, Blockchains, and Deep Learning Smart Networks*. London: World Scientific.

Swingle, B., Bentsen, G., Schleier-Smith, M. & Hayden, P. (2016). Measuring the scrambling of quantum information. *Phys. Rev. A*. 94(4):040302.

van Veenendaal, T.M., Backes, W.H., Tse, D.H.Y. *et al.* (2018). High field imaging of large-scale neurotransmitter networks: Proof of concept and initial application to epilepsy. *NeuroImage: Clinical*. 19:47–55.

Wang, Y., Li, Q., Liu, L. *et al.* (2019). TeraVR empowers precise reconstruction of complete 3-D neuronal morphology in the whole brain. *Nat. Commun.* 10(3474):1–9.

West, H. (2021). Enterprise IT Infrastructure Survey, 1Q21: Insights on end-user 2021 IT compute infrastructure priorities and adoption of quantum computing. IDC Report #US47687021.

Williams, S.R. & Atkinson, S.E. (2008). Dendritic synaptic integration in central neurons. *Curr. Biol.* 18(22). R1045–47.

Zhong, H.-S., Wang, H., Deng, Y.-H. *et al.* (2020). Quantum computational advantage using photons. *Science*. 370(6523):1460–63.

# Glossary

**Abelian:** Commuting (order of terms does not matter)

**Action:** Function used to calculate the equations of motion or path of a physical system

**Adiabatic:** Naturally evolving process to lowest energy configuration

**AdS/Brain:** AdS/CFT correspondence interpretation in neuroscience

**AdS/CFT correspondence (anti-de Sitter space/conformal field theory), gauge/gravity or holographic duality:** Claim that a gravity theory (bulk) is equal to a gauge theory or quantum field theory (boundary) in one less dimension

**Afferent:** Incoming conducting impulses directed towards the central nervous system

**Amplitude (probability amplitude):** The inner product between two state vectors in a quantum mechanical system (a complex number)

**Amplitude encoding:** A data vector represented by the amplitudes of a quantum state

**Anderson localization:** Absence of wave diffusion in a disordered medium (a useful property of electron localization in semiconductors)

**Anisotropic:** Different in different directions (versus isotropic: the same in all directions)

**Ansatz:** Guess, an educated guess, for example, of a wavefunction in quantum mechanics (exact methods are unavailable)

**Anti-de Sitter (AdS) space:** A toy model of real-life de Sitter space based on the negative hyperbolic geometry of a sphere (a maximally symmetric Lorentzian manifold with constant negative scalar curvature)

**Artificial neural network:** Computing system inspired by a biological neural network

**Attention (learning mechanism):** Machine learning method used in transformer neural networks as a tripartite mapping of query, keys, and values to assess data relevance

**Attractor:** (Complex systems) focal point around which a system organizes itself

**Autoencoder (automatic encoding):** Unsupervised learning technique (using Markov chains and principal component analysis) in which the system automatically learns a representation or encoding scheme for data with a reduced dimensionality representation

**Autoregressive neural network:** Neural network for time series (RNN alternative) modeling current values of a series as a function of past values

**Avogadro's number:** About $6.022 \times 10^{23}$ (0.6 billion billion); the number of molecules in 22.4 liters of gas at standard temperature and pressure

**Backpropagation (of errors):** Machine learning technique to optimize loss functions by calculating the error contribution of each neuron after a batch of data is processed

**Bell pair:** Particles entangled in a shared quantum state even over large distance

**Bifurcation:** Instability arising in a system when an attractor (organizing parameter) changes dramatically

**Black hole:** Dense region of spacetime with gravity so strong that nothing can escape, not even light

**Black hole information paradox:** Puzzle as to how information that goes into a black hole evaporates later as Hawking radiation

**Blind quantum computing:** Quantum computing protocol with hidden input, output, and task

**Bloch sphere:** Geometrical representation of the state space (Hilbert space) of the qubit

**Bloch wave:** Periodic wave

**Boltzmann distribution:** Probability that a system will be in a certain state given the state's energy and the system's temperature

**Boltzmann machine:** Machine learning network of visible and hidden layers of processing units using a Boltzmann distribution-based energy function to evaluate output

**Bond dimension (tensor rank):** Dimension of the index linking tensors

**Born machine:** Probabilistic model of machine learning using the Born rule to determine output probabilities (versus Boltzmann machine)

**Born rule:** Probability that a measurement of a quantum system will have a certain result (the probability density of finding a particle at a given point is proportional to the square of the magnitude of the particle's wavefunction at that point)

**Boson:** Force particle (photon) with integer spin (versus fermion)

**Boson sampling:** Statistical sampling of boson scattering output (classically intractable)

**Bound state:** A particle kept localized in a region of space by a potential

**Bouton:** Enlarged nerve ending forming a synapse

**Brain atlas:** Brain map of serial sections along anatomical planes by dimension (latero-lateral (x), dorso-ventral (y), rostro-caudal (z)), and section (coronal, sagittal, transverse)

**Brain–computer interface (BCI) or brain–machine interface (BMI):** A direct communication pathway between a wired brain and an external device

**Bump:** (Neuroscience) spatially localized concentrated increase in neural population firing

**Chaos:** Dynamical systems whose apparently random states are governed by deterministic laws and sensitivity to initial conditions

**Chaotic dynamics:** Evolution of dynamical systems per identifiable parameters

**Clifford algebra:** Geometric algebra of spacetime (a vector space with a quadratic form) giving a complete picture of spin representations of all spin groups and their relationships

**Clifford gates:** Basic quantum gates (Pauli matrices, Hadamard gate, CNOT gate) that can be simulated efficiently on a classical computer (i.e. in polynomial time)

**Clifford group:** Unitaries that preserve the Pauli group under similarity transformations

**Coherent state:** An oscillatory quantum state (quantum harmonic oscillator)

**Color code:** Topological quantum error-correcting codes using more computationally efficient gauge-fixing instead of magic state distillation to execute non-Clifford gates

**Complexity:** Attribute of systems that are nonlinear, emergent, open, unpredictable, interdependent, self-organizing, and multiscalar in time and space

**Computational complexity:** Difficulty of computing a problem, the minimum number of (quantum) gates required to prepare a state or solution of the computation

**Condensate:** Quantum collective wave; group state with the same phase and energy

**Condensed matter physics:** The study of the collective behavior of complex assemblies of electrons, nuclei, magnetic moments, atoms, or qubits

**Conformal field theory (CFT):** Quantum field theory that is invariant under conformal transformations (mappings do not change the angle between corresponding curves)

**Conjugate pair:** Observable quantity pairs that obey the Heisenberg uncertainty principle: position/momentum, energy/time

**Connectome:** Map (wiring diagram) of all neural connections in the brain

**Contraction (tensor):** Simplification in tensor multiplication

**Correlation function:** Required amplitude for particle propagation between two points

**de Sitter space:** Three-dimensional space of everyday reality

**Deep learning:** Machine learning networks with hidden layers to find higher-order relationships in data (shallow: 1–2 layers, deep: 3–8+ layers)

**Degrees of freedom:** System parameters; number of elements to characterize a system

**Dendritic integration:** *See* Synaptic integration

**Dendritic spikes:** Action potentials generated and aggregated by dendrites from postsynaptic density to soma

**Density matrix:** All information about a quantum state or system

**Density matrix renormalization group (DMRG):** Variational (sampling) technique for finding the lowest-energy matrix product state wavefunction of a Hamiltonian

**Diffeomorphism:** One-to-one relationship (isomorphism) between smooth manifolds

**Diffeomorphism invariant:** Invariant to diffeomorphism transformations (manifold changes). Example: gravity is a gauge theory because it is diffeomorphism invariant

**Diffusion:** Physical spread from high to low concentration, temperature, or pressure

**Diffusion equation:** Partial differential equation used to describe the macroscopic behavior of particles in Brownian motion and Markov processes such as random walks

**Dirac delta function:** Linear function from a space of all smooth functions (a linear activation versus a Heaviside step function activation)

**Discriminative learning:** Machine learning method that learns directly from labeled data

**Disentangler:** (Tensor networks) transformation into less entangled state

**Dressed electrons:** (Superconducting) non free-floating electrons (constrained in a metal)

**Eigenvector:** (Linear algebra) a non-zero vector that changes (is stretched) by a scalar factor (the eigenvalue) in a linear transformation

**Einstein field equations:** (General relativity) a set of equations relating the geometry of spacetime to the distribution of matter within it (very hard to solve)

**Electroencephalography (EEG):** Electrophysiological monitoring method to record electrical activity in different parts of the brain

**Endocytosis:** Draw in, e.g. neurotransmitter recycling (versus exocytosis)

**Entanglement:** (Quantum mechanics) correlated physical properties between particles

**Entanglement entropy:** Measure of interrelated information between two quantum systems

**Entropy:** The number of ways a system can be arranged, the degree of interrelatedness of subregions within a system, or the number of bits (qubits) required to encode and send a system state

**Escher *Circle Limits*:** Image of a circle with a few fish in the center growing to a near-infinite number of fish at the edge; AdS space analogy

**Excitatory postsynaptic potential (EPSP):** A synaptic potential rendering a postsynaptic neuron more likely to generate an action potential

**Exocytosis:** Expel outward, e.g. release of neurotransmitters (versus endocytosis)

**Extremal black hole:** Smallest possible black hole (in mass, charge, angular momentum)

**Fast scrambling:** System with rapid quantum information spread (e.g. black holes, the SYK model)

**Fault tolerance:** Preventing propagation of few-to-many errors

**Fermi liquid:** "Normal" metal phase with resistivity at low temperature

**Fermion:** Matter particle (electron) with spin ½ (versus boson)

**Feynman diagram:** Path integral formulation of quantum field theory (a graphical representation of amplitudes as a weighted sum of all possible system histories)

**Fish-counting metric:** (Informal) geodesic; shortest curve through the bulk

**Fisher information:** An observable random variable's information about an unknown parameter of a distribution

**Floquet theory:** Theory of periodically-driven systems (ordinary differential equations for solutions to periodic linear differential equations)

**Fock space:** Multi-particle Hilbert space

**Fock state:** Multi-particle state

**Fokker–Planck equation:** Partial differential equation of the time evolution of the probability density function of particle velocity under drag forces as in Brownian motion

**FTQC (fault-tolerant quantum computing):** Error-corrected quantum computers

**Gauge:** Mathematical formalism rendering systems in discrete scale tiers

**Gauge bosons:** Force particles that are the quanta of gauge fields

**Gauge field:** A (vector) field generated by the Lie algebra that describes the gauge theory

**Gauge fixing (choosing a gauge):** Procedure for simplifying the redundant degrees of freedom (characterization parameters) in a system

**Gauge group (symmetry group):** Lie group formed by possible gauge transformations

**Gauge invariance:** System property of a non-changing Lagrangian (system dynamics function) under local transformations

**Gauge theory:** A field theory in which the Lagrangian (state of a dynamic system) is invariant under local transformations of certain Lie groups

**Gauge transformation:** Transformations between possible gauges (levels) in a system

**Gaussian boson sampling:** Statistical sampling method (classically intractable)

**Gaussian state:** State whose distribution is Gaussian

**General relativity:** A geometry-based theory of gravity (versus Newton's mass-based theory) describing how to find the curvature or the spacetime warping effect (i.e. gravity) of a given amount of mass and energy

**Generative learning:** Unsupervised machine learning method that learns the distribution of unlabeled data to generate new samples

**Geodesic:** Straight line in curved space, shortest curve between two points

**Ghost imaging:** (Quantum teleportation) transmission in which the qubit interacts only with its correlated partner photon (not with the photon used to image it)

**Ginzburg criterion:** System criticality condition (critical exponent)

**Ginzburg-Landau theory:** (Superconductivity) the free energy of a superconductor near the superconducting transition (critical temperature) has the form of a field theory

**Glass networks:** Periodic switch-like behavior in biochemical networks

**GPT-3 (generative pre-trained transformer 3):** (Deep learning) autoregressive language model producing human-like text nearly indistinguishable from human-written

**Greenberger–Horne–Zeilinger (GHZ) state:** Entangled quantum state involving at least three subsystems (qubits or particle states)

**Green's function:** Mathematical operator used in correlation functions, can take the role of a propagator (Gaussian propagator)

**Grover's search algorithm:** Quantum algorithm to find a particular register in an unordered database

**H (*h*):** Planck's constant in Joules/second per cycle units, $6.626 \times 10^{-34}$ J·s, denoting the amount of energy change per change in frequency in quantum wave movement, expressed by the formula $E = hf$ (associated with the energy of the electromagnetic wave in Special Relativity's $E = mc^2$)

**H-bar ($\hbar$):** Reduced Planck's constant in units of Joules/second Radians, $1.055 \times 10^{-34}$ J·s/radian. Planck's constant divided by $2\pi$, hence the name h-bar, used as a more natural expression of angular frequency in mathematics and physics

**Haar randomness:** Stringent randomness condition (randomness drawn from a unitarily invariant ensemble of pure states)

**Hadamard coin:** Unitary operator action to update a binary property (spin or chirality)

**Hadamard gate:** Quantum gate which acts on one qubit to put it in a superposition state

**Hafnian:** Matrix function as the number of perfect matchings in the graph of an adjacency matrix (defined in Copenhagen (*Latin*: Hafnia))

**Hamiltonian:** Operator used to calculate the energy levels of a system

**Heaviside step function:** Step function-based activation (versus Dirac delta function)

**Heralded entanglement:** Announced entanglement generation

**High-dimensional entanglement:** Particles entangled in more than one dimension (e.g. time, space, polarization, propagation path)

**Hilbert feature space:** Data encoded as a Hilbert space feature map

**Hilbert space:** Infinite-dimension vector space of possible wavefunctions

**Holevo's theorem:** Theorem placing an upper bound on accessible quantum state information; used to facilitate quantum calculation

**Holographic principle:** The information stored in a spatial volume is encoded in its boundary in one less dimension

**Holography:** Three-dimensional image embedded in a two-dimensional surface

**Hopf bifurcation:** System critical point (e.g. resting-to-firing state) at which a periodic orbit appears/disappears due to a local change in stability

**Hubbard model:** Classically intractable model of superconducting (describing the interaction between electrons of opposite spin by a single parameter (e.g. the metal-Mott shift))

**Identity matrix:** (Linear algebra) an $n \times n$ square matrix with ones on the main diagonal and zeros elsewhere (main diagonal: top left to bottom right)

**Information theory:** Theoretical approach to the quantification, storage, and communication of information

**Inhibitory postsynaptic potential (IPSP):** A synaptic potential rendering a postsynaptic neuron less likely to generate an action potential

**Integrate-and-fire:** Threshold-based single-neuron model of spike activation (per the integration of weighted incoming synaptic inputs)

**Interference:** Phase difference between two wavefunction amplitudes

**Ising model:** Ferromagnetic model of phase transition with all spins aligned at low or high energy, and fluctuating in between

**Jackiw–Teitelboim (JT) gravity:** Gravity theory with one space and one time dimension

**Jansen–Rit model:** (Neuroscience) the coupling of two models with delays in the interconnections to simulate the synaptic connections within and between cortical areas

**Josephson junction:** Mechanism based on the quantum tunneling of superconducting Cooper pairs used in quantum computing chips

**Kernel:** (Machine learning) a data sort based on the distance between points in a high-dimensional feature space

**Kernel function:** Distance measure between pairwise points (vector inner products) used to construct the properties of a data distribution

**Kernel trick:** Iterating through data representations (kernels) for best fit

**Kondo effect:** Explanation of how electrons in a metal scatter off magnetic impurities, which produces an increase in resistivity at low temperature

**Kondo model:** A model for metals with magnetic impurities (a single localized quantum impurity coupled to a large reservoir of electrons)

**Kondo problem:** (Condensed matter physics) the inability of theoretical methods prior to the renormalization group to explain a rise in the resistivity of impure metal samples (e.g. gold) at low temperature since resistivity usually decreases when temperature decreases

**Kullback–Leibler (KL) divergence:** Relative entropy, probability distribution distance

**Ladder operator:** (Raising or lowering operator) an operator that increases or decreases the eigenvalue of another operator, used in combination to change the state of a particle

**Lagrangian:** Function describing the state of a dynamic system in terms of position coordinates, time derivatives, and potential and kinetic energy

**Langevin equation:** Stochastic differential equation of the time evolution of a system subset

**Laplacian:** Operator representing the flux density of the gradient flow of a function

**Large *N*:** A very large number of the items at hand; dimensions, observable values (e.g. scattering amplitudes), or system parameters (degrees of freedom)

**Large-*N* limit:** Quantum theory limit as the number of items gets close to infinity

**Levi-Civita connection:** Covariant derivative for differentiating tensors (as an operation on tangent bundles that differentiates vector fields)

**Lie algebra:** Local version of the Li group (global group object)

**Lie group:** A continuous group (allowing multiplication and division) that is a differentiable manifold (locally resembling Euclidean space)

**Light field:** Treating light as a 5D field (by analogy to the electromagnetic field)

**Light field microscopy:** Scanning-free 3D light-based microscopy

**Light sheet microscopy:** High-speed optical method for 3D reconstruction (only in-focus fluorophores are collected from the light sheet image of the sample)

**Lindblad equation:** Quantum version of the classical master equation (with system time evolution as a probabilistic combination of states)

**Lorentzian invariance:** Inertial-in-all-frames property of a spacetime manifold

**Lorentzian manifold:** (General relativity) manifold upon which tensor fields are defined to represent spacetime in a geometrical view of gravity

**Lyapunov exponent:** Exponent increasing exponentially with time (measuring the rate of separation of two trajectories) indicating chaos

**Lyapunov time:** Timescale on which a dynamical system is chaotic

**Machine learning:** Method in which computers perform tasks by relying on information patterns and inference as opposed to explicit instruction

**Majorana fermions:** Strongly coupled system with all-to-all random connections

**Many-body problem:** A quantum system with three or more entities (hard to model)

**Markov chain:** Stochastic model with event probability depending on the previous event

**Markov chain Monte Carlo:** Monte Carlo sampling method based on a Markov chain

**Matrix quantum mechanics:** Operator algebra formulation for multidimensional matrices

**MaxCut (maximum cut):** Optimization algorithm (partition function) that efficiently divides data, finding the optimal (maximal) cut through a dataset

**Mean-field theory:** Mean value of a field taken as a solvable approximation of an intractable system of underlying complexity

**Metric tensor (metric):** Complete description of the geometric structure of a spacetime system, including time, space, distance, volume, and curvature

**Mixed state:** A quantum state that can be written as a mixture of other states (versus pure state)

**Moment-generating function:** Equation for calculating moments (expectation values)

**Monte Carlo method:** Statistical approach of taking repeated random samples to profile a system

**Mott insulator:** Class of materials that should conduct electricity, but insulates at low temperatures due to electron–electron interactions

**Mott localization:** Condensed matter phase transition from metallic to insulating behavior due to strong Coulomb repulsion of electrons

**Motzkin model:** Streamlined quantum mechanical optimization model (no energy scale)

**Multi-scale entanglement renormalization ansatz (MERA):** Tensor network with alternating layers of disentanglers and isometries that coarse grain (consolidate) a system between microscale and macroscale

**Multistability:** Noise-driven switching between multiple weakly stable states

**Negentropy (negative entropy):** Measure of distance to normality

**Network neuroscience:** Graph-theoretic study of the brain

**Network science:** Graph-theoretic representation of a system's elements by nodes (vertices) and connections between them as links (edges)

**Neural code:** Hypothetical relationship between a neural stimulus and response

**Neural ensemble:** Collective behavior of a small group of neurons in uncorrelated states

**Neural field theory:** Large-scale model of collective brain behavior as a continuous field

**Neural mass model:** The mass action of a local population of neurons acting as a group

**Neural network:** Machine learning architecture inspired by the brain generally (typically consisting of alternating linear and nonlinear functions)

**Neurite (neuronal process):** A projection from a neuron's cell body

**Neuromorphic computing:** Computing circuits that mimic neuro-biological architectures

**Neuron reconstruction:** Conversion of imaging data to morphological description (with spatiotemporal topology)

**Neuroscience physics:** Neuroscience interpretation of foundational physics findings

**NISQ (noisy intermediate-scale quantum) devices:** Currently available quantum computers, ~50–100 qubits, without error correction

**No-hair theorem:** Black hole description based on mass, electric charge, and angular momentum (without any additional "hair")

**Non-abelian:** Non-commuting (order of terms matters)

**Non-Clifford gates:** Quantum gates with greater logical depth that cannot be simulated efficiently on a classical computer (e.g. $\pi/8$ gate)

**Non-Fermi liquid:** Metal phase deviating from resistivity at low temperature (not explained by traditional superconducting theories)

**Observable:** (Quantum mechanics) a measurable system attribute

**Omics:** High-throughput analysis characterizing the entirety of a biological phenomenon (e.g. genomics, proteomics, connectomics, synaptomics)

**Operator:** A function over a space of physical states to another space of physical states

**Optical neural network:** Neural network with all-optical components

**Optical quantum computing:** Quantum computing with all-optical components (single-photon sources, photonic integrated circuits, and single-photon detectors)

**Ordinary differential equation (ODE):** Equation with one unknown variable

**OSI (open systems interconnection) model:** Standard communications network model with 7-layers (physical, data link, network, transport, session, presentation, application)

**Out-of-time-order correlation (OTOC) functions:** Functions (operators) used to evolve a quantum system back or forward in time

**Page time:** Time evolution during which a black hole is reduced to half of its initial entropy or half of the surface area of its event horizon

**Parcellation:** Brain segmentation into functionally distinct regions

**Partial differential equation (PDE):** Equation with multiple unknown variables

**Partition function:** A function giving all aspects of a system

**Path integral:** Sum over all paths a particle can take through a space

**Pauli group:** 16-element group of the $2 \times 2$ identity matrix and all of the Pauli matrices for a quantum system

**Pauli matrices:** Three $2 \times 2$ matrices, describing angular momentum operators as observables of particle spin in Hilbert space (X, Y, Z); mainstay of quantum mechanical manipulations

**Pauli operator:** Spin operator derived from Pauli matrices (often used for quantum system measurement)

**Pauli-Z "plaquette" (face) operators:** (Lattice gauge theory) smallest closed loop function enclosing the region between four lattice sites

**Phase space:** Space with all possible states of a system represented

**Photonic quantum computing:** *See* Optical quantum computing

**Photonics:** Generation, manipulation, transmission, and detection of photons (quantum units of light)

**Piecewise function:** Function with multiple sub-functions for different domain intervals

**Planck's constant:** *See* **H ($h$)** and **H-bar ($\hbar$)**

**Plasma:** Highly ionized state of matter (e.g. quark-gluon plasma)

**Polarization:** Property of light as to its direction of travel (oscillation)

**Post-quantum cryptography:** Cryptographic algorithms not easily breakable by quantum computers (likely lattice not factoring based)

**Postsynaptic density:** In the receiving neuron, specialized protrusions from dendritic arbors (spines) as protein complexes that anchor neurotransmitter receptors and reconvert chemical signals to electrical dendritic spikes to forward to the soma (cell body)

**Presynaptic terminal:** In the sending neuron, bouton (enlarged area) at nerve ending that converts electrical action potentials to neurotransmitters to release into the synaptic cleft

**Probabilistic graphical model:** Probabilistic model in which a graph expresses the conditional dependence structure between random variables

**Probabilistic quantum models:** Using quantum-based methods to perform probability-related tasks such as machine learning classification

**Probability density:** The probability that a particle will be at a certain position at a certain time or have a certain momentum (calculated by squaring the wavefunction amplitudes)

**Pseudo-randomness:** Close-to-randomness approximation that can be used more efficiently in computation

**Pure state:** A quantum state that cannot be written on the basis of other states (versus mixed state)

**Quadratures:** (Quantum optics) operators that represent the real and imaginary parts of the complex amplitude of an oscillatory wave

**Quantization:** System energy level or other physical parameter limited to and instantiated as discrete values

**Quantum advantage:** Quantum computers performing tasks that classical computers cannot

**Quantum chaos:** Seemingly random but deterministic growth eras (e.g. ballistic and saturation phases)

**Quantum chromodynamics (QCD):** The field theory of the strong force

**Quantum circuit:** Quantum logic gates (sequential operations on qubits)

**Quantum clock network:** Global network of atomic clocks

**Quantum computing:** The use of engineered quantum systems to perform computation

**Quantum dynamics:** Motion, energy, and momentum exchange of quantum systems

**Quantum electrodynamics (QED):** The field theory of the electromagnetic field

**Quantum error correction:** Protecting quantum information from environmental noise

**Quantum error correcting code:** Error diagnosis code, for example identifying a bit flip or (phase) sign flip

**Quantum field theory:** A theory of fundamental particle interaction based on quantized fields and forces (a classical field is quantized as an operator-valued function acting on a Hilbert space)

**Quantum finance:** (Econophysics) quantum physics applied to problems in finance: option pricing, trading strategies, risk management, and portfolio optimization

**Quantum gate:** Building block of quantum computation in which a logical operation is performed on qubits (analogous to a classical gate)

**Quantum gravity:** Theory of gravity in domains with very small and very heavy objects (such as black holes and the Big Bang)

**Quantum information:** The state information of a quantum system

**Quantum internet:** Proposal for an ultra-fast ultra-secure internet with all-quantum components

**Quantum key distribution (QKD):** Quantum cryptography protocol to distribute random private keys among remote parties

**Quantum machine learning:** Machine learning algorithms run on quantum platforms

**Quantum matter:** Matter phases with quantum mechanical properties

**Quantum mechanics:** Framework for physical theories at the atomic scale ($1 \times 10^{-9}$ m) and below, formulated as many-particle (quanta) systems in Hilbert space

**Quantum memory:** Quantum mechanical version of computer memory

**Quantum Monte Carlo:** Application of Monte Carlo statistical sampling methods to quantum systems

**Quantum network:** (Global) network model of quantum computation, communication, or sensing

**Quantum neural networks (QNNs):** Neural networks based quantum mechanical principles

**Quantum neuroscience:** Application of quantum information science methods to neuroscience

**Quantum photonics:** Generating, manipulating, transmitting, and detecting light in regimes in which coherent control of individual quanta of the light field (photons) is possible

**Quantum quench:** Hamiltonian evolution per a sudden change in parameters

**Quantum-secure cryptography:** *See* Post-quantum cryptography

**Quantum state:** Information state of a quantum system (probability distribution of the outcomes of each possible system measurement)

**Quantum teleportation:** Sending quantum state information from one location to another (the quantum version of sending a fax)

**Quantum tomography:** Quantum state reconstruction method executed by measuring an ensemble of identical quantum states

**Quantum volume:** A benchmarking technique for NISQ devices based on approximating a specific class of random circuits and estimating the associated effective error rate

**Quantum walk:** Quantum version of classical random walk based on coin-flip operators (e.g. Hadamard coin) and lattice graph propagation (discrete-time or continuous-time)

**Quasi-particle:** Single particle excitation (an ideal particle used in models)

**Qubit (quantum information bit):** Two-level quantum system, basic unit of quantum information used for computation (analogous to the classical binary bit)

**Qubitization:** Preparing a quantum state (in qubits) for quantum computation

**Qudit (quantum information digit):** Multilevel quantum information unit existing in any number of states. A qubit is in a superposition of 0 and 1 before measurement; a qutrit in 0, 1, and 2, etc.

**Random field:** Function that takes a random value at each point in the domain

**Random matrix:** Matrix in which some or all elements are random variables

**Random surface:** Dynamically triangulated surfaces (random walks, branched polymers)

**Random tensor:** Generalization of random matrices (2D) to higher dimensions (3D+)

**Random tensor networks:** Tensor networks with each tensor chosen at random

**Random walk:** Markov process of left–right movement per a coin toss at each time step (versus quantum walk)

**Reaction-diffusion system:** Model describing the emergence of periodic patterns through local *reactions* that *diffuse* (spread out) over a domain

**Reduced density matrix:** Partial density matrix trace with fewer complex coefficients

**Reduced density operator:** Operator describing the state of a pure-mixed state system

**Reinforcement learning:** Machine learning paradigm in which intelligent agents maximize cumulative reward

**ReLU (rectified linear unit):** Machine learning activation function; the rectangular form acts more quickly than a sigmoid (s-curve shaped) function

**Renormalization group:** Mathematics enabling the investigation of a physical system at different scales

**Rényi entropy:** Generalized measure of four kinds of entropy: Shannon, Hartley, collision, and minimum entropy

**Reproducing kernel Hilbert space (RKHS):** Hilbert space described by a kernel function that reproduces every function in the space

**Restricted Boltzmann machine:** Machine learning method in which neurons are restricted to forming a bipartite graph in pair nodes from visible and hidden units

**Rich-club hub:** (Network science) a centralized hub that links distant regions of the network

**Rydberg atom arrays:** Experimental setup with atoms (alkali metals) in a highly excited state (Rydberg state) that is easy to measure (orders of magnitude larger than the ground state), has a long decay period, and an exaggerated response to electric and magnetic fields

**Ryu-Takayanagi formula:** Formalism that the entanglement entropy of a boundary region is equal to the area of a bulk minimal surface

**Sachdev–Ye–Kitaev (SYK) model:** Solvable model of strongly interacting quantum systems (Majorana fermions with random all-to-all interactions)

**Schmidt decomposition:** Fixing gauge degrees of freedom in a matrix product state

**Schrödinger equation:** Quantum mechanical wavefunction equation (hard to solve)

**Schwarzian:** Conformal mapping operator invariant under certain transformations

**Schwarzschild black hole:** Basic black hole with no charge or momentum

**Scrambling:** Measure of how quickly quantum information spreads out over an entire system so that a local measurement is not possible

**Shor's factoring algorithm:** Period-finding function with quantum Fourier transform

**Sign problem:** Negative values arising in probability distributions of quantum many-body calculations (typically unsolvable with classical methods)

**Small-world:** (Network science) graph property of shorter-than-random paths

**Softmax:** Function that exponentiates and rescales a set of numbers to sum to one

**Space crystal:** 3D structure with a repeating pattern in space, unaltered in time

**Special Relativity:** Theory equating mass and energy ($E = mc^2$), with time dilation effect

**Spike sorting:** Attributing action potentials to individual neurons

**Spike train:** Sequence of action potentials

**Spiking activation:** (Neuromorphic computation) threshold-based computation activation

**Spiking neural network:** Biologically realistic neural network architecture

**Spin:** Intrinsic form of angular momentum carried by elementary particles

**Spinors:** More complicated version of vectors or tensors needed to describe particle spin

**Squeezed state:** Quantum state squeezed (reduced) for less quantum noise

**Stabilizer codes:** Basic quantum error correction code (quantum version of linear codes); Pauli operators that measure entangled states and correct a corrupt quantum state (e.g. a bit flip or a spin flip) back to its original state (examples: toric code, surface code)

**Standard Model of particle physics:** Theory describing the electromagnetic, weak, and strong forces, but not gravity, and classifying all known elementary particles

**Statistical manifold:** Riemannian manifold whose points are probability distributions

**Stochastic calculus:** Calculus integrating stochastic (random) processes

**Strange attractor:** (Complex systems) complex fractal orbit with unstable divergence

**Strongly coupled system:** Quantum system with high-intensity particle interactions

**SU(*N*) special unitary group:** Subgroup of the unitary group (group of $n \times n$ unitary matrices). Example: the Standard Model is a unified symmetry group of SU(3) (strong force) × SU(2) (weak force) × U(1) (electromagnetic force)

**Superconductors:** Materials that conduct electricity without resistance

**Superfluid:** Fluid with zero viscosity that flows without the loss of kinetic energy

**Superposition:** Simultaneous coexistence of multiple incompatible classical realities (an unobserved particle exists in all possible states until collapsed in a measurement)

**Support vector machine:** Supervised learning method for binary classification problems

**Surface code:** (Stabilizer code) error correction code via lattice-entangled qubits

**Symmetry:** System property of looking the same at different scales

**Symmetry breaking:** Small fluctuations acting on a system crossing a critical point

**Symmetry group (gauge group):** Lie group formed by possible gauge transformations

**Synaptic integration:** (Dendritic integration) neuronal aggregation of thousands of incoming synaptic inputs from other neurons

**Synaptic plasticity:** The brain's ability to rewire synapse strength and structure

**Synaptome:** (Similar to connectome) comprehensive map of synapses in the brain

**Synaptosome:** (Synapse proteome) the set of synapse proteins in the brain by location

**Synaptotagmins:** Family of calcium sensor proteins facilitating neurotransmitter release

**Tensor:** A multidimensional array of numbers

**Tensor networks:** Tool to represent and solve many-body quantum states

**Thermal states:** States of a system at nonzero temperature

**Thermofield double (TFD) state:** Entangled state between two copies of a quantum state

**Theta neuron:** Biological neuron model based on oscillation-regulated bursts

**Time crystal:** Repeating structure that is periodic in time

**Tomography:** Imaging technique by reconstruction of wavefunction sections (e.g. fMRI)

**Toric code:** (Stabilizer code) error correction code with torus spin lattice topology

**Trace:** Sum of elements on the main diagonal of a matrix (upper left to bottom right)

**Traceless:** A matrix whose trace is zero (the main diagonal sums to zero)

**Tractography:** Three-dimensional representation of nerve tracts from diffusion MRI data

**Transformer neural network:** Machine learning model with an attention-based mechanism that simultaneously evaluates short-range and long-range correlations in input data as opposed to convolution (CNNs) or recurrence (RNNs)

**Transverse:** Data encoding in the plane perpendicular to the direction of travel

**Tree tensor networks (TTN):** Hierarchical tree structure formulation of tensor networks

**Trotterization:** Mathematical technique for approximating a continuous Hamiltonian (by the product of a large number of small discrete rotations on 1–2 qubits at a time)

**Turing instability:** Violation of the Turing pattern

**Turing pattern:** Spatially periodic pattern emerging between two diffusible substances irrespective of initial circumstances

**$2^n$ problem:** Property of quantum mechanical systems that the Hilbert space grows exponentially with system size (a spin-1/2 chain of length $n$ has $2^n$ degrees of freedom)

**Two-point correlation function:** The average (expectation value) of field operators at different positions; the amplitude for the propagation of a particle between A and B

**Unitarity:** Property of system evolving only by the unitary operator

**Unitary:** System evolution by the unit operator (advancing linearly by one regular unit)

**Unitary matrix:** (Linear algebra) an $n \times n$ complex square matrix whose conjugate transpose is also its inverse, and both are equal to the Identity matrix (matrix $U$ is unitary if $U^*U = UU^* = I$), which allows many transformations

**Unitary operator:** Operator advancing a quantum system by one unit

**Unitary transformation:** The action of unitary operator to evolve a quantum system forward

**U(N) unitary group:** A group of $n \times n$ unitary matrices

**UV complete:** A full bulk theory of quantum gravitation that can count black hole microstates in Lorentzian signature

**UV cutoff:** A model restricted to non-UV domains (i.e. long-range (IR) only)

**UV–IR correlations:** Short-range (ultraviolet (UV)) and long-range (infrared (IR)) correlations (UV and IR are used figuratively as the nearest and farthest reaches of a system, not literally as spectral wavelengths)

**Variational calculus:** The application of small changes (variations) to functions to find minima–maxima (geodesics)

**Variational method:** Statistical sampling method to approximate the ground state or excited state of a system by choosing a trial wavefunction, finding the lowest-energy expectation values, and repeating trial-and-error testing to establish the wavefunction profile

**Variational quantum algorithms:** Computational approximation methods for wavefunctions and quantum states. Examples: variational quantum eigensolver (VQE) and quantum approximate optimization algorithm (QAOA)

**Vector:** Arrow-based representation with a certain length and direction

**Viscosity:** Rate of perturbative excitation decay to system equilibrium

**Wave:** A propagating disturbance in a continuous medium or a physical field

**Wavefunction:** Quantitative description of a quantum state

**Wavelet:** Managed wave-like oscillations used in signal processing

**Wavelet transform:** Changing a wavelet in time extension but not shape (per the uncertainty principle time-frequency tradeoff)

**Wiener process:** Stochastic process used to study Brownian motion and diffusion

**Wormhole (Einstein-Rosen bridge):** Speculative structure linking points in spacetime, based on a special solution of the Einstein field equations

**Yang–Mills theory:** Non-abelian (non-commutative) gauge theory upon which the Standard Model of particle physics is based

# Index

**D**

**I**



**J**



**K**



**L**



**M**

**T**

CPSIA information can be obtained
at www.ICGtesting.com
Printed in the USA
JSHW042157110622
26918JS00001B/5

9 781800 610613